Clinical Phonetics and Linguistics

Edited by
Wolfram Ziegler and Karin Deger

Clinical Neuropsychology Research Group
Department of Neuropsychology,
City Hospital Bogenhausen, Munich

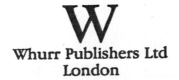

Whurr Publishers Ltd
London

© 1998 Whurr Publishers
First published 1998 by
Whurr Publishers Ltd
19b Compton Terrace, London N1 2UN, England

Reprinted 2003 (twice)

British Library Cataloguing-in-Publication Data
A catalogue record for this book is available from the
British Library.

ISBN: 1 86156 054 0

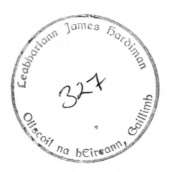

Printed and bound in the UK by Athenaeum Press Ltd,
Gateshead, Tyne & Wear

Contents

List of Contributors

Hermann Ackermann, Department of Neurology, University of Tübingen, Tübingen, Germany

Judith Aharon-Peretz, School of Education, University of Haifa, Mt Carmel, Haifa, Israel

Eckart Altenmüller, Institut für Musikphysiologie und Musiker-Medizin, Hannover, Germany

Shaheen N. Awan, Dept. of Communication Disorders and Special Education, Bloomsburg University, Bloomsburg, USA

Martin J. Ball, School of Behavioural and Communication Sciences, University of Ulster, Newtownabbey, Northern Ireland, UK

Janet Mackenzie Beck, Queen Margaret College, Department of Speech and Language Sciences, Edinburgh, UK

Regine Becker, Evangelic Geriatric Centre of Berlin, Berlin, Germany

Renée Béland, Centre de Recherche du Centre hospitalier Côte-des-Neiges, Montréal (Québec), Canada

Alim L. Benabid, Neurobiologie Préclinique, Centre Hospitalier Universitaire de Grenoble, Clinique Neurologique, Grenoble, France

Kirsten Meyer Bjerkan, Dept. of Linguistics, University of Oslo, Oslo, Norway

Inge Boers, Medical Psychology/Child Neurology Center, University Hospital Nijmegen, HB Nijmegen, The Netherlands

Caterina Breitenstein, Institute of Medical Psychology, University of Tübingen, Tübingen, Germany

Karen Bryan, Department of Human Communication Science, University College London, London, UK

Romola Bucks, The BRACE Centre, Clinical Research Centre and Memory Disorders Clinic, University of Bristol, Bristol, UK

John Clibbens, Department of Psychology, Faculty of Human Sciences, University of Plymouth, Plymouth, UK

Margaret Cooper, Department of Psychology, Faculty of Human Sciences, University of Plymouth, Plymouth, UK

Kenny R. Coventry, Department of Psychology, Faculty of Human Sciences, University of Plymouth, Plymouth, Devon, UK

Patrick. Cras, Department of Neurology (Born-Bunge-Foundation), University of Antwerp (UIA), Wilrijk, Belgium

Joanne M. Cuerden, The BRACE Centre, Clinical Research Centre and Memory Disorders Clinic, University of Bristol, Bristol, UK

Linda Daniel, Department of Speech and Hearing Sciences, University of North Texas, Denton, USA.

Ray Daniloff, Department of Speech and Hearing Sciences, University of North Texas, , Denton, USA.

Irene Daum, Institute of Medical Psychology, University of Tübingen, Tübingen, Germany

Ria De Bleser, Institut für Sprachwissenschaft, Universität Potsdam, Potsdam, Germany

Karin Deger, EKN, Clinical Neuropsychology Research Group, City Hospital Bogenhausen, München, Germany

Ernst G. de Langen, Abt. Sprachtherapie, Klinikum Passauer Wolf, Bad Griesbach, Germany

Grzegorz Dogil, Chair of Experimental Phonetics, University of Stuttgart, Stuttgart, Germany

Susan Edwards, Department of Linguistic Science, University of Reading, Reading, UK

Sylvia Elsner, Department of Neurology, University of Technology (RWTH), Aachen, Germany

Paul Fletcher, Department of Speech and Hearing Sciences, University of Hong Kong, Prince Philip Dental Hospital, Hong Kong

Andrea Geigenberger, EKN, Clinical Neuropsychology Research Group, City Hospital Bogenhausen, München, Germany

Michèle Gentil, Centre Hospitalier Universitaire de Grenoble, Clinique Neurologique, Unité de Pharmacologie, Clinique de la Pathologie du Mouvement, Grenoble, France

Fiona Gibbon, Department of Speech and Language Sciences, Corstorphine Campus, Queen Margaret College, Edinburgh, UK

Mária Gósy, Research Institute for Linguistics, Hungarian Academy of Sciences and Eötvös Loránd University, Hungary

Susanne Gräber, Department of Neurology, University of Tübingen, Tübingen, Germany

Wolfgang Grodd, Section Experimental MR of the CNS, Department of Neuroradiology, University of Tübingen, Tübingen, Germany

Claudine Guitton, Neuropsychologie Clinique de l'Enfant (INSERM), Hopital de la Salpetrière, Bâtiment Pharmacie, Paris, France

William J. Hardcastle, Department of Speech and Language Sciences, Corstorphine Campus, Queen Margaret College, Edinburgh, UK

Lee Harris, Southeastern Institute for Education in Music, University of Tennessee – Chattanooga, Chattanooga, USA.

M. Henoch, Department of Speech and Hearing Sciences, University of North Texas, Denton, USA.

Markus Hasselhorn, Department of Psychology, Technical University Dresden, Germany

Ingo Hertrich, Department of Neurology, University of Tübingen, Tübingen, Germany

Barry Heselwood, School of Applied Social Science, Leeds Metropolitan University, Leeds, UK

Gerd Hoch, Neurologische Klinik Bad Aibling, Bad Aibling, Germany

Susanne Holzleiter, Neurologische Klinik Bad Aibling, Kolbermoorer Straße, Bad Aibling, Germany

Sara Howard, Department of Human Communication Sciences, University of Sheffield, Sheffield, UK

Walter Huber, Neurolinguistics at the Department of Neurology, University of Technology (RWTH), Aachen, Germany

Wouter Hulstijn, NICI, Nijmegen, The Netherlands

Angela Hurd, Centre for Language and Communication Research SECAP, University of Wales Cardiff, Cardiff, Wales, UK

Tomohiko Ito, Tokyo Gakugei University, Japan

Mary S. Jackson, Canniesburn Hospital, Bearsden, Glasgow, UK

Tracey M. Jones, Department of Speech and Hearing Science, University of North Texas, Denton, USA.

Bernd Kardatzki, Section Experimental MR of the CNS, Department of Neuroradiology, University of Tübingen, Tübingen, Germany

Louise Kelly, Department of Linguistics, University of Edinburgh, Edinburgh, UK

Uwe Klose, Section Experimental MR of the CNS, Department of Neuroradiology University of Tübingen, Tübingen, Germany

Ahmet Konrot, Anadolu Üniversitesi, Egitim Fakültesi, Turkey

Handan Kopkalli-Yavuz, Anadolu Üniversitesi, Egitim Fakültesi, Turkey

John Laver, Faculty of Arts, University of Edinburgh, Edinburgh, UK

Christian Ledl, Neurologische Klinik Bad Aibling, Bad Aibling, Germany

Guylaine Le Dorze, École d'Orthophonie et d'Audiologie, Équipe de Recherche en Orthophonie, Université de Montréal, Montréal (Québec), Canada

Mark Leikin, School of Education, University of Haifa, Mt Carmel, Haifa, Israel

Marie-Thérèse Le Normand, Neuropsychologie Clinique de l'Enfant (INSERM), Hôpital de la Salpetrière, Bâtiment Pharmacie, Paris, France

Marjorie Lorch, Birkbeck College, University of London, London, UK

Ben Maassen, Medical Psychology / Child Neurology Center, University Hospital Nijmegen, Nijmegen, The Netherlands

Sharynne McLeod, School of Communication Disorders, University of Sydney, Cumberland College Campus, Lidcombe, NSW, Australia

Patricia Mavimbela, Department of Logopedics, Groote Schuur Hospital, Cape Town, South Africa

Jörg Mayer, Chair of Experimental Phonetics, University of Stuttgart, Stuttgart, Germany

Jane Maxim, Department of Human Communication Science, University College London, London, UK

Creighton J. Miller, Department of Special Education, Murray State University, Murray, USA

Nick Miller, Department of Speech, King George VI Building, University of Newcastle, Newcastle-upon-Tyne, UK

Padraic Monaghan, Centre for Cognitive Science, University of Edinburgh, Edinburgh, UK

Nicole Müller, Centre for Language and Communication Research SECAP, University of Wales Cardiff, Cardiff, Wales, UK

Moray Nairn, Queen Margaret College, Department of Speech and Language Sciences, Edinburgh, UK

Jean-Luc Nespoulous, Laboratoire de Neuropsycholinguistique Jacques-Lordat, Départment des Sciences du Langage, Université de Toulouse –Le Mirail, CHU de Toulouse – Purpan, France

Martis Okon, Department of Speech and Hearing Science, University of North Texas, Denton, USA

I. Papathanasiou, National Hospital for Neurology and Neurosurgery London, London, UK

Philippe Paquier, Department of ENT Surgery, Department of Neurology, University Hospital Erasme, Free University of Brussels (ULB), Bruxelles, Belgium

Carole Paradis, Centre de Recherche du Centre Hospitalier Côte-des-Neiges, Montréal (Québec), Canada

Sue Peppé, Department of Human Communication Science, University College London, London, UK.

Michael R. Perkins, Department of Human Communication Sciences, University of Sheffield, Sheffield, UK.

Sabine Perrin, Centre Hospitalier Universitaire de Grenoble, Clinique Neurologique, Unité de Pharmacologie, Clinique de la Pathologie du Mouvement, Grenoble, France

Hans Pihan, Department of Neurology, University of Tübingen, Tübingen, Germany

James R. Pirolli, 1020 Edgewood Ave NE, Atlanta, GA 30307, USA.

Monique Plaza, Neuropsychologie Clinique de l'Enfant (INSERM), Hopital de la Salpetriére, Batiment Pharmacie, Paris, France

David Poeppel, Biomagnetic Imaging Laboratory, Department of Radiology, University of California — San Francisco, San Francisco, USA.

Pierre Pollak, Centre Hospitalier Universitaire de Grenoble, Clinique Neurologique, Grenoble, France

Sabine Preis, Department of Pediatrics, University Düsseldorf, Düsseldorf, Germany

John Ryalls, Communicative Disorders, University of Central Florida, Orlando, USA

Vicki Reed, School of Communication Disorders, University of Sydney, Cumberland College Campus, Lidombe, Australia

Michael Riebandt, Department of Phoniatrics and Pedaudiology, University of Münster, Münster, Germany

A.Gerry Robertson, Beatson Oncology Centre, Western Infirmary, Glasgow, UK

Glenn Royall, Department of Speech and Hearing Science, University of North Texas, Denton, USA

Gabriele Scharf, Department of Neurology, Edith-Stein-Fachklinik für Neurologie, Bad Bergzabern, Germany

Kym Schulze, Dept. of Speech and Hearing Sciences, University of North Texas, Denton, USA

Manuela Schwarz, EKN, Clinical Neuropsychology Research Group, City Hospital Bogenhausen, München, Germany

James M. Scobbie, Queen Margaret College, Department of Speech and Language Sciences, Corstorphine Campus, Edinburgh, UK

Walter F. Sendlmeier, Institute of Communication Research, Technical University Berlin, Berlin, Germany

Richard Shillcock, Centre for Cognitive Science, University of Edinburgh, Edinburgh, UK

Tomohiko Shirahata, Faculty of Education, Shizuoka University, Japan

Sameer Singh, School of Computing, University of Plymouth, Plymouth, UK

David S. Soutar, Canniesburn Hospital, Bearsden, Glasgow, UK

Sybille Spieker, Department of Neurology, University of Tübingen, Tübingen, Germany

Stephanie F. Stokes, Department of Speech and Hearing Sciences, University of Hong Kong, Prince Philip Dental Hospital, Hong Kong

Karrie Surber, Department of Speech and Hearing Sciences, University of North Texas, Denton, USA

Sandra Terrell, Office of the Dean, Graduate College, University of North Texas, Denton, USA

Seyhun Topbaş, Anadolu Üniversitesi, Egitim Fakültesi, Isao Ueda, Osaka University of Foreign Studies, Osaka, Japan

John Van Borsel, Centrum voor Gehoor- en Spraakrevalidatie, Universitair Ziekenhuis, Gent, Belgium

Sjoeke van der Meulen, Deptartment of Phoniatrics, University Hospital Utrecht, Utrecht, The Netherlands

Jan van Doorn, School of Communication Disorders, University of Sydney, Cumberland College Campus, Lidcombe, Australia

Pascal van Lieshout, Academic Hospital Nijmegen, ENT-clinic, Department of Voice and Speech Pathology, Nijmegen, The Netherlands

Peter van Vugt, Unit of Neurolinguistics, University of Antwerp (UIA), Universiteitsplein, Belgium

Bill Wells, Department of Human Communication Science, University College London, London, UK

Gert Westermann, Centre for Cognitive Science, University of Edinburgh, Edinburgh, UK

Tara L Whitehill, Department of Speech and Hearing Sciences, University of Hong Kong, Prince Philip Dental Hospital, Hong Kong

Renata Whurr, National Hospital for Neurology and Neurosurgery London, London, UK

Gordon K. Wilcock, The BRACE Centre, Clinical Research Centre and Memory Disorders Clinic, Blackberry Hill Hospital, Bristol, UK

Dirk Wildgruber, Section Exp. MR of the CNS, Department of Neuroradiology, University of Tübingen, Tübingen, Germany

Klaus Willmes, Department of Neurology, University of Technology (RWTH), Aachen, Germany

Alan Wrench, Department of Speech and Language Sciences, Queen Margaret College, Corstorphine Campus, Edinburgh, UK

Wolfram Ziegler, EKN, Clinical Neuropsychology Research Group, City Hospital Bogenhausen, München, Germany

Marsha Zlatin-Laufer, SUNY at Stony Brook, Setauket, New York, USA

Preface

This volume contains a collection of papers presented at the Fifth Annual Meeting of the International Clinical Phonetics and Linguistics Association (ICPLA) in Munich on 16–18 September 1996. This conference provided a forum for almost 90 oral and poster presentations from the fields of clinical phonetics and clinical linguistics, and attracted a great number of scientists and clinicians from many different countries.

The 55 chapters of this book give a representative account of the issues discussed at ICPLA '96. They cover a wide range of topics, from infant babbling to language in dementia, from pragmatic disabilities to cleft-palate articulation, and from slow potentials to nasalance measures. Some of the chapters contribute to fundamental issues in speech and language disorders, others to clinical issues like assessment and treatment. The reader is therefore presented with a large variety of research questions, patient groups, syndrome taxonomies, experimental paradigms, and measurement techniques.

What sense does it make to collect manuscripts from such profoundly different research areas within a single volume? The common denominator of all contributions to this book is their intention to increase our understanding of communication disorders and to improve the methodologies for diagnosing and treating these disorders. Due to the diversity of topics, the reader becomes acquainted with the research questions of colleagues working in completely different fields and with the particular methods they use in investigating these questions. Paradigms like, for instance, cross-linguistic comparisons, have already found their way into fields as different as cleft palate speech (Chapter 19), phonological disorders in children (Chapter 10) and apraxia of speech in adults (Chapter 44). Likewise, other approaches presented here may also turn out to be transferrable to new clinical or research applications. Readers may therefore profit from the multitude of approaches, finding an opportunity to look beyond the horizon of their own fields, and learning from the many paths that may be followed in the study of disordered communication.

Despite their great heterogeneity, the contributions to this volume can be grouped under a limited number of headings. Not unexpectedly, phonological and articulation disorders in children and motor speech disorders in adults, leading topics of earlier ICPLA meetings, make up a major proportion of the proceedings of this conference. There are also entirely new accents, however – for example on brain imaging studies of speech and language processing in normals, on non-linguistic factors influencing language acquisition, or on prosodic disorders. We used these and other major topics as a skeleton to structure the present volume, hoping that readers may thereby find their way through the many thoughtful contributions collected here. Moreover, selected subsections of the volume are introduced by invited 'keynote chapters' that are intended to provide readers with a comprehensive overview of particular topics (Chapters 1, 35, and 42).

We wish to thank all authors for their contribution to this volume. We are also indebted to Maria Neubauer for her help in collecting and editing the manuscripts and in preparing the list of contributors and the subject index.

Wolfram Ziegler
Karin Deger

PART I
DISORDERS OF SPEECH AND
LANGUAGE ACQUISITION

GENERAL ASPECTS

Chapter 1
Perspectives on Grammatical Impairment in Children

PAUL FLETCHER

Introduction

The modern study of specific language impairment (SLI) could be said to start with the work in the early 1970s of a group working in the Institute for Childhood Aphasia at Stanford University. One of those researchers was David Ingram, who with Donald Morehead published 'The development of base syntax in normal and linguistically deviant children' (Morehead and Ingram, 1973). This paper could be claimed to have inspired modern investigations into grammatical impairment in these children. At a recent conference on language impairment to which we both contributed, David Ingram asked me what advance in knowledge had been made on his and Morehead's 1973 findings in the years since. I am not sure if the question was meant entirely seriously, but it is thought provoking. It can serve as a useful starting point for an assessment of the state of the art in the study of grammatical impairment. After all, more than two decades have passed since this pioneering work. During that time there has been extensive research on the effects of SLI on grammar in English-speaking children. In the last six or seven years we have also begun to learn about grammatical impairment in languages other than English. It would have been very surprising if all of this work had not added value to work that emerged more than 20 years ago. I would like to react to Ingram's question by reviewing the original study and then evaluating recent perspectives on SLI to determine where we now stand in this field. Finally I will consider where we might usefully go in the future.

The Morehead and Ingram study

It seems appropriate to take a close look at Morehead and Ingram (1973) (henceforth Morehead and Ingram) if we are to make any judgement about advances since the publication of their paper. Let us examine the method first. This study of grammatical ability, based on language samples from 15 SLI and 15 language age-matched normals, sets the scene for what follows in SLI research on a number of counts. We deal with each of the major features of the methodology in turn.

Cross-sectional study

It is worth highlighting, at the outset, a major difference in methodology between the Morehead and Ingram study (together with almost all subsequent studies of SLI) and a major strand of normal language acquisition studies. Specific language impairment may usefully be seen as a special case of language acquisition, where the basic question is: given that the vast majority of children learn the language of their speech community in the pre-school years, apparently without effort, what is it that inhibits a similar facility in the case of SLI children? While the methodology of choice in a wide range of studies of normal children has involved case-based longitudinal studies, SLI research has favoured cross-sectional group studies. The main reason for this is variation in the rate of development in normal children, which makes the identification of impaired individuals unreliable until late in the pre-school years (Bishop and Edmundson, 1987).

Sample size

Sample sizes in SLI group studies tend to be small. Subsequent studies have seldom exceeded the figure of 15 per group in the Morehead and Ingram study (but see Rice and Wexler (1996); Schelleter, Fletcher, Ingham, King and Sinka (1996)), and indeed have often gone below. A sample size of 10 is common and occasionally studies have even lower numbers. Sample-to-population inferences may be a problem with group sizes such as this.

Mean length of utterance (MLU) matching

Mean length of utterance, usually measured in morphemes, has been used in matching by many subsequent studies. The justification is as follows: comparisons between SLI children and their chronological age peers that show grammatical differences between language-impaired and language-normal (LN) groups may simply reflect a language delay. All we can conclude from such a result is that the SLI group is developing language more slowly than is its age matches. If, however, a study uses MLU to ensure that the SLI and LN groups are equivalent in language age, any grammatical differences that emerge can be argued to reflect grammatical deficits in the SLI children.

The inevitable consequence of language-age matching is that it produces two groups that are a long way apart in chronological age and hence in experience of the world. These are the chronological ages of the groups in the Morehead and Ingram study:

- LI: age range 3;6 to 9;6, mean age 6;7
- LN: age range 1;7 to 3;1, mean age 2;4

Language samples as database for analysis

In using language samples as the basis for their grammatical analysis, Morehead and Ingram were following the trend in studies of normal language acquisition initiated by Roger Brown at Harvard a decade earlier. They had three conditions for data collection: free play with experimenter or parent, elicitation while playing with toys, and elicitation while viewing a standard child's book. The use of spontaneous language samples of between 100 and 200 utterances became a standard procedure in this field after Morehead and Ingram.

Detailed grammatical analysis using current grammatical model

The procedure used for analysis is essentially the Aspects model of Chomsky (1965), adapted for application to children's language. Subsequent studies have, after a period, updated their grammatical models in line with developments in linguistics.

One important feature missing so far from this summary of the Morehead and Ingram methodology is the description of subjects. No precise details are given in the paper of how and why subjects were selected, although this was and remains an important issue for this area of research. The SLI children in the study are described as 'deviant' and as being 'selected from the deviant population . . . at the Institute for Childhood Aphasia'. They are further said to be 'restricted to children who lacked sufficient intellectual or physiological impairment to account for their difficulties in acquiring language'.

We do, however, have the basis here for the exclusion criteria that have since been widely used to identify SLI children: briefly, no hearing impairment, no known neurological impairment and cognitive abilities within normal limits. These criteria are somewhat controversial and the cognitive criterion, in particular, has come under attack recently. The usual requirement for a child to be included in an SLI group in published studies, so far as intellectual ability is concerned, is a non-verbal IQ performance within one standard deviation of the mean. (Verbal IQ performance will inevitably be depressed.) The use of the IQ criterion has recently been questioned from two directions. First, whereas the potential involvement of hearing impairment or neurological damage or a syndrome such as autism in language learning is clear, since these factors may have a direct causal involvement in language deficit or disorder, the relationship between a relatively mild intellectual deficit as represented by a non-verbal IQ of, say, 75 and any particular feature of specific language impairment is not so apparent (Fey, Long and Cleave, 1994). Second, experimental work has made it clear that SLI children who meet the exclusion criterion for IQ nevertheless do display cognitive deficits in non-verbal functioning (Johnston 1992).

As our knowledge of SLI children's cognitive and neurological deficits improves, it may well be that this category of disorder either disappears or, more probably, becomes considerably refined and sub-classified. In the meantime and for the rest of this paper I will, while acknowledging the problems with subject selection and definition, adhere to the usual definition.

Within this methodological framework, what did Morehead and Ingram discover and what current relevance do their findings have? There are two major results that continue to have resonance:

1. *'[SLI children] develop quite similar linguistic systems [to those of normal children] with a marked delay in the onset and acquisition time.'*

This finding suggests, and almost all studies since indicate, that SLI children may develop language slowly but in the course of their development they do not construct 'wild grammars' from the input they receive. 'Deviance' in the sense of forms that are unattested in either the adult language or in normal language acquisition is rare. A caveat here is that the preponderance of cross-sectional studies, with relatively small numbers of subjects, means that we could easily be missing SLI individuals who at some point in their development hypothesized unusual constructions, but for the most part this result holds up in the face of later research.

2. *'Moreover, once the linguistic systems are developed, deviant children do not use them as creatively as normal children for producing highly varied utterances.'*

Somewhat surprisingly in view of the focus of much subsequent research on SLI in English, a second conclusion of the paper relates to the diversity of SLI children's utterances in comparison with their normal counterparts. As we shall see later, much of the research that has followed the Morehead and Ingram methodological model over the two decades since it was published has dwelt on SLI children's deficiencies in inflectional morphology, particularly verb inflections. Morehead and Ingram explicitly exclude inflectional morphology as a problem in their cohort:[1]

> . . . deviant children, when studied at their particular level of linguistic development, are not seriously deficient in the organization of phrase structure rules, types of transformations . . . or inflectional morphology. (p. 226)

The question of how SLI children deploy the grammatical resources available to them, which is what appears to be at issue here, was not extensively addressed in later research. Morehead and Ingram appear to be arguing for a pervasive deficit, which has the effect of limiting the range and diversity of structures that can be produced by SLIs, using the grammatical infrastructure available to them.

If we now fast-forward to the 1990s, how does the Morehead and Ingram work fare? True, their methodology has not been greatly changed, although there is an increasing awareness of the need to go beyond the analysis of spontaneous speech data into experimental work. Later work also concurs with the view that language acquisition develops slowly in SLI children and that they do not construct 'wild grammars'. There is an influential body of work, however, which holds that the effects of SLI on the grammatical system are selective, not pervasive. Inspired by a Chomskyan perspective on how language is acquired, this work focuses on the acquisition of functional categories, particularly (but not solely) those represented in English by verb inflections.

Are grammatical deficits selective?

The selectivity of grammatical deficit is an issue with important theoretical and practical ramifications. The Chomskyan language acquisition device (LAD) is modular, operates only on positive evidence and relies on crucial data from input to trigger parameter settings in relation to functional categories such as tense and agreement. If the fault-lines of a deficit in children with SLI demarcate a 'natural class' of categories from the grammar, this would tend to support the Chomskyan view of how the LAD is structured and the role that it plays in acquisition. A selective deficit such as this would also have serious practical implications. If the 'hard-wiring' that children bring to language learning is not adequate for the task, remediation may be difficult for them, if not impossible.

One detailed attempt to account for language impairment in terms of a defective language acquisition device comes in the work of Gopnik and her associates (see Matthews, 1994). Beginning with a report on a three-generation family in England, half of whose 30 members are impaired, this research has now been extended to other languages (particularly Greek and Japanese). The claim (with particular reference to

past tense deficits) is that impaired subjects lack inflectional morphological rules. They remain within the normal range with respect to certain other linguistic abilities, however, as well as their general cognitive
abilities. Ullman and Gopnik (1994: 111) are quite clear about the
source of the problem with past tense in the affected members of the
family that they investigated: a 'genetic dysfunction' is blamed for the
lack of normal development of mechanisms necessary for the acquisition of this part of the grammar of English. Whatever the accuracy of this
claim about the members of the family studied by Gopnik, the vulnerability of past tense in English-speaking SLI individuals is regularly
attested, most recently in a study with the relatively large sample size of
37. In this study (Rice and Wexler, 1996), problems with tense (which
in the authors' terms includes markings of finiteness on main and
auxiliary verbs in English) are interpreted as a clinical marker of SLI in
children.

Verbs and argument structure

In the face of what may be seen as an over-emphasis of functional categories in current research, is there any recent evidence that would
bear on the Morehead and Ingram conclusion that the effect of SLI on
the grammar is pervasive? In an effort to identify more extensive effects
of language impairment on grammar, a group at the University of
Reading[2] has been examining SLI children's facility with inflectional
morphology and their knowledge of verb argument structure alternations. The narrowly syntactic aspects of verb complementation can
be argued to be as potentially vulnerable to the effects of SLI as the
building of morphological paradigms. Children are required to learn
language-specific facts about the complementation of verbs. The most
straightforward example concerns obligatory complements: the verb
shave in English does not require a direct object, whereas in Cantonese
it does. As it turns out, children with SLI tend not to omit obligatory
verb complements, at least so far as we can tell from the analysis of language samples. However there are other language-specific syntactic facts
concerning verbs, such as their participation in alternations. The complementation potential of the verb break, for example, allows the theme
to be expressed as direct object, as in *he broke the cup*, or as subject as
in *the cup broke*. Only certain verbs, in which an agent causes a change
of state for an object, allow this alternation. In English it does not apply
for *fall*, for instance. Overgeneralizations of the form *Johnny falled my
bricks* indicate that young normal children are sensitive to the potential
of certain verbs to alternate in this way, even though they may not yet
have restricted the alternation to the appropriate set of verbs.
  Specific language-impaired children's knowledge of argument structure alternations can serve as one test case for a selective grammatical

deficit hypothesis that is limited to functional categories. An alternative hypothesis, the modern equivalent of the second of the Morehead and Ingram conclusions, is that SLI grammar exhibits a more general deficit, affecting a range of areas in syntax and morphology. If this is the case then a deficit in verb inflections should be accompanied by deficits in other areas.

To determine whether this association existed between a functional category deficit (past tense in this case) and argument structure alternations, Fletcher *et al.* (1996) examined past tense[3] ability as well as argument structure alternations in 24 SLI children aged 5;1–8;9 from schools for language-impaired children and from language units in normal schools, in the south of England. A group of 48 normal children provided chronological age-matched and language-matched normal controls. The procedures used for assessing the children's morphological status involved free conversation, and narratives elicited by video cartoon. To assess verb alternations a series of illustrative action scenes were filmed and shown to the children, who were required to describe what happened in the scenes, when prompted with the relevant lexical verb in citation form.

One set of four verbs (*bounce, open, move, wave*) involved alternations between inchoative – e.g. *the ball is bouncing* – and causative – e.g. *the boy is bouncing the ball.* For the video scene designed to elicit the inchoative version of *bounce,* the viewer sees frames showing a ball bouncing across a patio, with no agent visible. For the scene designed for the causative version, the film clip shows the boy initiating the action. In addition to the inchoative/causative alternation, two other types of verbs displaying complement structure alternations were investigated: locative/contact verbs (e.g. *load, scrape*), and dative/benefactive verbs (e.g. *give, make*).

Provision of past tense in obligatory contexts (which we have seen is a widely used dependent measure in the research literature) was assessed in order to examine inflectional performance. The performance of both chronological age-matched (CA) and language-age matched (LA) children on past tense provision was on average above 90% (a level usually taken to indicate that children have fully acquired the form). The SLI children split into two sub-groups. One sub-group of 12 subjects, whom we designate SLI-M, had an average success rate on past tenses of 29%. The other sub-group, SLI+M, also with 12 subjects, had an average past tense provision rate of 89% – very close to a level at which we would be prepared to say they had learned the rule for regular past in English.

When we look at the performance of the two sub-groups of SLI children on verb alternation tasks, the conclusion is inescapable that inflectional problems and problems with verb alternations are highly correlated. If we take just the inchoative/causative alternations, which were the most successful overall at eliciting responses from normal and impaired subjects, we find a significant difference between the SLI+M sub-group and the SLI-M sub-group. If a child provided responses with the theme as object (e.g. *the boy is bouncing the ball*) and the theme as subject (e.g. *the ball is bouncing*) to the appropriate pictures, he or she was credited with knowledge of the alternation. The average score for the SLI+M sub-group was 3.18 alternations (out of a maximum of 4), while for the SLI-M sub-group it was 1.36 (U = 21, p = 0.002).

More generally, if we consider just those verbs for which all adults were credited with alternating argument structures in the task, and ask how the child groups fared against this adult criterion, we find the CA matched group doing best, with 75% of the group achieving adult performance levels. (These data include performance on both causative/inchoative and locative/contact verbs.) In the LA matched group, 50% of the children reached the adult criterion, while 58% of the SLI+M group did so. This is in contrast to just 8% of the SLI-M group. It seems reasonable to conclude from this that a morphological deficit (as measured by past tense provision) will be accompanied by a verb argument structure deficit (as measured via the alternations elicited via the film clips the children watched). It does appear that the impairment of the grammar of at least some SLI children goes beyond the functional categories that have been the focus of so much research. (It is also clear from these data that there are school-age SLI children for whom grammar may no longer be a difficulty, although they may well continue to have other problems such as pragmatic difficulties. This question was not addressed as part of this research, but see Craig, 1995.)

A persisting generalization about SLI in English concerns inflection, and the details of grammatical deficit in relation to functional categories, particularly those realized by verb inflection, have been assiduously pursued by researchers. This is partly because inflectional deficits undoubtedly do exist in these children, partly because identifying inflectional error is (relatively) straightforward in easily procurable data, such as free conversation, and partly because functional categories, particularly those associated with verb inflection, have had a significant role in recent grammatical theory. If we design the correct tools for exploring other areas of the grammar, however, it seems that we can identify other deficits that correlate with the inflectional gaps. Even without experimental investigation, additional grammatical features that are symptomatic of language impairment have been isolated. Gavin, Klee and Membrino (1993), using a discriminant analysis technique on grammatical profiles derived from spontaneous speech, identified the underdevelopment of the noun phrase as one of three variables (the others being errors in the verb phrase and an over-use of one-word utterances) that characterize their SLI group. If SLI has effects on grammar that encompass inflection, verb argument structure and noun phrases, then an alternative to the selective grammatical deficit hypothesis begins to appear tenable. It is likely that English-speaking children with SLI are exhibiting a generalized set of symptoms reflecting a system that is generally degraded, with no selective deficit that targets any one area of the grammar. As we indicated at the outset, differing ages of subjects, and distinct ways of identifying them, mean that great caution is required in relation to any generalization about SLI, but at present the 'general degradation' view seems more plausible than a selective deficit position. To that extent we may say that Morehead and Ingram are vindicated.

Are grammatical deficits grammatical?

This is a way of asking whether it is appropriate to conceptualize the problems that we see in SLI children as 'grammatical deficits'. Is there some alternative to a perspective that relates errors that we identify to a defective grammatical system, whether the effect of SLI on the system is selective or general?

Specific language impairments in other languages

The first, somewhat indirect, approach to this question leads us to an area in which there have been clear advances since 1973: the study of SLI in other languages. Comparisons between children learning language A and children learning language B are notoriously problematic; we inevitably face linguistic systems that are not necessarily commensurable and also the knotty problem of comparability of subjects. Some work that goes a long way towards dealing with these often underestimated problems is that on the Italian language by Leonard and his associates from 1987 (e.g. Leonard, Sabbadini, Leonard and Volterra, 1987; Leonard, Bortolini, Caselli, McGregor and Sabbadini, 1992).

The focus of the enquiry in these studies is agreement, not tense. The results demonstrate that for certain forms of verbs, Italian SLI children perform as well as both CA and LA matched controls. For third person singular present verb forms the mean scores for the three groups (SLI, CA matches and LA matches) were all above 90%. All groups were performing at the same level. The SLI children did not perform as well as the control groups on all verb forms however. On third person plural present the SLI group provided the correct form in 50% of obligatory contexts on average, most frequently substituting the third person singular form in its place. Whereas it is not possible from these data to say that the Italian SLI children had no difficulty with verb agreement, the striking discrepancy between their facility with third person singular agreement and the English SLI's problems with English third person singular agreement deserves more detailed scrutiny. The

English SLI children (who had a similar MLU range to the Italian children and were similar in age) achieved a third person singular score of only 34%. What could explain this discrepancy? At this point that we need to consider explanations for the effects of SLI other than the LAD deficit approach.

Leonard's response to his data has been to consider processing limitations as a possible basis for the grammatical deficits we have so far considered. The 'surface' hypothesis suggests that the physical properties of the morphemes that code third person singular present agreement in the two languages may be responsible for the discrepancy in performance between the two groups of SLI. The word-final non-syllabic consonant that, in English, is added to a stem to signal agreement is relatively non-salient compared to the stressed, syllabic vowel form that signals third person singular agreement in Italian. The learnability problem for the child learning English or Italian is the formation of morphological paradigms for verb forms. As Leonard (1994: 100) puts it: 'limited processing capacity makes inflections with difficult surface characteristics more vulnerable to loss when combined with the operations of paradigm building'. In the procedure described by Pinker (1984), children go from word-specific paradigms based on present and past forms of particular words to general paradigms in which the morphological material common to a number of words is abstracted. To explain the difference in performance between the two SLI groups it is assumed that the relative phonetic salience of Italian third person agreement forms is more facilitative of paradigm construction than the English form. English children need more frequent exposure to the forms to overcome the limitations of their reduced processing capacity.

This account has some immediate appeal in terms of the differences between English and Italian, and also more generally in its potential for dealing with the thorny problem of partial knowledge of grammatical rules, as reflected by variable but gradually improving use of an inflection over a lengthy period. The interaction of an inefficient processing device and a paradigm builder that could produce partial inflectional generalizations over a subset of vocabulary would help to account for the long period of acquisition that we see. (For data on changes in SLI children's use of English morphemes over time see Johnston and Schery (1976: 241), reprinted in Kent (1994: 214)). As Leonard points out, however, a more detailed account of what the limited processing capacity hypothesized for the SLI child entails is required if the processing account is ultimately to have credibility. We await some independent specification of the relative complexity of the various linguistic and non-linguistic operations that a limited processing capacity might affect (see also Rice and Wexler, 1996: 1252–3).

The possibility that the differences found by Leonard between English-speaking SLI and Italian-speaking SLI are due to processing problems should give pause to those who assume that the grammatical acquisition device itself is malfunctioning. Nevertheless, grammatical agreement problems in the English-speaking SLI children still remain, even if the reasons for these problems may be at root perceptual. The resulting deficits can still be regarded as grammatical – deficiencies in grammatical representation.

There is one more study that I would like to briefly sketch before drawing things together and considering what the future might hold. This study (King, 1996) suggests that not all limitations in grammatical performance reflect limitations on grammatical knowledge.

Optional complements of verbs in SLI children[4]

As we saw earlier, the areas of obligatory complements and potential alternations are obvious areas to consider when examining what the language learner needs to know about lexical verbs in order to deploy them appropriately. In considering 'construction types', as Morehead and Ingram did, it may also be appropriate to look at optional complements. 'Optional' in this case is a grammatical term, signifying a phrase, either an NP (nominal phrase) or a PP (propositional phrase), that can occur as a complement of a verb but which is not gramatically necessary. In conversational contexts, of course, the grammatically 'optional' complement may well be contextually or pragmatically required.

Table 1.1. Complementation types, SLI and LN Groups (n = 11) (63 sentences per subject)

	Intransitive		
	0	PP	
SLI	95	145	(240)
LN	67	215	(282)
	Transitive		
	NP	NPPP	
SLI	282	96	(378)
LN	222	135	(357)
	Clausal complements		
	CL	NPXP	
SLI	53	19	(72)
LN	48	3	(51)

In an analysis of conversational language samples, the deployment of verb complementation types in school-age SLI children and LA-matched normally developing children was investigated. The two groups did not differ in their (very low rate of) omission of obligatory verb complements. Once it was clear that they maintained grammaticality, we were interested to know if there were differences in their deployment of verb complement types. As an inspection of Table 1.1 will reveal, some interesting disparities emerge.[5]

The complementation types are arranged in three sets:

Intransitive
  zero complementation – *the little boy's crying*
  PP complementation – *he ran into the garden*

Transitive
  NP – single obligatory complement – *Billy built a tower*
  NPPP – two obligatory complements – *put the bike in the shed*
  one obligatory and one optional complement – *she filled the bucket with water*

Clausal complements
  CL – complements containing finite verbs – *pretend you're a pirate*
  NPXP – small clauses, lacking finite verbs – *mummy helped me dress*

One difference is that the SLI children are actually more proficient at complementation types (CL and NPXP) that could be considered in some sense more complex than the other four types. But then, as we said earlier, the SLI children are older – they have been around longer than their LA counterparts and perhaps they simply have a more extensive verb vocabulary – this is a reflection of lexis rather than grammar. The second observation comes from observing non-clausal complementation types. The data can be interpreted as indicating that SLI children will adopt a communicatively minimalist strategy to the task of provision of their side of a conversational turn. These children use more zero complementation types and fewer PPs with intransitive verbs. The strategy would appear to be: if it's an intransitive verb, let's just use the verb; say 'we're leaving' rather than 'we're leaving for the station'. Again, in the transitive categories, SLIs use significantly fewer NPPP sequences. This discrepancy could be interpreted in a similar way. If you need to use a transitive verb, supply only the direct object: say 'I saw Jane', rather than 'I saw Jane in the playground', or 'I saw Jane at the party'. The SLI children's tendency to omit optional complements while maintaining grammaticality suggests a processing limitation rather than any representational difficulty.

Advances

It is fair to say that the original paper by Morehead and Ingram continues to be relevant, most obviously in its methodology, the major features of which have persisted to date. Most subsequent studies have also agreed that SLI children do not construct 'wild' grammars and that their acquisition route resembles, in general terms, that of normals, although the rate of development is much slower. The second Morehead and Ingram finding, however, of a general effect of SLI reflected in limitations on 'construction types' has not been picked up to the same extent. Some recent findings discussed in this paper suggest that this Morehead and Ingram conclusion may be worth pursuing more systematically.

Of course in many respects we know more than we did. We certainly have a wealth of descriptive information on the types of grammatical behaviour that distinguish SLI from LN in English. We also now have information on a limited range of other languages, mostly European: German, Dutch, Swedish, Italian and also Hebrew. The third area of advance concerns explanatory accounts. Morehead and Ingram make no effort to explain their findings. We now have available explanatory accounts, or what purport to be explanatory accounts, from within linguistic theory and from other fields, although we have not looked at them in any detail here. There is the defective LAD account of selective deficits, language production processing accounts (e.g. Bishop, 1994), receptive processing accounts presented by studies of phonological working memory (Gathercole and Baddeley, 1990) and accounts of SLI children's inefficiency at processing a rapidly changing acoustic signal (Tallal et al., 1996). These all have their problems. The defective LAD account is challenged by non-selective deficits and possibly by interlanguage differences. The language production processing account is plausible on the face of it, but lacks precision and experimental support. The phonological working memory and auditory temporal processing hypotheses, both of which have some experimental support, suffer from the drawback that it is not clear how they can be linked to all the grammatical deficiencies that have been the subject of our discussion.

Where next?

There are four areas we might want to consider in terms of future development.

- The SLI category is too general and needs refining. Whether this greater delicacy of subject definition comes from independent variables such as age, from the extension of our knowledge of potential causal variables such as cognitive ability, or neurological status, or from behavioural classification, or from some combination, its demise as a cover-all category is just a matter of time.
- Our knowledge of the rate and route of development of SLI, of the

strategies adopted in inefficient language learning, and of individual differences among SLI children has been greatly inhibited by the general lack of longitudinal studies. It is usually argued that, as we may not be reliably able to distinguish SLI from the bottom end of the normal language acquisition distribution before four years or so, we will never know about the early stages of development of language-impaired individuals, or in what respects they differ from one another. Two points to make in response are: (a) it would still be interesting to have the longitudinal information from the time these individuals are diagnosed, and (b) as we know from familial aggregation studies that speech and language disorders run in families, it would surely be worth our while to monitor the younger siblings of identified LI children.

- I would argued that spontaneous language sample data are always valuable but they are not as much under the investigator's control as we would like them to be. These samples are also biased towards some features of the grammar and against others. Accordingly, in common with other researchers in this area, we have begun to use experimental approaches. This trend is likely to continue.

- It is important not to lose sight of the relationship between research on the characteristics of SLI and remediation. The better we are able to describe (and eventually explain) language impairment, the more useful our work is to the practitioner. Take for example the grammatical-but-minimal approach to verb complementation of the older group of SLI children. The implication here is that we do not concentrate on grammar as a mechanism that may have gone wrong or may not be complete but on how the grammatical resources available are to be maximally used for informational and communication purposes in the settings that face the child. Grammar is the central part of the communication system, but it is a servant, not a master, and while we might define grammar in formal terms for research purposes, it is the functional role of grammar in daily life that we may want to concentrate on in remediation in a clinical context.

References

Bishop D (1994) Grammatical errors in specific language impairment: competence or performance limitations? Applied Psycholinguistics 15: 507–50.

Bishop D and Edmundson A (1987) Language impaired 4-year-olds: distinguishing transient from persistent impairment. Journal of Speech and Hearing Disorders 43: 227–41.

Chomsky N (1965) Aspects of the Theory of Syntax. Cambridge, Mass: MIT Press.

Craig H (1995) Pragmatic impairments. See Fletcher and MacWhinney (1995) 623–40.

Fey M, Long S, Cleave P (1994) Reconsideration of IQ criteria in the definition of specific language impairment. In R. Watkins and M. Rice (eds) Specific Language Impairments in Children. Baltimore: Paul H Brookes Publishing Co, 161–78.

Fletcher P, MacWhinney B (1995) The Handbook of Child Language. Oxford: Blackwell.

Fletcher P, Ingham R, King G, Schelleter C, Sinka, I (1996). Final Report, ESRC Project R000234135, Verb-Related Impairments in Children with Specific Language Impairment.

Gathercole S, Baddeley, A (1990) Phonological memory deficits of language disordered children: is there a causal connection? Journal of Memory and Language 29: 336–69.

Gavin, W, Klee T and Membrino I (1993) Differentiating specific language impairment from normal language development using grammatical analysis. Clinical Linguistics and Phonetics 7: 191–206.

Johnston J (1992) Cognitive abilities of language impaired children. In Specific speech and language disorders in children. In Fletcher P, Hall D (Eds) Specific Speech and Language Disorders in Children. London: Whurr Publishers, pp 105–16

Johnston J and Schery T (1976) The use of grammatical morphemes by children with communication disorders. In Morehead D, Morehead A (Eds) Normal and Deficient Child Language. Baltimore: University Park Press, pp 239–58.

Kent R (1994) Reference Manual for Communicative Sciences and Disorders: Speech and Language. Austin, TX: Pro-Ed.

King G (1996) Verb complementation in language-impaired schoolage children. In Aldridge M (Ed) Child Language. Clevedon: Multilingual Matters, pp 84–91.

Leonard L (1994) Some problems facing accounts of morphological deficits in children with specific language impairments. In Watkins RV and Rice ML (Eds) Specific language impairments in children. Baltimore, Md: Paul H Brookes Publishing Co.

Leonard L, Sabbadini L, Leonard, J and Volterra, V (1987) Specific language impairment in children: a cross-linguistic study. Brain and Language 32: 233–52.

Leonard L, Bortolini U, Caselli MC, McGregor K and Sabbadini L (1992) Morphological deficits in children with specific language impairment: the status of features in the underlying grammar. Language Acquisition 2: 151–79.

Matthews J (Ed) (1994). Linguistic aspects of familial language impairment. McGill Working Papers in Linguistics 10: 1–2.

Morehead D, Ingram D (1973) The development of base syntax in normal and linguistically deviant children. Journal of Speech and Hearing Research 16: 330–52. Reprinted in Morehead D and Morehead A (Eds) (1976) Normal and Deficient Child Language. Baltimore: University Park Press, pp 209–38.

Pinker S (1984) Language Learnability and Language Development. Cambridge, MA: Harvard University Press.

Rice M, Wexler K (1996) Towards Tense as a clinical marker of specific language impairment in English-speaking children. Journal of Speech and Hearing Research 39: 1239–57.

Schelleter C, Fletcher P, Ingham R, King G, Sinka, I (1996) English-speaking SLI children's use of locative/contact and causative alternations. Paper presented at Child Language Seminar, Reading, England, April.

Tallal P, Miller S, Bedi G, Byma G, Wang X, Nagarajan S, Schreiner C, Jenkins W, Merzenich M (1996) Language comprehension in language-learning impaired children improved with acoustically-modified speech. Science, 271, 5 January, 81–4.

Ullman, M and Gopnik M (1994) The production of inflectional morphology in hereditary specific language impairment. See Matthews J (1994) 81–118.

Notes

1   Morehead and Ingram do not, however, define what they include under the heading of inflectional morphology. It is possible that they do not intend past tense, for example, to be included under this heading. If so, one rather puzzling discrepancy between their work and later work would be explained.

2   Paul Fletcher, Richard Ingham, Gabrielle King, Christina Schelleter and Indra Sinka. The work reported here is supported by the UK Economic and Social Research Council.

3   Here and subsequently, 'past tense' refers to regular past tense.

4   The work reported here was supported by the UK Medical Research Council.

5   Table 1.1 is based on 63 analysable utterances from 11 subjects per group. A category 'Other Complement Types', which accounted for only six sentences out of a total of 1380, is omitted from this Table.

Chapter 2
Testing Children's Language Abilities – A Description of a New Language Test: Reynell Developmental Language Scales [1]

SUSAN EDWARDS

Introduction

The Reynell Developmental Language Scales (Reynell 1977) (henceforth RDLS) is a test used extensively by speech and language therapists in English-speaking countries (and in translation elsewhere) to screen children between the ages of 1;06 and 7;00 and to gauge progress of children attending therapy. These scales offer a means of comparing a child's comprehension and production of speech with scores that have been standardized on a large sample of British children. The Comprehension Scale continues to be widely used, unlike the Expressive Scale which therapists find difficult to score objectively and whose results they find uninformative. Hence, in 1995 the publishers NFER-Nelson invited tenders for a contract to revise and restandardize the RDLS and a team of academics in the Department of Linguistic Science at the University of Reading was awarded the contract.

In this paper a brief account of the construction of the test will be given, followed by a summary of the test contents. Finally, some highlights from the results will be presented. A full description of the background to the construction of the test, a description of contents, statistical information, directions for use and other such details can be found in The RDLS III Manual (Edwards, Fletcher, Garman, Hughes, Letts and Sinka, 1997).

Background

The aim was to produce a test that would measure aspects of children's understanding and production of language between the ages of 1;06 and 7;00 years, discriminating performance on a developmental continuum. Although the project would eventually yield a radically revised test, it was also important to retain the feel and the philosophy of the original versions of the test. Accordingly, the two scales that measure comprehension and expressive abilities separately were retained, some items from the original Comprehension Scale were modified and included and the use of pictures and objects as test materials was also adhered to, although much of the toy material and all of the pictures were replaced.

As with the first two versions of the RDLS, the emphasis in the new edition is on vocabulary and connected speech: the phonological system is not explored separately. There are similarities with the original version but there are important differences. The test reflects current views of language in that language is conceived as a modular system not only in the sense that language may function independently of other cognitive abilities but also in the sense that, at least to some extent, it is possible to separate the so-called levels of language. Research supports clinical experience that children may have deficits in one or more aspects of language and it was considered a useful aim to endeavour to increase the linguistic transparency of each section. So, for example, sections in both scales explore a child's ability to understand and produce single nouns, verbs and various phrasal and clausal constituents. Failure in a section can be used to guide a clinician to further detailed testing of specific aspects of a child's language skills and results provide guidance for therapy.

It was clearly not possible to explore all aspects of language production and comprehension in such a test and choices had to be made. These were motivated by our collective clinical and research experiences and by other work that has been produced in the two decades since the first edition of RDLS was published. Work on normal language development (e.g, Chapman, 1988; Crystal, Fletcher and Garman, 1989; Dale and Fenson, 1996; Fenson, Dale, Reznick, Bates, Thal and Pethick, 1994; Fletcher, 1985; Sutter and Johnson, 1990; Wells, 1985) and work that highlights aspects of the language system that differentiate normal development from delayed development (e.g. Fletcher and Peters, 1984; Leonard, Sabbadini, Leonard and Volterra, 1987; Rice, Wexler and Cleave, 1995; Schelleter, Fletcher, Ingham, King and Sinka, 1996) was consulted and referenced at appropriate places throughout the manual.

Drafting items

After the range of linguistic features to include had been decided, items had to be constructed that would elicit (for the Expressive Scale) or test (for the Comprehension Scale) those and only those aspects of language under investigation. This practical aspect proved to be one of the most difficult parts of the construction of the test. In clinical work (and we suspect much research) one is able to repeat or reformulate the stimulus but, in order to build in a clear and distinct method of scoring, test procedures were restricted so that every stimulus was given once and once only.

To guide the choice of vocabulary items we made detailed use of *A Lexical Development Norms Database* (Dale and Fenson, 1996). For the later stages of the test we consulted data on 5-year-olds taken from the Gordon Wells' Bristol study (Raban, 1988). Guidance for the structures tested came from two sources. We followed a developmental perspective, again guided by the available published data, but within this developmental perspective we selected those aspects of speech that are thought to differentiate normally developing children from those with language problems (Bates, Dale and Thal 1995, Fenson et al. 1994, Miller and Paul 1995, Wells 1985).

Trialing

A number of procedures and possible test items were discussed and pre-trialed with normally developing children and with some children attending speech and language therapy as it was important to check that testing procedures would also work with this population as well as with children whose language was developing normally. Using these preliminary results and feedback from speech and language therapists, two trial versions were constructed with approximately 50 per cent of all the items as anchor items in each version. This enabled us to trial around 180 items while keeping each version the same length as the final version, 120 items. Subjects for trialing were selected from schools, nurseries, playgroups, mother-and-toddler clubs and a few through personal contacts. The selection criteria were that the children should be developing normally, should not have attended speech and language therapy and that they should have English as their first language.

Our field-workers tested 363 children during September 1995. We checked all record forms, noting items that were problematic for scoring, and we collected feedback from the field-workers about each section of the test. Results from the trialing showed that there was a developmental progress across sections and that the Comprehension Scale discriminated well at the early stages. The Expressive Scale, however, while discriminating well in the older age range, was less satisfactory for the very youngest children. Eighteen-month-old children were not scoring very much on the test and scores were mainly confined to the single-word section. If these children were using language beyond naming single objects then these testing procedures were not capturing it.

These findings might superficially seem to contrast with reports of child language development in the literature. For example, Bates, Dale and Thal (1995) found that 11% of parents of 18-month-old children reported that their children often combined words and another 46% said their children sometimes did this. At 24 months most parents reported that their children often combined words although approximately 10% were failing to do so. Wells (1985), while observing large individual differences, reports on children using connected speech before the age of two years – about the time when children in our data start scoring. However, these studies examine reported and recorded spontaneous speech while our results measure test performance and it is therefore not surprising that the children under two years old we tested were barely scoring. After all, despite wide variation in development, what children might say and what they can be persuaded to say during a test are likely to be different.

Constructing the scales for standardization

The data were analysed to produce a range of information on items, section scores and test versions including a discrimination index and facility scores for each item. Items were pruned to produce two single scales (Comprehension and Expressive) for the standardization version of the test using both the statistical results and information received from the field workers on administration.

In view of the low scores obtained by the 18-month-old children and in line with current clinical practice it was decided that the Expressive Scale would start at two years while 18 months remained the lower limit for the Comprehension Scale.

There are 62 items in each scale. The Comprehension Scale tests a child's understanding of single nouns and verbs, expanded noun phrases, locative relations and thematic role assignment. The penultimate section explores the child's understanding of complex constructions such as passives, relative clauses and negation. The final section tests a child's ability to extract information from a complex picture and to answer inferential questions. The Expressive Scale, which starts with naming common objects, includes tasks to elicit phrasal and clausal utterances, bound grammatical morphemes marking plurality and tense, question forms, and complex clausal subordination. Explicit instructions for administration are given and examples of acceptable answers for the Expressive Scale (including acceptable pronunciations) are included to maximize reliability.

Standardization

For standardization, the test was administered to 1076 children between the ages of 18 months and 7 years across the British Isles over a three-month period in 1996. The field workers were mainly students but qualified speech and language therapists were also used. Urban and rural locations were used, spread across the British Isles, including some sites in Scotland, Wales, Northern Ireland and the Republic of Ireland. Selection criteria were the same for both trialing and standardization. No child participated in both the trialing and the standardization.

Recruitment of school-aged children was eased by the co-operation of a large number of headteachers, whereas the number of pre-school-aged children who participated in the standardization was fewer than those originally identified. Nevertheless, the results given in RDLS III, can be considered to be robust and representative. The total cohort used in standardization of 1076 subjects across six years compares favourably with cohorts of other standardized tests. (For example, the English version of the WISC (Wechsler 1992) was standardized on 824 children between the ages of 6 and 16). A sub-group of 191 children between the ages of 4;0 and 7;6 years (84 boys and 107 girls) was given two further test, the Test for the Reception of Grammar (Bishop, 1982) and the British Picture Vocabulary Scales (Dunn, Whetton and Burley, 1997)

Results

Results via feedback from the fieldworkers were encouraging: children enjoyed doing the test and the speech and language therapists employed reported that the test could be administered in practice and was potentially useful. Furthermore, the statistical analyses revealed that the scales discriminated well across the age range tested. In this short section it is necessary to give brief and selected details from the results: further details can be found in Edwards et al. (1997).

The data were first analysed using general linear modelling to check whether factors other than age contributed to the scores. A slight effect was found to be associated with both the site of testing and the tester. However, the size of this contribution was small compared with the contribution of age and did not affect the validity of the test. Reliability coefficients using the Kuder-Richardson formula and based on all the children gave coefficient scores of 0.97 for the Comprehension Scale and 0.96 for the Expressive Scale. Reliability was high throughout the age range for the Expressive Scale but less so after six years of age for the Comprehension Scale. These results reflect the difficulty of discriminating comprehension skills in children of school age. Interestingly the Expressive Scale discriminates well across the full age range.

Cross-validation

A subgroup of the sample (191) was tested with two other tests that are widely used by speech and language therapists. Both test aspects of comprehension although differ in the aspects of language tested. The TROG tests a child's understanding of meaning conveyed by various grammatical constructions and the BPVS is a vocabulary test. These tests measure related but different aspects of language from those measured by RDLS III and this partial relationship is reflected in the correlations obtained and shown in Table 2.1.

Table 2.1. Correlations between RDLS III, BPVS and TROG.

	RDLS exp.	BPVS	TROG
RDLS comp.	0.62	0.68	0.70
RDLS exp.		0.75	0.67
BPVS			0.75

Gender differences

Despite the claim made over 30 years ago that, in language development, there is a real sex difference in favour of girls (McCarthy, 1954: 580) other opinion, perhaps led by a re-examination of some early studies (Macaulay, 1978) has tended to take the opposite view. Wells (1985: 345) states categorically that according to data collected on the Bristol project there is 'no evidence of a consistent and significant difference between sexes in either route or rate of development'. This conclusion was based on two subsets of the data. First, a sub-sample of 40 children aged 39 months was examined for patterns of initiations and second, t-tests were applied to the results of data from 60 children aged 40 months, and 65 children aged 65 months. No significant difference was found (Woll, Ferrier and Wells, 1975; Woll, 1979).

In contrast to these findings, results from the standardization of RDLS III reveal some gender differences. The difference between boys and girls was marked in the younger age groups where there is a significant difference for both the Expressive and the Comprehension

Scales. For example, there are significant differences between comprehension scores of boys and girls between the ages of 1;9 and 2;11 (N = 182, t = 13.76, df = 14, p<0.001) and between the scores of boys and girls between 1;09 and 3;11 (N=300, t=14.73, df=14, p<0.001) and between 4;0 and 5;6 (N = 460, t = 7.41, df = 18, p< 0.001) for Expression. Although further analyses are necessary, these preliminary findings would appear to be at odds with other claims although consistent with the results of the first edition the RDLS (Reynell, 1977) and suggest that there might be real differences in the rate of language development for boys and girls. Whereas the sample size at the lower end of the RDLS is small compared with the school-aged children, it compares favourably with the Bristol samples. The amount and type of data analysed varies considerably from the data used in the Bristol project and these results do not necessarily demonstrate a faster rate of language development in girls. However, this would seem to be an area worth investigating again. While waiting for this issue to be clarified, the prudent clinician might wish to take these differences into account.

Traditionally, a speech and language therapist will use a range of procedures in assessment including informal observation, standardized tests and analyses of spontaneous speech samples. In view of the potentially different information gained from test results and spontaneous speech data it would seem to be crucial to continue this practice. Of course, the methodology employed in the collection, transcription and analysis of spontaneous speech data needs to be as reliable as possible and it is therefore important to follow consistent procedures (Garman and Edwards, 1995). In selecting a standardized test the clinician also needs to consider the reliability and robustness of that test. The RDLS III, which has been standardized on a large representative sample of English-speaking children, offers an attractive way of assessing children's expressive and comprehension abilities. It is clinically useful, detailed enough to discriminate reliably between children's performance, it reflects developmental progress, gives standardized scores and motivates clinical decisions. The format is attractive to busy clinicians, and engaging enough to capture a child's attention, and we predict that it will become an important addition to routine clinical assessment.

References

Bates E, Dale P, Thal, D (1995) Individual differences and their implications for theories of language development. In Fletcher P, MacWhinney B (Eds) The Handbook of Child Language. Oxford: Blackwell.

Bishop D (1982) TROG: Test for Reception of Grammar. Abingdon, UK: Thomas Leach.

Chapman R (1988) Language acquisition in the child. In Lass N, McReynolds L, Northern J, Yoder D (Eds) Handbook of Speech-Language Pathology and Audiology. Toronto: B.C.Decker, pp 309–53.

Crystal D, Fletcher P, Garman M (1989) The grammatical analysis of language disability. 2nd edn. London: Whurr Publishers.

Dale P, Fenson L (1996) Lexical developmental norms for young children. Behaviour Research Methods, Instruments and Computer 28: 125–7.

Dunn LM, Whetton C, Burley J (1997) British Picture Vocabulary Scale (Second edition). Windsor: NFER-Nelson.

Edwards S, Fletcher P, Garman M, Hughes A, Letts C, Sinka I (1997) The Manual of The Reynell Developmental Language Scales III. Windsor: NFER-Nelson.

Fenson L, Dale P, Reznick J, Bates E, Thal D, Pethick S (1994) Variability in early communicative development. Monographs of the Society for Research in Child Development, 59, serial no, 242.

Fletcher P (1985) A Child's Learning of English. Oxford: Blackwell.

Fletcher P, Peters J (1984) Characterising language impairment in children: an exploratory study. Language Testing 1, 33–49.

Garman M, Edwards S (1995) Syntactic assessment of expressive language. In Grundy K (Ed) Linguistics in Clinical Practice London: Whurr Publishers.

Leonard L, Sabbadini L, Leonard J, Volterra V (1987) Specific language impairment in children: a cross-linguistic study. Brain and Language 32: 233–52.

Macaulay R (1978) The myth of female superiority. Journal of Child Language 5: 353–63.

McCarthy D (1954) Language Development in Children. In Carmichael L (Ed) Manual of Child Psychology. New York: Wiley.

Miller J, Paul R (1995) The Clinical Assessment of Language Comprehension. Baltimore: Paul Brookes Publishing.

Raban B (1988) The Spoken Vocabulary of Five-Year-Old Children. Reading: Reading and Language Information Centre, The University of Reading.

Reynell J (1977) Manual for the Reynell Developmental Language Scales (Revised). Windsor: NFER.

Rice M, Wexler K, Cleave P (1995) Specific language impairment as a period of extended optional infinitive. Journal of Speech and Hearing Research 38: 850–63.

Schelletter C, Fletcher P, Ingham R, King G, Sinka I (1996) English-speaking SLI children's use of locative/contact and causative alternations. Paper presented at The Child Language Seminar, Reading, April.

Sutter J, Johnson C (1990) School-aged children's metalinguistic awareness of grammaticality in verb form. Journal of Speech and Hearing Research 33: 84–95.

Wells G (1985) Language Development in the Pre-School Years. Cambridge: CUP.

Wechsler D (1992) Wechsler Intelligence Test for Children. 3rd edn. Sidcup: Harcourt Brace Jovanovich.

Woll B (1979) Sex as a variable in child language development. Bristol Working Papers in Language 1: 71–86.

Woll B, Ferrier L, Wells G (1975) Children and their parents: who starts talking, why and when? Paper presented at the Language and the Social Context Conference, Stirling, January 1975.

Note

1   The generous contributions of the project manager, Indra Sinka, consultants and contributors Paul Fletcher, Michael Garman, Arthur Hughes and Carolyn Letts and the statistical adviser Tony Woods are freely and gratefully acknowledged.

Chapter 3
Speech Perception and Comprehension of Dysphasic Children

MÁRIA GÓSY

Introduction

The term 'developmental dysphasia' is applied to children's language development where starting to speak is delayed beyond the normal range (Wyke, 1977. Evidence suggests that such children are particularly impaired in acquiring correct pronunciation and syntactic and morphological rules, although well-defined syndromes of impaired language development have not yet been determined. Auditory processing deficits have also been demonstrated in dysphasic children, but only a very restricted number of scientific experiments and descriptions concerning these processes are available (cf. Tallal, 1976; Ludlow, 1980). Children are generally labelled dysphasic when they fail to speak by three years of age. However, those who are still in the holophrasic period of language development at the age of two are definitely risk children for dysphasia. According to Ingram's definition, developmental dysphasia occurs despite normal intelligence and average family background, with the characteristics of slow language development, articulation deficits, poor syntactic structures, restricted mental lexicon and poor rhythmic ability (Ingram, 1976). Unfortunately, this definition does not contain any reference to deficits of speech perception and comprehension.

Little research has been aimed at determining the cause of developmental dysphasia in children and few hypotheses have been suggested. The great variety in the language development of dysphasic children means that various significant features of the syndrome are provided instead of a detailed description of the phenomenon. Tallal and Piercy say that the deficits of the speech perception processes might cause developmental dysphasia, and their experimental findings seem to support their hypothesis (1977). It is possible that developmental dysphasia might be caused by several diverse factors (see, for example, Bartak and Rutter, 1975; Ludlow, 1980; Geschwind and Galaburda, 1985; Paul and Shiffer, 1991).

Our aim was to analyse the speech perception and comprehension processes of dysphasic children at the age of three and between the ages of six and eight. The results of the experiments were intended to answer the following questions:

1. What do we know about the verbal decoding processes of three-year-old dysphasic children?
2. Do older dysphasic children show deficits in their speech perception and comprehension processes?
3. Are there differences between the performances of these children of various ages?

Subjects, method, material

Two series of experiments have been carried out with dysphasic children of various ages using the GMP standardized test-package for the evaluation of children's decoding processes (the test had been developed by the present author, Gósy, 1989; 1995, and is used widely throughout Hungary).

Experiment I

One hundred young dysphasic children took part in the first experiment. Their mean age was 3;0 and varied between 2;10 and 3;2, 68 boys and 32 girls. Beside their age the following criteria had been used in order to select them for the experiment: (a) normal birth circumstances, (b) normal IQ, (c) no neurological problem reported, (d) no autistic features detected, (e) no previous treatment by a speech therapist. All these children were in the 'holophrasic' phase of first language acquisition, i.e. their vocabulary was limited to a small number of words (below 20), they expressed their wishes by non-verbal gestures but they were able to decode adults' verbal utterances to a certain degree.

These children were tested by the GMP20 subtest of the test-package that aims at obtaining information about the children's hearing, speech perception (if available), comprehension and articulation ability (if available). Subtest GMP16 was used to detect the children's sentence comprehension. A set of picture pairs was used (standardized for three-

and four-year-olds) to test sentence comprehension where one of the two met the semantics of either a simple or a complex Hungarian sentence. The children had to choose one of each pair according to the sentence they had been given. The duration of the test procedure was generally 15 minutes.

Experiment II

Forty-two dysphasic children took part in the second experiment (cf. Table 3.1). The selection criteria for these children were as follows: (a) normal birth circumstances, (b) normal IQ, (c) no neurological problem reported, (d) normal hearing, (e) no articulation defect, (f) on the basis of their speech therapists' evidence they started to speak around the age of three.

Table 3.1. Proportion of children

Test groups	Ages	Proportion of children (%)	
		girls	boys
preschool children	5;10–6;6	28.5	71.5
first graders	6;10–7;6	17.6	82.4
second graders	7;10–8;6	27.2	72.8

Seven subtests of the original test-package were chosen for the sake of this experiment; the speech material varied from isolated words to sentences and to a longer text. The speech material of five subtests was distorted according to the actual purpose of the subtest (like words and sentences were covered by white noise, the signal/noise ratio was 4 dB; pass-band filtration: 36 dB/octave between 2200 and 2700 Hz; electrically speeded-up sentences: the average speech tempo was 13.5 sounds/second). Meaningless sound sequences were used for detection of the children's serial perception ability. Text comprehension was tested by various questions concerning the details and the interrelations of a tape-recorded short story. Sentence comprehension was checked by means of the standardized subtest (see Experiment I) for six- and seven-year-olds. The selected subtests of the test-package (GMP2, 3, 4, 5, 10, 12 and 16) aim at measuring the acoustic, phonetic and phonological levels of the speech perception process, serial perception and sentence and text comprehension.

The test method also varied according to the purpose of the subtest, depending on the subprocess to be tested (Table 3.2). The distorted speech material and the short story were tape-recorded and were used at a comfortable volume without headphones. The sound sequences and the test sentences of the sentence-comprehension material were pronounced by the examiner. All children were tested individually. The duration of the test procedure was generally 12 minutes.

Table 3.2. Methods of the subtests used in the experiments

Subtest	Material	Method
GMP2	noisy sentences	repetition
GMP3	noisy words	repetition
GMP4	filtered sentences	repetition
GMP5	fast sentences	repetition
GMP10	sound sequences	repetition
GMP12	short story	multiple questions
GMP16	sentences	picture decision

Results

Experiment I

On the basis of the subjective hearing screening, 3% of the 3-year-old dysphasic children proved to have severe hearing loss whereas 35% had slight hearing loss. Only 62 of the tested 100 3-year-olds showed normal hearing. These results were confirmed later by objective audiological examinations (at the Pedoaudiological Department of the Heim Pál Children's Hospital in Budapest). Overall speech comprehension was judged to be appropriate to the age requirements in 52% of all children whereas 48% of them showed backwardness.

Sentence comprehension results showed enormous individual differences among the tested children. The standard performance of the sentence comprehension test at the age of three is 70%, i.e. the children have to be able to comprehend correctly seven sentences out of 10. The mean result of our dysphasic children's correct responses is 39.4%, the range is 0–80%. One child performed slightly better than the age requirement, eight children showed the expected performance while 91 of them underperformed. The dysphasic children performed significantly poorer than their normally developed controls although their sentence comprehension was significantly better than their text comprehension. An extremely interesting aspect of these data is the performance of the nine children who understood the sentences at the same level as normally developed children do. What can be the explanation for their result? Without appropriate speech production experience these children were able to decode complex structures and complex morphology (Hungarian has a very rich morphological structure) within one sentence with actual semantics. These results seem to support the view that the 3-year-old dysphasic children (a) may have more relatively complex language knowledge than it is supposed and (b) their decoding processes may work without any interrelations with the production processes. These findings lead to the question of whether these children's further perception and comprehension development proceeds undisturbed or will show slower development compared to their speech production. In order to answer this question the second set of experiments was carried out with older 'dysphasic' children.

Experiment II

The speech production of the subjects of this experiment did not deviate in any respect from those of normally developed children of the same ages. However, results of their speech perception and comprehension performance did not meet the age requirements. Identification of filtered, noisy and fast sentences as well as of meaningless sound sequences by these children showed significant backwardness ($p < 0.001$), i.e. their phonetic and phonological knowledge, necessary for the operations of the tested subprocesses, was underdeveloped (Figure 3.1).

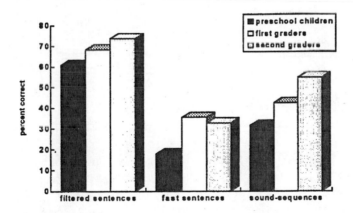

Figure 3.1 Speech perception performance of the tested dysphasic children.

The filtered sentences were identified best, although performance here was poorer than the standardized value, which is a 100% correct response for all tested age groups. The identification of the fast sentences and the meaningless sound sequences by the tested children showed the standardized performance of normally developed 3- and 4-year-olds ($p < 0.0001$). The required value of the fast sentence identification task is 90% correct for preschool children and 100% for school-children, while the required value is 100% in all age groups in the case of meaningless sound sequences. The range of (a) the preschool children's data is 20-100% for filtered sentences, 0–70% for fast sentences and for meaningless sound sequences; (b) the first graders' data are 0–100% for filtered sentences, 0–80% for fast sentences and 0–90% for meaningless sound sequences; (c) the second graders' data are 40–100% for filtered sentences, 20–60% for fast sentences and 20–90% for the sound sequences.

A significant difference was found between the correct identification of noisy sentences and noisy words ($p < 0.001$) although the largest actual difference occurs with the preschool children and the smallest one with the second graders (Table 3.3). The dysphasic children's performance was close to that of normally developed 4- and 5-year-olds ($p < 0.0001$). There is a gradual development in the identification of noisy sentences through age groups but this is not the case for the words. It is possible that this phenomenon is due to the speech therapists' work that concentrates on structures.

Table 3.3. Identification of noisy words and sentences

Test groups	Correct identification (%)			
	words mean	range	sentences mean	range
6-year-olds	77.8	50-90	53.5	20-90
7-year-olds	75.8	50-90	56.4	10-90
8-year-olds	77.2	40-100	65.4	10-90

The dysphasic children's sentence comprehension was significantly better than their text comprehension but all the data show a significantly poorer performance compared to that of normally developed children of the same ages ($p < 0.0001$), cf. Figure 3.2. The standardized sentence comprehension produced 80% correct scores for preschool children and 100% correct scores for schoolchildren. The standardized text comprehension scores were 70% correct for all responses among preschool children, 90% for first graders and 100% for second graders. So, in the case of normally developed children there is only a 10% difference between sentence and text comprehension; a higher value means not only poorer performance but various undesirable consequences (e.g. reading and spelling difficulties). Mean values of the dysphasic children's comprehension show a difference of more than 10% between sentence and text comprehension. The mean value of the dysphasic preschool children's sentence comprehension is poorer than the regional value by about 30% whereas their text comprehension is poorer by about 40% than the required value. First graders' performance is poorer by about 40% both in sentence and text comprehension.

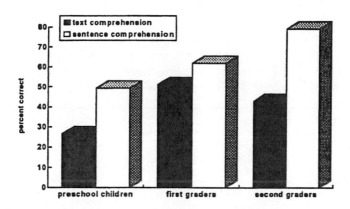

Figure 3.2. Comprehension differences in the tested dysphasic children.

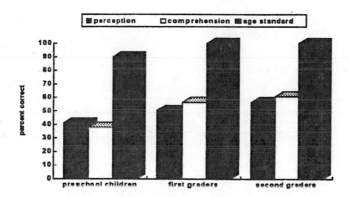

Figure 3.3. Speech perception and comprehension performance of dysphasic children compared to the standard values.

Second graders show a poorer performance by about 20% in sentences and 60% in text comprehension. These data confirm that sentence comprehension shows a gradual development across ages, but text comprehension does not. More complex strategies are needed to decode a text than to decode a sentence, and these strategies appear to be underdeveloped with the dysphasic children. We can assume that these strategies are functions of an undisturbed language acquisition process rather than intelligence, logic or thinking.

Figure 3.3 demonstrates the average data of the speech perception and comprehension processes for all test groups. The data show that (a) our dysphasic children's decoding processes are significantly

underdeveloped, and that (b) the difference between their performances and those of the normally developed children is very large.
Taking mean values into consideration, our preschool children are
three years behind both in speech perception and in comprehension;
the first graders are behind by three years in speech perception and by
two years in comprehension and the second graders are behind by four
years in speech perception and by three years in comprehension. This
means that despite some development in these processes, the children
show a relatively stable level of backwardness in relation to their biological age.

Conclusion

The results suggest that all our dysphasic children showed deficits in
their decoding mechanism. However, some children performed appropriately in some of the subprocesses. There were no large age differences among the tested children; text comprehension showed practically no development. These children need extra treatment to correct
their auditory decoding processes.

Figure 3.4 shows the performances of a dysphasic boy who had been
going through systematic and special speech therapy treatment from
the age of 5. This boy, whose vocabulary consisted of five holophrases
at the age of three, performed perfectly on almost all tests by the age of
seven. We must conclude that developmental dysphasia contains
deficits in the speech perception and comprehension processes with
enormous individual differences. In order to prevent the children from
experiencing further problems like reading difficulties, special therapy
is needed as early as possible.

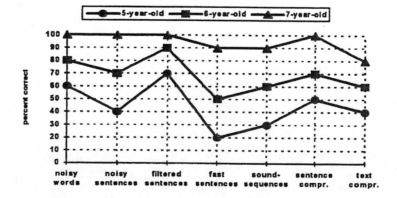

Figure 3.4. The improvement of the speech perception and comprehension of
a dysphasic boy on special treatment.

References

Bartak L, Rutter M (1975) Language and cognition in autistic and 'dysphasic' children. In O'Conner N (Ed.): Language, Cognitive Deficits and Retardation. London: Butterworth, pp. 97–134.

Geschwind N, Galaburda, AM (1985) Cerebral lateralization: biological mechanism, associations, and pathology: I. A hypothesis and a program for research. Archives of Neurology 42: 428–59.

Gósy M (1989) GMP – Beszédészlelési és beszédmegértési teljesítmény. Tesztcsomag. (GMP – Speech Perception and Comprehension Performance Test-package). Budapest: Logo-Press.

Gósy M (1995) GMP – Diagnosztika. (GMP – Diagnostics) Budapest: Nikol.

Ingram TTS (1976) Speech disorders in childhood. In C. and E. Lenneberg (Eds) Foundations in Language Development. New York: Academic Press, pp. 235–61.

Ludlow CL (1980) Children's language disorders: Recent research advances. Annals of Neurology 7: 497–507.

Paul R, Shiffer ME (1991) Communicative initiations in normal and late-talking toddlers. Applied Psychology 12: 419–33.

Tallal P (1976) Rapid auditory processing in normal and disordered language development. Journal of Speech and Hearing Research 19: 561–71.

Tallal P, Piercy M (1977) Defects of auditory perception in children with developmental dysphasia. In Wyke (1977) Developmental Dysphasia. London and New York: Academic Press, pp. 63–83.

Wyke, AM (Ed) (1977) Developmental Dysphasia. London and New York: Academic Press.

GRAMMAR AND LEXICON

Chapter 4
Vulnerability of Conjunction and Verb Tense Use in the Narrative Speech of Dyslexic Children

MONIQUE PLAZA, CLAUDINE GUITTON,
MARIE-THÉRÈSE LE NORMAND

Introduction

Failures concerning linguistic skills have been observed in dyslexic children. Phonological awareness, syntactic processing and lexical access, in particular, have been evaluated. The spontaneous and/or narrative speech of dyslexic children have been less well documented. Narrative production gives some idea of the level of semantic diversity and complexity of which children are capable when linguistic structure is not being modelled for them by adults. Indeed, in order to tell a narrative, the child must draw upon his or her linguistic structural knowledge and competence. The few studies that assess narrative production by dyslexic children tend to support theories of a language deficit in dyslexia (Davenport, Yingling, Fein, Galin and Johnstone, 1986; Feagans and Short, 1984; Murphy, Pollatsek and Well, 1988).

This study focuses on two language features: the compounding of lexicon used by dyslexic children and the modality of verb tense. We examine how 20 French children with reading difficulties (a) used basic grammatical morphemes in their narrative speech elicited by a picture book and (b) processed verb tense. The use of two control groups (good readers of the same chronological age, and younger reading-level matched children) allows hypotheses to be formulated about whether the observed difficulties may be causes or consequences of reading failure.

Method

Material

Children's narrative productions were elicited with a picture book, *Frog Where Are You?* (Mayer, 1969).

Procedure

Children were seen individually. They were asked to tell the story as clearly as possible. The experimenter did not intervene during the session. All the recordings were audiotaped and transcribed ortho-graphic-ally using the convention of the CHAT system to facilitate analysis by the CLAN computer program (MacWhinney and Snow, 1991). For each transcript (1) we scored (a) the number of different words and tokens, the type and the number of verbs, pronouns, nouns, determiners, adjectives, conjunctions, prepositions, adverbs and frozen forms used by the child and (b) the ratio of each word type in relation to the total of different words and to the total of tokens; (2) we assessed each transcript to investigate the modality of verb tense in the child's speech.

Subjects

The subjects were 60 French children. Twenty children (mean age: 8;6) exhibited specific reading difficulties (mean reading level: beginning Grade 2), 20 children were children of the same age developing norm-ally (mean age: 8;4), and 20 children were younger reading-level-matched children (mean age: 7;6).

Statistical data

Comparisons between dyslexic children and the two control groups were carried out using an analysis of variance (ANOVA).

Results

(1) Compared with the chronological age-matched control group, dyslexic children showed significant deficits in: (a) type-token ratio ($p < 0.0001$), (b) verb, noun, conjunction and adverb diversity, (c) con-junction and preposition token ratio, and (d) general verb tense and use of past tense. They also exhibited a greater use of frozen forms than the control group and they produced a similar number of tokens for telling the 25 episodes of the story.

(2) Compared with the reading-level matched control group, dyslexic children showed significant deficits in: (a) type-token ratio ($p < 0.01$), (b) conjunction diversity ($p < 0.03$), (c) conjunction token ratio ($p < 0.01$), and (d) general verb tense and use of past tense ($p < 0.01$). They also exhibited a greater use of frozen forms than the control group and they produced a similar number of tokens for telling the 25 episodes of the story.

Discussion

The lexical deficit

Dyslexic children appeared to exhibit a significant deficit in lexical diversity: they used comparatively fewer word types than the two control groups. Such a vocabulary deficit has been observed in previous studies (Bryant, Bradley, Maclean, and Crossland, 1989; Stanovich, Cunningham and Feeman, 1984; Wolf and Goodglass, 1986).

The first question is 'what kind of relationships exist between reading failures and vocabulary deficits?' It may be assumed that lexical production deficit is a consequence of reading failure since literacy allows vocabulary to develop dramatically. Nevertheless, in our study dyslexic children perform at a lower level than the younger reading-level matched children do. This discrepancy allows us to hypothesize that the lexical deficit may be associated with earlier language deficiencies.

The second question is whether these language deficiencies are general or specific. Most contemporary views favour the specific (modular) hypothesis and claim that phonological skills are more likely proximal causes of poor reading achievement (Khami and Catts, 1989; Stanovich, 1988; Morais, 1994). According to the phonological hypothesis, lexical production deficit should represent a difficulty in word retrieval related to a difficulty in representing or retrieving phonological information. Such a deficit is also closely related to a verbal working memory weakness.

The conjunction deficit

The lexical deficit was particularly significant in conjunction use. Dyslexic children did not use conjunctions as easily as the two control groups of children, particularly the conjunctions *mais* (but) and *quand* (when).

Conjunctions are grammatical function words that underlie intersentential connections. Connectives are complex linguistic features. On the one hand, they do not have a referent in an extralinguistic context and so they begin to work for children as indexical items without autonomous meaning (Orsolini, 1993). On the other hand, connectives are used for both semantic and pragmatic functions (Bloom, Lahey, Hood, Lifter, and Fiess, 1980). Developmental studies show that children initially conjoin sentences by simple juxtaposition without a surface conjunction (Miller, 1981).

The meaning of the conjunction *mais* (but) has been defined in terms of contrast such as in semantic opposition or negation between two elements, violation of expectation or exception, in which one clause qualifies or limits the other. Children at all ages use *but* to fulfil both semantic and pragmatic functions (Peterson, 1986).

The conjunction *quand* (when) is a co-temporal connective that marks simultaneity. *When* appears as a simpler temporal notion than *first, before* or *after* (Silva, 1991).

It can be concluded that dyslexic children used conjunctions less, and particularly two complex connectives involving contrast and simultaneity. This conjunction deficit is assumed to involve the syntactic level, since dyslexic children in our study tended to use very simple sequential intersentential connections (involving *and, and then, there, there is*) and to avoid relative clauses and embedded sentences. Current research assessing syntactic organization in the narrative speech of dyslexic children, compared to a control group of young beginning readers, permits the assumption that such syntactic impairment is more than a consequence of the reading disability.

The verb tense deficit

Dyslexic children used the past tense significantly less than the two groups and they favoured the present tense.

A study concerning the acquisition of narrative language in German revealed that children and adults exhibited a similar pattern of tense with a predominance of the present tense (Bamberg, 1987). In our study, dyslexic children favoured the present tense and used significantly less preterit and imperfect than the two control groups.

Preterit and imperfect are strongly related to literacy and academic achievement. These verb tenses require the child to look for appropriate conjugated forms and to possess grammatical knowledge. Preterit is a particularly complex tense that preschool children do not use easily. In our study, the control-groups of good readers tended to use preterit as a stylistic composition and they made some errors in conjugation. By contrast, dyslexic children did not try to use preterit and imperfect and they favoured the more automatized present tense.

Conclusion

In summary, dyslexic children exhibited a lexical deficit, a conjunction deficit and a verb tense deficit. Dyslexic children tended to avoid the more complex forms in their narrative speech and to have recourse to simpler automatized forms. They exhibited greater use of the frozen forms *ya* and *yavait* (contracted forms of *il y a*, 'there is' and *il y avait*, 'there was'), the form *et puis* (and then) that allowed them to introduce propositions and then tended to compensate for conjunction deficit. They also favoured the present tense, which is more descriptive.

The reasons for this lower performance are probably twofold. On the one hand, it appears as a dramatic consequence of the decoding failure and of the academic difficulties. Nevertheless, the fact that dyslexic children performed at a lower level than the younger reading-matched control group in lexical production, conjunction and verb tense use could reveal a more specific impairment with written language and literacy. It can be hypothesized that this difficulty is of a metalinguistic nature, and concerns metaphonological and metasyntactic skills. Dyslexic children seem to display difficulties not only with grapheme-phoneme correspondence rules, but also with syntactic verbal-written correspondence rules.

In order to examine this important issue, future data will compare the lexical competence of dyslexic children involved in different tasks (elicited narrative, denomination, designation), their syntactic processing, and their phonological skill.

References

Bamberg M (1987) The acquisition of narratives: learning to use language. Berlin: Walter de Gruyter.

Bloom L, Lahey M, Hood L, Lifter K, Fiess, K (1980) Complex sentences: acquisition of syntactic connectives and the semantic relations they encode. Journal of Child Language 7: 235–61.

Bryant PE, Bradley L, Maclean M, Crossland J (1989) Nursery rhymes, phono logical skills and reading. Journal of Child Language 16: 407–28.

Davenport L, Yingling CD, Fein G, Galin D, Johnstone, J (1986) Narrative speech deficits in dyslexics. Journal of Clinical Experimental Neuropsychology 8(4): 347–61.

Feagans L, Short EJ (1984) Developmental differences in the comprehension and production of narratives by reading-disabled and normally achieving children. Child Development 55 (5) 1727–36.

Khami AG, Catts HW (1989) Reading Disabilities: a Developmental Language Perspective. Boston: Little, Brown.

MacWhinney L, Snow K (1991) The CHILDES Project: Tools for Analyzing Talk. Hillsdale, NJ: Lawrence Erlbaum.

Mayer M (1969) Frog Where Are You? New York: Picture Puffins, Dial Books for Young Readers.

Miller JF (1981) Assessing Language Production in Children. London: Edward Arnold.

Morais J (1994) L'Art de Lire. Paris: Odile Jacob.

Murphy LA, Pollatsek A, Well AD (1988) Developmental dyslexia and word retrieval deficits. Brain and Language, 35 (1): 1–23.

Orsolini M (1993) Because in children's discourse. Applied Psycholinguistics 14: 89–120.

Peterson C (1986) Semantic and pragmatic uses of 'but'. Journal of Child Language 13 (3): 583–90.

Silva M (1991) Simultaneity in children's narratives: the case of when, while, and as. Journal of Child Language 18: 641-662

Stanovich KE (1988) The right and wrong places to look for the cognitive locus of reading disability. Annals of Dyslexia 38: 154–77.

Stanovich KE, Cunningham AE, Feeman DJ (1984) Intelligence, cognitive skills and early reading process. Reading Research Quarterly, 19: 278–303.

Wolf M, Goodglass H (1986) Dyslexia, dysnomia and lexical retrieval: a longitudinal study. Brain and Language, 28: 154–68.

Chapter 5
The Processing of Past Tense in Norwegian Specifically Language Impaired Children[1]

KIRSTEN MEYER BJERKAN

Introduction

The question of how lexical and morphological features are stored in the brain has long been a much-debated issue in linguistics. Tests of the processing of regular and irregular inflections, and especially regular and irregular (or weak and strong) past tense forms of verbs, have been important sources of information. The question addressed in these studies has been whether regular and irregular forms should be treated as intrinsically different from each other, or whether they should be seen as the same kind of entities. In order to find out more about this matter, a Norwegian past tense test was conducted with normally developing (ND) children and adults and with specifically language impaired (SLI) children.

Specifically language impaired children show significant limitations in language ability but have normal non-verbal intelligence, normal hearing abilities, normal physical development and no severe emotional disturbances that could cause language problems (Rom and Leonard, 1990). All aspects of language may be problematic, but morphology often tends to be particularly difficult for SLI children.

Much of the earlier work on verb processing has been carried out with English-speaking children. Norwegian verbal morphology differs from that of English in some respects, so the study of Norwegian children may provide a new angle to the explanation of past tense acquisition.

Norwegian verbal morphology

Like English, Norwegian has two main verb classes, weak, and strong (also called regular and irregular) but unlike English it has two weak classes. The formal distinction between weak and strong verbs is that weak verbs have a syllabic suffix in the past tense, whereas strong verbs do not. The verbs in the weak class with the highest type frequency (called the *large weak class*) have a suffix starting in a vowel (*-et* or *-a*), and the verbs in the *smaller weak class* have a suffix starting in a consonant (*-de* or *-te*). Each of these three verb classes is exemplified in Table 5.1 below.

Table 5.1. The main verb classes in Norwegian

	Large weak class	Small weak class	Strong
Stem (=imperative)	dans 'dance'	spis 'eat'	drikk 'drink'
Infinitive	danse	spise	drikke
Present	danser	spiser	drikker
Past tense	danset	spiste	drakk
Past participle	danset	spist	drukket
Present participle	dansende	spisende	drikkende

Two models of acquisition and processing

There are currently two main models that aim to explain the acquisition and processing of past tense, the *dual mechanism account* and the *single mechanism account*.

The dual mechanism account is related to a generative or symbolic framework (e.g. Marcus, Pinker, Ullman, Hollander, Rosen and Xu, 1992; Prasada and Pinker, 1993; Xu and Pinker, 1995). According to this model, the morphological component is divided into two subparts or mechanisms. First, there is a lexicon, where all word stems and strong forms are stored, and secondly there is a rule component that generates weak forms. The retrieval of strong forms from the lexicon is probabilistic and sensitive to frequency of exposure. The higher frequency a form has, the stronger is its representation in the lexicon and the less likely it is to be overgeneralized. The retrieval of a strong form from the lexicon blocks the application of the regular rule.

The single mechanism account is related to a connectionist framework (e.g. Plunkett and Marchman, 1993) and is also in accordance with a cognitive grammar approach (e.g. Bybee, 1988; 1995; Langacker, 1987). Here, only one mechanism is at play for all kinds of inflections. This mechanism is sensitive to input factors like type and token frequencies and to the phonological properties of verb forms. All past tense forms (with the connection to their input forms) are memorized to a certain extent, but given a certain amount of phonologically similar forms, generalizations are created across these forms.

These two accounts differ, then, with regard to the role that they ascribe to frequency factors and phonological properties of verbs.

Under the dual mechanism account, these factors play a minor role, since they are not relevant for the application of the regular, default rule, but only for the lexical retrieval mechanism. Under the single mechanism account, however, these factors are relevant for all kinds of inflection, on both strong and weak verbs.

Method

Ragnarsdóttir, Simonsen and Plunkett (in preparation) have constructed a test to investigate past-tense inflection in Norwegian and Icelandic ND children. The test consists of 60 verbs, half of them weak and half of them strong. The two weak classes are represented with the same number of verbs.

Simonsen has conducted the test with ND Norwegian children at the ages of 4, 6, and 8, with approximately 30 subjects in each group. In this study the same test was conducted with 30 normal-speaking adults and to SLI children at the age of 6 and 8, with four children in each group.

Results

Correct scores

The mean number of correct answers for each subject group is shown in Table 5.2 below. As can be seen, there was a clear developmental effect in the overall performance.

Table 5.2. Percentage of correct answers for each subject group

ND 4-year-olds	51%
ND 6-year-olds	72%
ND 8-year-olds	90%
ND Adults	94%
SLI 6-year-olds	57%
SLI 8-year-olds	76%

The mean number of correct answers increased with age. The ND children had just about half of the verbs correct at the age of 4. At the age of 8 they were close to the adult score, which is quite high. Among the SLI children, the 6-year-olds were better than the ND 4-year-olds, but quite far behind the ND 6-year-olds. At the age of 8, they performed only slightly better than the ND 6-year-olds.

The performance was not, however, the same across verb groups, as illustrated in Figures 5.1 to 5.6 below.

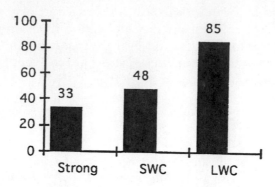

Figure 5.1. ND 4-year-olds.

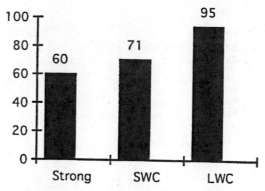

Figure 5.2. ND 6-year-olds.

The ND 4- and 6-year-olds scored significantly better on the large weak class than on the other groups ($p<0.05$). The performance on the small weak class seemed to cluster with that of the strong verbs, and there is no significant difference between them. The only difference between the 4- and 6-year-olds is that the 6-year-olds had higher scores on all verb groups.

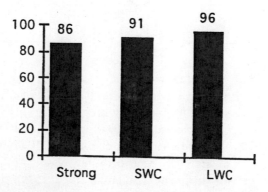

Figure 5.3. ND 8-year-olds.

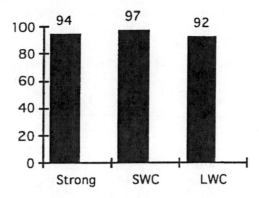

Figure 5.4. Adults.

The ND 8-year-olds and the adults obtained a high score on all verb classes. The 8-year-olds performed slightly better on the large weak class, as did all the other groups of children, but there was no significant difference between the different verb classes for the 8-year-olds. Interestingly, the adults performed best on the small weak class, and worst on the large weak class.

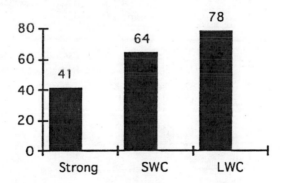

Figure 5.5. SLI 6-year-olds.

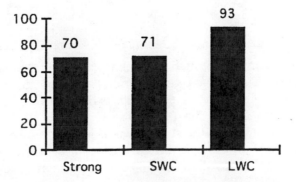

Figure 5.6. SLI 8-year-olds.

The SLI children showed the same profile as the younger ND children (i.e. the 4- and 6-year-olds), in that they performed considerably better on the large weak class than on the two other classes. For the 8-year-olds the strong verbs reached the same level as the small weak class, but both of these classes were far behind the large weak class.

Error types

The errors made by the subject groups give a broader picture of which verb patterns they know. Only overgeneralization errors will be discussed here. Each of the three verb classes constitutes a potential pattern, which may form the basis for overgeneralization. Overgeneralization to the large weak class means productive use of the suffix -et or -a. Both strong verbs and verbs from the small weak class were overgeneralized to this class. An English equivalent of this error would be *shoot–shooted* instead of *shoot–shot*. Overgeneralization to the small weak class means productive use of the suffixes -de or -te. There is no exact English equivalent, since English has only one weak class.

Overgeneralization to strong verb patterns is strong inflection of weak verbs. An English example would be the inflection of the verb snow as *snow–snew* (analogous with *grow–grew*), or *reach–raught* (analogous with *teach–taught*).

Taking type frequency into account, we would expect the large weak class to be the most productive one. This is indeed what we found for most of the informant groups, but it was not the only productive pattern, as shown in Table 5.3.

Table 5.3. Overgeneralization errors

	Gen > LWC	Gen > SWC	Gen > STR
SLI 6 years	58%	40%	2%
SLI 8 years	50%	35%	15%
ND 4 years	76%	21%	3%
ND 6 years	59%	31%	10%
ND 8 years	39%	47%	14%
Adults	14%	60%	26%

Overgeneralization to the small weak class and the strong class increases with age. The ND 8-year-olds overgeneralize more to the small weak class than to the large one, and the adults hardly overgeneralize to the large weak class at all. The SLI children show a higher percentage of overgeneralizations to the small weak class than do the younger ND children. The SLI 6-year-olds actually have more overgeneralizations to the small weak class than the ND 6-year-olds, but they have fewer generalizations to the strong pattern. The SLI 8-year-olds also resemble the ND six-year-olds, but they have slightly more overgeneralizations to strong patterns.

Discussion

SLI versus ND children

When we compare the test performance of the SLI children and the ND children, we find that the SLI children have the same total scores as younger ND children. That is, the SLI 6-year-olds have almost the same overall score as the ND 4-year-olds, and the SLI 8-year-olds have the same score as the ND 6-year-olds. Thus, on the basis of correct inflections, we could say that the SLI children are delayed by almost two years.

There is, however, a difference between the SLI children and the normals who are two years younger in the kinds of overgeneralizations they make. The ND 4-year-olds overgeneralize almost exclusively to the large weak class, whereas the SLI 6-year-olds also use the small weak class productively to a large extent. The SLI 8-year-olds overgeneralize slightly more to the small weak class, and to the strong classes, than do the ND 6-year-olds.

Hence, even though the SLI children perform like children who are two years younger in terms of correct scores, they seem to have a higher general knowledge of the possible verb patterns in the language and are able to use more patterns productively.

This increasing use of more verb classes as a basis for generalizations, which is seen in both the SLI and the ND children, can be explained by a 'critical mass' effect: the smaller children may not have a sufficiently large vocabulary to be able to discover all the patterns of the different verb classes.

The single versus dual mechanism account

According to the dual-processing model, the large weak class is derived by rule and should be the default form. This was observed among the 4-year-olds: they performed considerably better on this class than on the other classes, and they overgeneralized predominantly to this class. The large weak class cannot, however, be regarded as a default form for any of the other informant groups. All of them overgeneralize quite frequently to the small weak class and also to the strong class. Norwegian has no one default pattern of verbal inflection.

According to Prasada and Pinker (1993), all overgeneralizations are possible but only if the item in question is highly similar to items that already exist. The productive use of the strong pattern is not a problem within this model, because all the weak verbs that are inflected as strong, rhyme with strong verbs. However, the very high frequency of overgeneralization to the small weak class is a problem, since the verbs in question are not necessarily similar to already existing verbs in the small weak class.

Within the single-processing model, the same mechanism is at work in all kinds of inflections. If weak and strong inflection were two completely different phenomena we would expect the large weak class to function as a default form for all age groups. As we have seen, this is not the case. All the different verb classes are used productively and the small weak class is the most productive one for the ND 8-year-olds and the adults. These data give support to the single mechanism account according to which the same mechanism is at work in all kinds of inflection.

References

Bybee JL (1988) Morphology as lexical organisation. In Hammond M, Noonan M (Eds) Theoretical Morphology: Approaches in Modern Linguistics. New York: Academic Press, pp 119–41.

Bybee JL (1995) Regular morphology and the lexicon. Language and Cognitive Processes 10: 425–55.

Langacker R (1987) Foundations of cognitive grammar. Vol. 1, Theoretical prerequisites. Stanford, CA: Stanford University Press.

Marcus GF, Pinker S, Ullman M, Hollander M, Rosen TJ, Xu F (1992) Overregularisation in language acquisition. Monographs of the Society for Research in Child Development 57.

Plunkett K, Marchman V (1993) From rote learning to system building. Acquiring verb morphology in children and connectionist nets. Cognition 48: 21–69.

Prasada S, Pinker S (1993) Generalisation of regular and irregular morphological patterns. Language and Cognitive Processes 8: 1–56.

Ragnarsdóttir H, Simonsen HG, Plunkett K (in preparation) The acquisition of past tense morphology in Icelandic and Norwegian children. An experimental study.

Rom A, Leonard LB (1990) Interpreting deficits in grammatical morphology in specifically language-impaired children: preliminary evidence from Hebrew. Clinical Linguistics and Phonetics 4: 93–105.

Xu F, Pinker S (1995) Weird past tense forms. Journal of Child Language 22: 531–56.

Note

1   I would like to thank Marianne Lind, Inger Moen and Hanne Gram Simonsen for helpful comments on this work.

Chapter 6
Rapid Lexical Learning: Video versus Live Presentation of Text

SANDRA TERRELL, RAY DANILOFF, GLENN
ROYALL, KYM SCHULZE

Introduction

Video tapes and computer programs are being used with increased frequency as a method of instruction in the classroom to replace or supplement traditional live teaching. Claims for such instructional technology are that these technologies are more efficient and less expensive than live instructors. Despite these claims, empirical studies of the effectiveness of machine versus human instruction are relatively limited for language learning.

Research has shown that all three techniques are effective methods of instruction. Bourne and Ekstrand (1982), Rice and Haight (1986), Rice and Woodsmall (1988), and Rice, Buhr, and Nemeth (1990) have all found that children acquire novel words after one or two uninstructed exposures to televised programmes. McKeown (1985), Carnine, Kameenui and Coyle (1984) have shown that, when a live instructor reads children stories they learn both new words and their meanings relatively quickly. Finally, computers are a useful method for improving a child's capacity both to learn and retrieve words (Chertkow, Bub, and Seidenberg, 1988; Forster, 1981; Wiener, 1991).

Few studies have compared the effectiveness of machine versus human modes of presentation of new vocabulary. O'Connor and Schery (1986) and Lemish and Rice (1986) compared human versus machine modes of presentation of new words and declare them roughly equivalent.

Recent studies focusing on word learning suggest that, even at 2 years of age, lexical acquisition uses basically the same abilities of social cognition and cultural learning that children demonstrate in other social-cognitive domains and that these abilities are more powerfully used in the process of lexical acquisition than previously thought (Tomasello and Barton, 1994). Another study revealed that 2-year-old children are sensitive to discourse novelty in word learning and are able to learn words in a wide variety of pragmatic contexts (Akhtar, Carpenter and Tomasello, 1996). Oetting, Rice and Swank (1995) extended studies of QUIL to older children (6 to 8 years) and discovered that although the gain is less dramatic than during the preschool years, the ability to learn words incidentally from oral contexts gradually increases, with word type continuing to affect word learning (object label advantage). Weismer and Hesketh (1996) found that children with SLI were less proficient than MA matched peers at comprehending and producing novel words; vocabulary level was not significantly correlated with novel word learning in this study. Collectively, these studies imply that there is a broad variety of ages at which word-learning takes place. Various age and ability groups may differ in the rate that they acquire words but they are similar in the manner of acquisition and the social-cognitive abilities used for word learning.

Although previous research indicates that children can learn with computers, videos, and human teachers, studies exploring the relative effectiveness of electronic versus live human methods of teaching new words are limited. Terrell and Daniloff (1996) compared the effectiveness of computer video display tube, videotape, and live adult reading modes of instruction in teaching children vocabulary. A small, significant advantage for live voice reading was established. The current study extends the work of Terrell and Daniloff (1996). Quick incidental word learning, QUIL, is compared in children exposed to story-book reading using (a) live reading (LR) and (b) computer (VDT) modes of presentation. This study was designed to probe the influence which (a) the written text and (b) indices of language performance, have upon QUIL performance of preschool children.

Table 6.1. Contextual factors analysed

S -   Rated salience of pictured word: highly salient words are pictorially readily identified because of spatial delimitation (discreteness), structurally well-integrated (spatially coherent), and identity/function well-cued by text.

                                                                       *5 point scale (0-4)

SL -   Rated sentence length: very long, long, moderate, short in length.

                                                                       *4 point scale (0-3)

NW -   Number of words to be learned in each sentence.

TPT -   Number of times that word used was specifically pictured (text-picture-tie).

SC -   Rated syntactic complexity of sentences containing words.

                                                                       *5 point scale (0-4)

Procedures

The general procedures used followed those of Terrell and Daniloff (1996). Twenty-six children were given a pre-test of word identification and, following exposure to a narrated illustrated text via either (a) live reading (LR) or (b) computer (VDT) presentation, a post-training test.

Subjects

Twenty-six children were assigned to two instructional mode groups: 13 children, mean age = 51.5 months, SD = 5.9 months, in the book group (BG); and 13 children in the computer group (CG), mean age = 51.7 months, SD = 6.3 months. The children were enrolled in a university developmental preschool programme. Each child passed immittance and pure tone hearing screening at 15 dB HL in both ears and did not present a history of pervasive middle-car medical problems. Each child was further screened for expressive language (CELF-R), receptive language (CELF-R), vocabulary development (PPVT-R), and articulation proficiency (Arizona test).

Materials

A copiously colour-illustrated book of *Peter and the Wolf* was used as the text. Thirteen pictured nouns from the written text (such as *grandfather, pond, hunter, gun*) were selected for training; each occurred 10–13 times in the written text and in three or more illustrations. Thirteen very-low-frequency-of-occurrence words were substituted for the 13 common nouns: grandfather = codger, gun = musket, pond = tarn, as shown in Table 6.1. The text with 13 coloured illustrations was scanned into a computer – both the illustrations and the vocal narration of the text by a male reader. The same male reader read the text live to the BG children. The video/audio scanned text was presented at conversational audio level from a 19" colour monitor to the CG children. Each was seated a metre away at eye level from the VDT screen. The male graduate-assistant reader provided no explicit visual, manual, or auditory cues regarding the 13 illustrated nouns.

Test procedures

The children were given pre- and post- word-recognition tests, three to four weeks apart, to assess pre- and post- training knowledge of the test words. Each child faced a felt board with four snippets of colour pictures cut from illustrations in the text. One of the foils represented the correct target word as spoken by the male reader, two were non-target

pictures of words presented in at least one of the illustrations and mentioned in the text, and one picture illustrated a noun not mentioned in
the text. Each child was asked to point to the picture that represented
the word spoken by the male speaker.

In a test session, a BG child sat side by side at a table with the male
reader who read aloud the text accompanying each colour illustration,
turning pages to new text and pictures until the entire text was read.
The examiner used no verbal asides, gestures, or prompts in the 10–12
minute test session. In the CG group, the child and male experimenter
sat facing the colour VDT and speakers of an AV computer. The experimenter triggered each new colour picture and audio narration in
sequence until the child had heard all of the spoken narrative and had
seen all of the coloured pictures.

Results

Contextual factors that were analysed included (a) the experimenters'
ratings of the syntactic complexity of each sentence containing a test
word (SC), (b) the rated length of each sentence in number of words
(SL), (c) the percentage of occurrences of a test word in the text for
which there was an explicit pictorial representation (i.e. an accompanying text-picture-tie (TPT)), (d) the rated salience of each picture with
respect to the word (S), and (e) the number of test words in sentences
containing one or more (NW), see Table 6.2. Salience was a construct
that included such factors as picturability, intrinsic interest of the item,
relative frequency of the picture's occurrence in storybooks and the
transparency of the sentence relative to the inferrability of the identity
or function of the noun.

Table 6.2. Textual-pictorial context factors

Textual-Pictorial Context Factors words used	S	SL	NW	PT(%)	SC
musket	3.50	1.67	2.83	0.33	3.33
marksman	3.50	1.50	2.65	.625	3.00
larch	2.88	1.25	2.38	0.25	2.75
mallard	2.88	1.37	2.63	0.25	2.37
loup	2.75	1.00	2.75	0.12	2.75
lariat	2.57	1.14	2.43	0.57	2.71
codger	2.38	1.13	1.87	0.62	2.25
tarn	2.25	1.375	2.375	0.50	0.25
feline	1.71	1.28	2.43	0.43	2.57
portal	1.63	1.13	2.25	0.25	2.25
glade	1.25	0.88	1.88	0.62	1.88
thrush	1.25	1.25	2.25	0.00	0.13
domicile	1.22	1.11	2.22	0.44	2.44

Prior to training, children knew or guessed correctly (chance guessing rate = 1/4) about two words, on average, in each group. The computer group knew slightly, but significantly more (p≤ 0.02). Following training, both groups learned about 2.3 new words (17%) of the 13 (during one testing) presented in the *Peter and the Wolf* story (Figure 6.1). Scores ranged from 0 to 7 words learned. The differences in learning scores between groups were not significant (p≤ 0.25). Three words learned especially well by both groups were *codger* (9/26), *marksman* (8/26), and *musket* (8/26); three not learned well were *domicile* (2/26), *glade* (2/26), and *portal* (0/26). Statistics suggest that 26 children recognizing 13 words with a one in four probability of a randomly selected correct identification should produce 64 correct guesses – that is, 4.8 correctly guessed identifications for each word. The six words mentioned above are well above and well below the chance rate of guessing, per word.

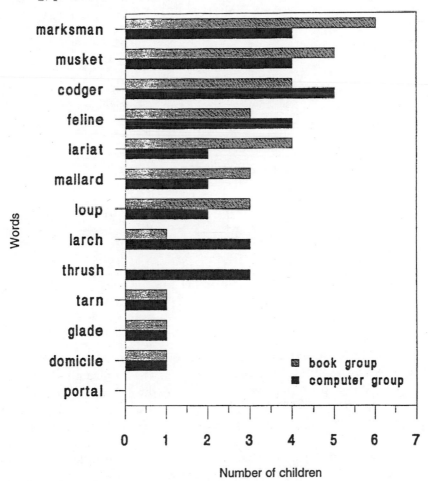

Figure 6.1. Number of children learning each word.

The average of 2.3 words per child learning rate was comparable to that observed by Terrell and Daniloff (1996) with their 'read' text, but in contrast to that study, there was no significant difference between modes of presentation in this study. Correlations of QUIL scores with screening test scores (Table 6.3) revealed that only age produced a significant, and positive (p≤ 0.03) correlation with QUIL scores in either group of children. On the other hand (Table 6.4), correlation of QUIL scores with contextual factors, revealed no significant correlations for the CG children; the correlations with salience (S) and number of words (NW) were significantly positive (p≤ 0.0055, 0.044 respectively) while syntactic complexity (SC) was significantly negatively correlated with QUIL scores (p≤ 0.009) for the BG children only. That is, context sensitivity emerged only for live reading of the text.

Table 6.3. Correlation of word-learning score and screening scores

Screening Variables	Book group	Computer group
CELF-E	NS	NS
CELF-R	NS	NS
PPVT	NS	NS
ATAP	NS	NS
Age	p<0.03	p<0.01

Spearman Rho (ρ) Correlation coefficient

Table 6.4. Correlation of word learning score with context

Textual-Pictorial Context Factors Mode of Instruction	S	SL	NW	TPT	SC
Book	p<0.005	NS	p<0.044	NS	p<0.009
Computer	NS	NS	NS	NS	NS

Discussion

This study demonstrates that children at roughly 4 to 6 years of age, on average, have the ability to learn 2.4 of 13 new low-frequency words from picture-text presented via live voice reading (LR) or colour visual/audio presentation (VDT) of pictures with the same reader's voice. The BG–CG modes of presentation are on average equivalent. However, only for BG children were correlations with contextual factors such as salience, syntactic complexity and number of test items per sentence significant. Although the live reader simply turned pages and read the text, the BG children revealed a correlation of QUIL scores with textual factors. It would appear that social-pragmatic factors are at play in live reading that are not systematically elicited by a computer mode of instruction – the computer mode is the more 'anonymous' instructor. This personal element would probably have been amplified had the live reader used gestures such as head turning, gaze, picture-text pointing, or smiles. These kinds of activities could not be effected in the computer mode we employed. We suggest that educators/therapists be aware of the human element missing during computer-based instruction such as ours. Finally, our results demonstrated that language and picture vocabulary screening scores within normal ranges do not correlate significantly with QUIL performance, whereas age did so over the 4-to-6 year span of age studied here, suggesting that maturation did modestly affect learning.

References

Akhtar N, Carpenter M, Tomasello M (1996) The role of discourse novelty in early word learning. Child Development 67: 635–45.

Bourne LE, Ekstrand BR (1982) Psychology: its Principles and Meanings. New York, NY: Holt, Rinehart & Winston.

Carnine D, Kameenui EJ, Coyle G (1984) Utilization of contextual information in determining the meaning of unfamiliar words. Reading Research Quarterly 19: 188–203.

Chertkow H, Bub D, Seidenberg M (1988) Priming and semantic memory loss in Alzheimer's disease. CHCN Working Papers, Centre de Recherche, Centre Hospitalier Cote-de-Neiges.

Forster K (1981) Priming and the effects of sentence and lexical contents on naming time: evidence for autonomous lexical processing. Quarterly Journal of Experimental Psychology 33: 465–95.

Lemish D, Rice M (1986) Television as a talking picture book: a prop for language acquisition. Journal of Child Language Vol 13 (2) June: 251–74.

McKeown MG (1985) The actuisition of word meaning from context by children of high and low ability. Reading Research Quarterly 20: 482–96.

O'Connor L, Schery TK (1986) A comparison of microcomputer-aided and traditional therapy for developing communication skills in normal toddlers. Journal of Speech and Hearing Disorders 51: 356–61.

Oetting JB, Rice ML, Swank LK (1995) Quick incidental learning (QUIL) of word by school-age children with and without SLI. Journal of Speech and Hearing Research 38: 434–45.

Rice ML, Buhr JC, Nemeth M (1990) Fast mapping word learning abilities of language-delayed preschoolers. Journal of Speech and Hearing Disorders 55: 33–42.

Rice ML, Haight PL (1986) 'Motherese' of Mr Rogers: a description of the dialogue of educational television programs. Journal of Speech and Hearing Disorders 51: 282–7.

Rice ML, Woodsmall L (1988) Lessons from television: children's word learning when viewing. Child Development 59: 420–9.

Terrell S, Daniloff R (1996) Children's word learning using three modes of instruction. Perception and Motor Skills 83: 779–87.

Tomasello M, Barton M (1994) Learning words in nonostensive contexts. Developmental Psychology 30(5): 639–50.

Wiener R (1991) Computerized speech: a study of its effect on learning. Technological Horizons in Education Journal 18: 100–2.

Weismer SE, Hesketh LJ (1996) Lexical learning by children with specific language impairment: Effects of linguistic input presented at varying speaking rates. Journal of Speech and Hearing Research 39: 177–90.

Note

The authors wish to acknowledge the assistance of Edward Gonzalez.

PHONOLOGY

Chapter 7
The Role of Phonotactic Range in the Order of Acquisition of English Consonants[1]

RICHARD SHILLCOCK AND GERT WESTERMANN

Introduction

This paper is concerned with quantifying the factors that affect the order of acquisition in phonological development in English. As Menn and Stoel-Gammon (1995) observe, the question of the order of acquisition of the phonemes of English is problematic: acquisition varies between children learning the same language; related allophones are acquired at different times; acquiring a phoneme may not mean that the relevant phonemic contrasts have been acquired; the position of the target phoneme in the syllable, together with the other contents of the syllable, affects pronunciation. Nevertheless, the literature does contain observed orders of acquisition of English, together with claims concerning the factors determining that order. Below, we first employ multiple regression analysis to determine the extent to which a reported order of acquisition can be accounted for by phonological and distributional factors. We then compare this conventional statistical modelling with a connectionist modelling approach. In the light of the caveats listed above, the current explorations will determine whether a particular reported order of acquisition is susceptible to a parsimonious statistical description – can a large part of the variance be accounted for by only a few variables? The account, if successful, will stand as a falsifiable model that may then be tested against more detailed observational data taking into account the dimensions of the problem discussed by Menn and Stoel-Gammon.

Statistical modelling

We select, partly on the grounds of its clinical status, an order of acquisition of the consonants of English presented by Grunwell (1985); this order abstracts away from syllable position and gives a timescale by which particular segments might be expected to be reliably deployed by English-speaking children.

A number of different variables have been suggested as determining order of acquisition: articulatory factors; acoustic properties; function in the phonological system; subsegmental phonological structure; functional load. In addition, whether a particular segment in a particular position is correct may be influenced by factors such as interaction with morphological structure; interaction with lexical and syllabic context; lexical stress. We describe, below, a precise quantification of 'function in the phonological system' (Ingram, 1988) in terms of phonotactic range, and assess its contribution against that of various phonological factors. We also dissect the precise content of the phonotactic range variable.

Representative statistics concerning the distribution of segments in English speech were obtained from an idealized phonetic transcription of the London-Lund and CHILDES corpora. (See, Shillcock, Hicks, Cairns, Levy and Chater (in press) for a description of the conversion of the original orthographic transcriptions into phonetic ones.) Phonotactic range was defined as the number of different segment bigrams in which a particular segment participates, above a criterial probability (0.001); for /t/, the bigrams included /tə/, /tr/, /tɪ/, /lt/, /st/, /nt/, and so on. For the 22 consonants of English, this measure ranged between 0 (for /ʒ/) and 29 (for /t/); that is, /ʒ/ occurred only in very infrequent contexts, whereas /t/ occurred in more high frequency combinations than any other segment, meaning that /t/ played a more central role in the phonology in these purely distributional terms. Various other distributional statistics were also obtained from the same corpora, involving, for instance, defining phonotactic range over trigrams of segments or excluding the function words from consideration.

The role of subsegmental structure was represented in terms of the nine elements of Government Phonology (Kaye, Lowenstamm and Vergnaud, 1985; Harris and Lindsey, 1993; Shillcock, Lindsey, Levy and Chater, 1992). Each of the 22 consonants was represented by a feature vector of these elements.

Linear regression analyses were carried out to determine the factors affecting Grunwell's reported order of acquisition measured in months. Different combinations of the distributional variables and the presence or absence of particular subsegmental structure typically accounted for more than half of the variance in the dependent variable, the order of acquisition. In the most successful analysis using the simple phonotactic range variable, three variables accounted for 77% of the variance in the order of acquisition ($R^2 = 0.765$, $F(3,18) = 19.48$, $p<0.0001$). In order of importance, the variables were:

- the subsegmental element 'R' – 'apicality, coronality, coronal formant locus'. Segments containing this element were acquired later (b = 0.579, $p<0.0001$);
- phonotactic range. Segments with a larger phonotactic range were acquired earlier (b = –0.522, $p<0.002$);
- the subsegmental element '?' – 'occlusion, abruptness, alone, glottal stop'. Segments containing this element were acquired earlier (b = –0.362, $p<0.02$).

The best model of the order of acquisition was obtained from the distributional statistics taken from the adult speech addressed to children up to 28 months in the CHILDES corpus. Using distributional statistics from only the content words did not provide a better account of the data. The number of different subsegmental elements involved in the specification of a particular segment was not a significant predictor of the data.

Prompted by the connectionist modelling, below, we partitioned phonotactic range into its 'forward' (e.g. /tə/, /tr/, /tɪ/, ...) and 'backward' (e.g. /lt/, /st/, /nt/...) components. The forward phonotactic range from the CHILDES corpus produced the best model of the data, accounting for 79% of the variance ($R^2 = 0.794$, $F(3,18) = 23.09$, $p<0.0001$), with the independent variables in the same order of importance as above.

In summary, phonotactic range, and especially forward phonotactic range, is a better determiner of order of acquisition than simple segment frequency; the more central the role of the segment in the phonology, in terms of combining with other segments, the earlier it is acquired. The presence of the element 'R' – implicated in /t/, /d/, /n/, /s/, /l/, /ʃ/, /z/, /r/, /ʒ/, /θ/, /ð/ – was associated with later acquisition, whereas the element '?' – implicated in /m/, /p/, /b/, /t/, /d/, /n/ /ŋ/, /k/, /g/, /l/ – was associated with earlier acquisition. We might speculate that coronality/apicality ('R') involves a considerable range of gestures – the tip and blade of the tongue can be variously positioned – thereby presenting the child with the relatively difficult tasks of matching gesture and sound and of mastering the movements involved, leading to slower acquisition of the relevant segments. We might also speculate that the physical gestures associated with occlusion ('?') are complete, finished gestures (as opposed to ones that require to be reached and held) and are also constrained by the physical shape of the vocal tract; such gestures may be easier to acquire, facilitating the acquisition of the relevant segments.

Thus, a good account of the order of acquisition (abstracted away from syllable position) can be achieved by taking into account only the identity of the adjacent segments and the subsegmental composition of the target segment. Note that the version of the corpus from which we drew our statistics was not marked for syllable position (indeed, resyllabification effects could have been derived only from the original speech).

Connectionist modelling

We also modelled the order of acquisition with a connectionist neural network. For these simulations, the segments in the idealized transcription of the London-Lund corpus were represented by a subsegmental feature-vector based on Government Phonology. Since three of the nine features of this encoding can take the value 0.5, they were split so that each segment could be expressed by a vector of 12 binary values.

The neural network architecture is shown in Figure 7.1. It is a modification of the network used by Cairns, Shillcock, Chater and Levy (in press), the only difference being that 40 hidden units were used instead of 60. The network consisted of three layers with a fully recurrent hidden layer. The continuous transcription of the corpus was presented to the input layer, one phonemic feature-vector at a time. The output layer was divided into three slots: one was trained to recall the previously presented segment, one to duplicate the current segment, and one to predict the next segment in the sequence. This prediction task corresponded to learning the forward phonotactics of each segment. For

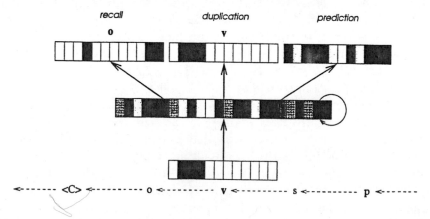

Figure 7.1. The recurrent neural network, showing consecutive phonemes presented to the input nodes, and the recall, duplication and prediction of the same phonemes at the output nodes.

example, for the segment /t/ the network was supposed to learn the sequences /tr/, /tɪ/, /ti/, and so on, in the continuous input.

The network was trained with the backpropagation through time algorithm (Rumelhart, Hinton and Williams, 1986). The training proceeded according to the incremental learning procedure proposed by Elman (1993) in that the size of the time-window was increased, from an initial size of 4, by 1 every 50 000 epochs until a final size of 10 was reached at epoch 300 000. The size of the time-window was limited by resetting the recurrent connections in the network to 0.

Training the network consisted of presenting the first 500 000 segments of the corpus in sequence. At different stages of training the network was tested on a set of 10 000 consecutive segments taken from a section of the corpus that was not contained in the training data.

A segment (being presented to the network and duplicated in the middle slot of the network output) was considered to have been 'acquired' by the network once its forward phonotactics, i.e. the prediction of the range of possible segments to follow the current one, had been learned. According to this view, a phoneme has been acquired if it can be deployed reliably, and this involves knowing the contexts in which it occurs. In this study, only the predictive, 'forward' phonotactics were considered. In measuring this acquisition of phonotactics, the prediction feature-vectors from a particular segment were averaged over all its occurrences in the training data, and this measure was compared with the relevant distributional statistics for the segment, taken from the corpus. The degree of acquisition was measured as the degree of similarity (cosine) between this averaged prediction-vector and the corresponding vector from the corpus statistics.

A threshold of 0.95 for the cosine between the two vectors was defined as the criterion for successful acquisition of the phonotactics of the target phoneme, and hence acquisition of the phoneme itself, recording the number of training epochs it took for each segment to reach this threshold. This measure yielded the following order of acquisition of consonants by the network: /v/, /d/, /l/, /n/, /t/, /m/, /r/, /ð/, /b/, /k/, /f/, /h/, /s/, /z/, /g/. The threshold was not reached within 500,000 epochs for /p/, /θ/, /ʃ/, and /ʒ/. This order of acquisition was correlated, marginally significantly, with the human acquisition order reported by Grunwell (r = 0.389, p = 0.10).

In order to distinguish the effects of frequency and phonotactic range in the model's acquisition of phonemes, we examined the course of learning for frequent and infrequent segments with a wide and a narrow phonotactic range, this time including vowels in our analysis. Table 7.1 shows the four segments used in this analysis.

The course of acquisition of the phonotactics for these four phonemes was recorded. Whereas the phonotactics for the phonemes with a wide phonotactic range (/i/ and /z/) were learned very quickly,

Table 7.1. The four selected phonemes

		Frequency	
		high	low
Phonotactic range	wide	I	z
	narrow	A[1]	h

[1] The segment employed here is, in fact, specific to the Government Phonology transcriptions of diphthongs and long monophthongs, and appears only as the first segment in /aɪ/, /aʊ/ and /ɑː/. Despite the non-standard status of this segment, it still allows us to test the effects of the distributional differences between the segments on the network's learning.

those with the narrower phonotactic range learning took considerably longer: only after more than 200 000 epochs were the phonotactics for /A/ learned equally well as those for /z/, although the frequency of /A/ in the data was twice that of /z/. For the network, a wide phonotactic range facilitated the acquisition of the target phoneme better than high frequency of the target phoneme, although frequency seemed to have an effect too; the rather infrequent /z/ had a U-shaped learning curve in comparison with the more frequent /i/. These results confirmed those from the statistical modelling discussed above.

An analysis of the predictions of specific segments by the network showed that they depended upon both segment frequency and phonotactic range. The network learned the phonotactics best for segments with a wide phonotactic range; what was being learned was the superposition of all possible segments that could follow the current one, taking into account their frequency. Individual segments (i.e. no superposition of feature-vectors for different segments), albeit possibly the wrong ones, were best predicted from high-frequency segments. The correct individual segments were best predicted from frequent segments with a narrow phonotactic range.

In summary, although the connectionist modelling did not capture the acquisition data as transparently or as accurately as the conventional 'symbolic' statistical modelling, it did provide interesting ways of construing the process of phonological acquisition and inspired the splitting of the phonotactic range variable into its forward and backward components in the statistical modelling reported above. The connectionist approach characterized phonological acquisition as learning the appropriate context of use and operationalized it as the accurate prediction of the next segment. The default prediction of the next segment is simply the superposition of all the segments in proportion to their frequency, and what must be learned is a departure from this pattern. This departure is a large one for predictions involving only a narrow phonotactic range, and hence learning is slower.

Conclusions

The predictors of the order of phonological acquisition that we have identified – phonotactic range, and the subsegmental elements 'R' and '?' – have implications for diagnosis of delayed or distorted phonological production, for the construction of stimulus materials for therapy, and for the order of improvement, spontaneous or guided. The information contained in simple bigrams emphasizes the fact that normal development may proceed by access to spoken language through a minimal length window, at least initially (cf Elman, 1993). The three predictors of the order of acquisition that we discuss above may be confirmed or falsified by more detailed observational data but they constitute the default hypothesis concerning a theoretical account of new data.

References

Cairns P, Shillcock R, Chater N, and Levy J (in press). Bootstrapping word boundaries: A bottom-up corpus-based approach to speech segmentation. Cognitive Psychology

Elman JL (1993) Learning and development in neural networks: the importance of starting small. Cognition 48: 71–99.

Grunwell P (1985) Phonological Assessment of Child Speech (PACS). Windsor, UK: NFER-Nelson.

Harris J, Lindsey G (1993) The elements of phonological representation. In Durand J and Katamba F (Eds) New Frontiers in Phonology. Harlow, Essex: Longman.

Ingram D (1988) The acquisition of word-initial /v/. Language and Speech 31: 77–85.

Kaye JD, Lowenstamm J, Vergnaud, J-R (1985) The internal structure of phonological elements: a theory of charm and government. Phonology Yearbook 2: 305–28.

Menn L and Stoel-Gammon C (1995) Phonological development. In Paul Fletcher, Brian MacWhinney (Eds) The Handbook of Child Language. Blackwell, Oxford

Rumelhart DE, Hinton GE, Williams RJ (1986) Learning internal representations by error propagation. In Rumelhart DE, and McClelland JL (Eds) Parallel Distributed Processing: Explorations in the Microstructure of Cognition, Volume 1: Foundations. Cambridge, MA: MIT Press, pp 318–62.

Shillcock RC, Hicks J, Cairns P, Levy J, Chater N. (in press). A Statistical Analysis of an Idealised Phonological Transcription of the London-Lund corpus.

Shillcock RC, Lindsey G, Levy J, Chater N (1992) A Phonologically Motivated Input Representation for the Modelling of Auditory Word Perception in Continuous Speech. Proceedings of the 14th Annual Cognitive Science Society Conference, 1992, Bloomington, pp. 408–13.

Note

1   The first research described was partly supported by ESRC (UK) grants R000 23 3649 and R000 22 1435. Gert Westermann was supported by grant no. 2.95.29 from the Gottlieb Daimler- und Karl Benz-Stiftung. Thanks are due to Jim Scobbie and John Hicks for advice and help.

Chapter 8
Evidence from Vowel Disorders for the Nature of Minimal Phonological Units in Acquisition[1]

MARTIN J. BALL

Introduction

Phonological development encompasses a wide range of linguistic phenomena, such as the acquisition of word and syllable structure, phonotactic constraints, and the wide range of prosodic features that characterize adult connected speech. However, great interest has always been expressed by developmental phonologists in the acquisition of the basic contrastive system of consonants and vowels.

In recent times it has been assumed by many that a phonological system (in the strict sense of the term 'system') is not acquired in a unit-by-unit (i.e. 'phoneme-by-phoneme') way but through a set of features that may be thought of as the building blocks of contrastive units (the consonants and vowels). Distinctive feature theory has undergone much refinement since the early works of Jakobson, Fant and Halle (1952), Jakobson and Halle (1956) and Chomsky and Halle (1968). Nevertheless, it is probably true to say that distinctive features as binary oppositions – as described in those early works – are still the most commonly encountered in phonological theory, albeit with modifications such as proposed in feature geometry (see Roca, 1994). In the field of phonological development, therefore, the dominant paradigm in feature acquisition studies appears to be binary feature system (see Jakobson, 1968 (original 1941) for the classic study in this mould; also Blache, 1978).

It is worth spending some time in examining whether binary feature systems are the best way of characterizing phonological contrasts. If they are not, particularly if they are not from a psycholinguistic (or cognitive linguistic) point of view, then we may wish to explore alternatives and start looking for evidence for these in the phonetic record. In previous work (e.g. Ball, 1996) I have discussed unary primes as alternatives to binary distinctive features. These primes are found in phonological approaches such as dependency phonology (DP) (see Anderson and Durand 1986, 1987; Anderson and Ewen, 1987; Durand, 1990; Lass, 1984) and Government Phonology (GP) (e.g. Harris, 1994; Harris and Lindsey, 1995). In this same study, evidence was brought forward from normal phonological acquisition to support an analysis via primes, and in this account I wish to examine evidence from vowel disorders to see whether this too supports such an analysis.

A component analysis of vowels

Before going further, we must examine what a component-based phonology might look like. We will restrict this to an analysis of vowels, set within a Government Phonology framework as described in Harris (1994). Harris shows GP primes on a feature geometry tree in Figure 8.1:

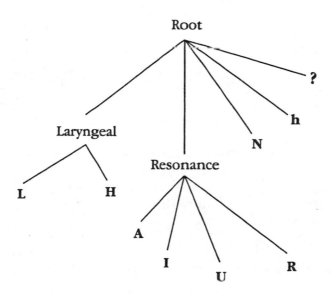

Figure 8.1. Government phonology feature geometry tree.

(The meaning of the components **?**, **h**, **N** is not important for the following discussion.) The **R** prime refers to coronal segments, while the other three primes (which we also find with the vowels) cover respectively labials (**U**), palatals (**I**) and uvulars/pharyngeals (**A**). The tree in Figure 8.1, however, omits the prime @ that represents centrality in vowels. Harris (1994) uses this for dorsal (but non-palatal) in consonants, i.e. to represent velar.[2] We are left, then, with a five-unit analysis, though the precise number of primes is still a matter of debate within GP. It may well be that some smaller grouping of primes for place of articulation in consonants is better motivated at the developmental stage, with perhaps a later division of coronal and dorsal nodes into the **R** and **I**, and @ and **A** primes. An initial three-component analysis would also tally with the three vowel primes that appear well motivated in acquisition.

In GP, vowels which are represented by the simple three vowel elements are as follows:

A	[a][3]
I	[i]
U	[u]

Combinations of elements will provide a wider vowel set, of course. However, in combinations, one element is normally deemed to be the 'head' (or governor) and others are dependent on the head. In GP formalism the head element is underlined; where no element is underlined, then the elements are in non-governing relationship. If we examine some English vowels, we can see this process in operation:

[I, @]	/ɪ/
[A, I, @]	/ɛ/
[I, A]	/æ/
[U, A]	/ɒ/
[U, @]	/ʊ/
[@]	/ʌ/
[A, @]	[ɐ]

As can be seen, those short vowels of English that are generally considered to be lax vowels as well, are governed by the neutral element @. Looking at long vowels, it should be noted that in GP these are considered to occupy two segment slots (like diphthongs), and can be characterized as shown in Figure 8.2.[4]

Evidence from vowel disorders

In Ball (1996) evidence from the normal acquisition of vowel systems was presented to support phonological primes of the types argued for

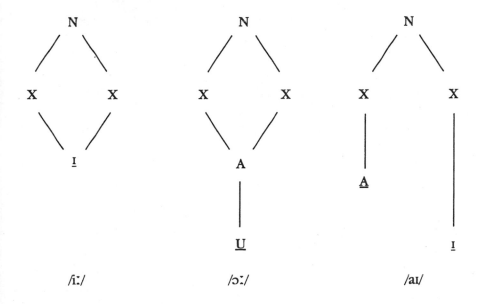

Figure 8.2. Long vowels and dipthongs in GP.

in DP and GP. For the clinical linguist it is obviously important that we can apply a similar analysis to disordered vowel systems. There is currently a paucity of information in this area as compared with research into disordered consonant systems. Nevertheless, work in both disordered phonology generally and the phonology of the hearing impaired in particular does provide us with some data that we can examine.

Hearing impairement and vowels

Cowie and Douglas-Cowie (1992) describe a range of typical vowel problems in both prelingually deaf speakers, and postlingually deafened ones. The postlingual patterns are of most interest to us here, as there is a greater regularity of substitution patterns than with the prelingually deaf. For postlingual vowel errors, Cowie and Douglas-Cowie (1992) note several patterns. The first two of these, interestingly, involve converse vowel movements: of non-close front vowels towards a more close position, and of non-open front vowels towards a more open position. Competing patterns are also observed with back vowels: first of raising vowels towards a more close position, but also of lowering towards an opener position. Clearly, these patterns can readily be interpreted as movement towards a simpler, single prime (I, A, or U), away from the more complex vowels that would contain two or more primes.

Other substitution patterns, found with both prelingually and postlingually hearing-impaired subjects show movement towards a schwa position. It may be therefore that in these instances we are seeing a breakdown of the vowel primes altogether, being replaced by the default @ unit.

Phonological disorder and vowels

Among recent works on vowel disorders are Gibbon, Shockey and Reid (1992), Pollock and Hall (1991), Pollock and Keiser (1990), Reynolds (1990), Stoel-Gammon and Herrington (1990) and Walton and Pollock (1993). Naturally, these few studies will give conflicting results, and we cannot yet expect the general patterns that have been identified in consonant substitutions.

Pollock and Keiser (1990) and Stoel-Gammon and Herrington (1990) both examine atypical vowel systems in phonological disordered American English children. Whereas a wide variety of substitution patterns was found in both studies, there was a marked tendency for what Stoel-Gammon and Herrington term 'the corner vowels' to be produced correctly early and for substitutions to involve movement to these corner vowels. It was also noted that diphthongs were often subjected to monophthongization, and for rhotic vowels to cause considerable difficulties. Clearly, the corner vowel pattern supports an analysis in terms of three primes **I, A,** and **U.** Monovalent phonologies would also characterize diphthongs and rhotic vowels as more complex than monophthongs and non-rhotic vowels, but this would also be the case in more traditional feature approaches.

Simplification of diphthongs is also reported in Gibbon et al (1992) for a British English child, along with a loss of contrast among high front vowels, and among high back vowels. This suggests that, while the child has begun to use complex units based on the **A** prime, the same ability with the **I** and **U** primes has yet to be fully developed. It is difficult to see how a traditional feature approach could account for this case.

Reynolds (1990) presents data from the biggest study of vowel disorders in British English speakers and we do not have space here to examine the results in detail. However, if we look at the main pro-cesses reported for monophthongs, we find a general tendency to move towards, or to, the so-called corner vowels, in other words our basic vowel primes. Reynolds uses a variety of terms for these processes as he was not working within our framework. For example, his lowering and fronting processes generally yield an **A** prime, while the pattern of diphthong simplification is also noted.

Finally, we can note the work of Pollock and Hall (1991). This study examined five speakers with Developmental Apraxia of Speech (DAS). As might be expected, there was considerable variability in the data, but the pattern of movement towards **A** is noticeable in all three of those subjects who exhibited marked vowel errors. Problems with diphthongs and rhotic vowels are also present, but there was too much variability with the high vowels to determine whether the **I** and **U** primes could be usefully employed to analyse the data.

We clearly need more data from vowel disorders of various types to determine whether an approach using monovalent phonological primes is more insightful than binary distinctive features, or even the mixed binary-unary approach found in some current feature geometry accounts (see Roca, 1994 for descriptions of these). Nevertheless, the studies we have reviewed suggest that in both phonological acquisition and disorder, the three primes of **I, A,** and **U**, together with the default @ and the notion of simple and complex units, can account for many of the common patterns encountered in the data.

Conclusion

We have seen how the nature of minimal units of phonology is still open to debate. We have seen how the privative phonological prime with phonetic interpretability is a good candidate and that studies of phonological acquisition and vowel disorders can be seen to support at least some version of this unit.

References

Anderson J, Durand J (1986) Dependency Phonology. In Durand J (ed.), Dependency and Non-Linear Phonology. London: Croom Helm.

Anderson J, Durand J (Eds) (1987) Explorations in Dependency Phonology. Dordrecht: Foris.

Anderson J, Ewen C (1987) Principles of Dependency Phonology. Cambridge: CUP.

Ball MJ (1996) An examination of the nature of the minimal phonological unit in language acquisition. In Bernhardt B, Gilbert J, Ingram D (Eds) Proceedings of the UBC International Conference on Phonological Acquisition. Somerville, MA: Cascadilla Press, pp 240–53.

Blache S (1978) The Acquisition of Distinctive Features. Baltimore: University Park Press.

Chomsky N, Halle M (1968) The Sound Pattern of English. Cambridge, MA: MIT Press.

Cowie R, Douglas-Cowie E (1992) Postlingually Acquired Deafness. Berlin, Mouton de Gruyter.

Durand J (1990) Generative and Non-linear Phonology. London: Longman.

Gibbon F, Shockey L, Reid J (1992) Description and treatment of abnormal vowels in a phonologically disordered child. Child Language Teaching and Therapy 8: 30–59.

Harris J (1994) English Sound Structure. Oxford: Blackwell.

Harris J, Lindsey G (1995) The elements of phonological representation. In Durand J, Katamba F (Eds) Frontiers of Phonology. London: Longman, pp 34-79.

Jakobson R (1968 (original 1941)) Child Language, Aphasia, and Phonological Universal. The Hague: Mouton.

Jakobson R, Fant G, Halle M (1952) Preliminaries to Speech Analysis. Cambridge, MA: MIT Press.

Jakobson R, Halle M (1956) Fundamentals of Language. The Hague: Mouton.

Lass R (1984) Phonology. Cambridge: Cambridge University Press.

Pollock KE, Hall PK (1991) An analysis of the vowel misarticulations of five children with developmental apraxia of speech. Clinical Linguistics and Phonetics 5: 207–24.

Pollock KE, Keiser N (1990) An examination of vowel errors in phonologically disordered children. Clinical Linguistics and Phonetics 4: 161–78.

Reynolds J (1990) Abnormal vowel patterns in phonological disorder: some data and a hypothesis. British Journal of Disorders of Communication 25: 115-48.

Roca I (1994) Generative Phonology. London: Routledge.

Stoel-Gammon C, Herrington P (1990) Vowel systems of normally developing and phonologically disordered children. Clinical Linguistics and Phonetics 4: 145–60.

Walton JH, Pollock KE (1993) Acoustic validation of vowel error patterns in developmental apraxia of speech. Clinical Linguistics and Phonetics 7: 95–111.

Notes

1 An earlier version of some sections of this paper appeared in Ball (1996).

2 @ was omitted from the tree because it represents a default value or 'blank canvas' (Harris, personal communication).

3 The vowel here is presumed to be somewhere between cardinal vowel 4 and 5. In this and other lists of symbols, IPA values are followed. In Harris (1994) and Harris and Lindsey (1995) the Americanists' tradition is followed.

4 N in the following figures stands for nucleus, not the nasal element.

Chapter 9
Variability in Phonological Disorders: Can we Search for Systematicity? Evidence from Turkish-Speaking Children

SEYHUN TOPBAŞ AND AHMET KONROT

Introduction

A review of the literature showed that in identifying phonological systems of phonologically disordered children, similar.classifications were made by several authors. Some have noted a pure delay (Fletcher, 1990); some have noted unusual errors; some have noted idiosyncratic or variable errors as typical characteristics of phonologically disordered children and a delay on overall phonological development (Ingram, 1976; Grunwell, 1985; Fey and Gandour, 1982;Compton, 1975; Leonard, 1985; Dodd, 1993). Similarly Dodd (1993) hypothesized that there are three subgroups of phonologically disordered children: those who make errors characteristic of younger normally developing children, those whose speech is characterized by the consistent use of non-developmental phonological error patterns, and children whose speech is characterized by inconsistent phonological errors. These three subgroups have also been identified in a population of phonologically disordered Cantonese-speaking children (So and Dodd, 1994). Their studies suggested that the deficits underlying the different subtypes of disorder may result in similar surface error patterns irrespective of the language being learned.

In this paper data from Turkish, a language that has not been the subject of clinical cross-linguistic studies up to the present time, will be reported. A comprehensive classification of phonological disorders has not been carried out in Turkish. Data from normal and phonologically disordered children learning different languages can provide important evidence concerning the nature of the disorder, the classification of phonological disorders, the effects of the ambient language, individual variation and concerning intervention approaches.

The purpose of this study is to analyse the phonological error patterns in phonologically disordered Turkish children, to see whether the error patterns reflect those of their normally developing peers and to find out whether the phonologically disordered children's error patterns are systematic or not.

Brief Turkish phonology

Modern standard Turkish is spoken in Turkey. Basic word order is subject-object-verb (SOV). Being an agglutinating language, suffixation has to be applied to every word root. The morphological system is very regular and transparent. The standard orthography assigns one symbol per phoneme. There are eight vowel /i, y, ɯ, ʊ, ɛ, œ, ʌ, ɔ,/ and 21 consonant /p, b, m, n, t, d, tʃ, dʒ, k, g, ɣ, f, v, h, s, z, ʃ, ʒ, l, ɾ, ɟ/ phonemes in Turkish. The basic syllable pattern of Turkish does not permit consonant clusters except in word-final position. There are allophonic variations such as vowel and consonant harmony in Turkish. Vowel length (although controversial) is asserted as being not phonemic in modern Turkish. Thus, all vowels are accepted as short.

Method

Subjects

Ten monolingual Turkish-speaking children (five boys, five girls), aged 5 to 7 years, were included in this study. They were diagnosed at other clinics and referred to our clinic for therapy. None of them was reported as physically, audiologically or cognitively problematic but they were diagnosed as having articulation disorders, unintelligible speech or speech delay. Their receptive language was within normal limits as ascertained by the Peabody Picture Vocabulary Test (Turkish version), the only standardized language test in this language. Their expressive language performance was screened by age-appropriate criterion-referenced tests developed by the first author. The expressive language performance of the subjects seemed age-appropriate although two of them had word-finding difficulties. Thus, subjects had no recognized aetiology for their disorder.

Procedure

The data used in this study were obtained from recordings that were audio taped during the assessment phase. Data collection was based on spontaneous speech samples elicited using picture compositions and examiner- or child-selected topics. The picture compositions comprised a set of 22 composite themes developed to provide a representative sample of Turkish phonology (consonants, vowels, clusters, phonotactics) and culture. Picture compositions were scenes available for narrating stories containing objects, animals, people and activities.

Analysis

The total data corpus consisting of 1531 words was based on consensus-transcriptions of two phoneticians. Narrow phonetic transcription was employed using IPA and PRDS symbols and diacritics (revised to 1989). Unintelligible words were eliminated. The data were then analysed in terms of surface error patterns and compared to normally developing children (Topbaş, 1991; 1992; Acarlar, 1994). A phonological assessment procedure, the Turkish Phonological Assessment Kit (TSDT), was used for this purpose. This kit was mainly guided by selected procedures from Ingram (1976; 1981) and PACS (Phonological Assessment of Child Speech: Grunwell, 1985). Minor modifications were necessary due to the characteristics of Turkish language. In order to determine that a process had occurred, the process had to be used in at least four different words. A process was considered 'frequent' if it was used in at least 10 per cent of overall target process occurrences. Consonants were analysed in syllable-initial (SI)/word-initial (WI), syllable-initial /within word (WW), syllable-final(SF)/within-word, syllable-final/word final(WF) positions. The processes used were then categorized in terms of usual, unusual or idiosyncratic processes.

Results

The error patterns observed were grouped under three basic subgroups:

(a) The processes that are commonly used among normally developing children, but which were not suppressed at around the expected age (Topbaş, 1991; Acarlar, 1994) and which were still used after the age of 5, were grouped under persisting normal processes as described by Grunwell (1985). This type of error pattern can be considered as delayed development (Grunwell, 1985; Dodd, 1993; Dodd, Hambly and Leahy, 1989) since most of these processes are suppressed at about 3 years of age in Turkish children (Table 9.1). SF consonant deletion, SF cluster reduction, liquid deviation, stopping of fricatives and affricates were used by all of the children. /j/ deletion and velar fronting, SI voicing, alveolar assimilation and SI consonant deletion were the next most frequent processes used among children. Affrication of fricatives, palatalization as backing, nasal assimilation, WI /h/ deletion, syllable deletion were used by six children, and velarization as backing, labial assimilation and reduplication were used by almost half of the children. Other processes occurred less in the children's speech.

(b) The processes that are rarely used among normally developing children and that were somehow variable were grouped as unusual processes as described by Leonard (1985). This group showed a disordered development (Dodd, 1993). These processes were further analysed for underlying systematicity (consistency) and consistency was found. Consistency means that the error patterns can be explained or interpreted systematically by rules (Table 9.1). Among these processes, syllable reduction was used by all of the subjects. Syllable reduction in this data can be defined as a complete change in the structure of polysyllabic words by reducing consonants or both syllables and consonants. Due to the agglutinating nature of Turkish, word length in some trisyllabic words was usually preserved but the structure of the word was changed.

For example, a trisyllabic word with CVC+CV+CVC structure was changed to CV+CVC by deleting not a whole syllable but consonants (example (1)) or CV+CV+CV.

(1)   Syllable reduction
      subject 1:   /k/ → [t] fronting
      /portakal/ →   [pɔtʌt] orange >>
                              ↓
                  [pɔtʌt (al)] → [-al] → ∅

To elaborate controversially, a child who drops the syllable nucleus may still be considered to signal the existence of that syllable by using a 'processed' consonant. Consonant metathesis, coalescence and denasalization were the next most frequent processes used by the children. Stopping of /ɾ,j/ was seen in two subjects. Normal Turkish children seldom use these processes. For example, metathesis may be seen before the age of three. This process can be seen in adult language as well with respect to intervocalic adjacent consonants in -C,C- structures (/toprak / → [torpak]; /kibrit/ → [kirbit]). Reduplicating and assimilating new forms frequently occurred in some children's speech. Reduplicating the syllables with other inter-

Table 9.1. Persisting normal, unusual and idiosyncratic processes in phonologically disordered Turkish children.

Persisting Normal Processes	1	2	3	4	5	6	7	8	9	10
Reduplication	v	v		v			v			v
Syllable deletion	v	v	v	v			v	v		
SF Consonant deletion	v	v	v	v	v	v	v	v	v	v
SI Consonant deletion	v								v	v
/i/ Deletion	v	v	v	v	v	v	v	v	v	v
WI /h/ Deletion	v		v				v	v	v	v
WF Cluster reduction	v	v	v	v	v	v	v	v	v	v
Assimilation processes										
Labial assimilation		v	v				v		v	v
Alveolar assimilation	v			v	v	v	v		v	v
Velar assimilation							v			
Nasal assimilation	v			v	v		v		v	v
Liquid Deviation										
SF /l, r/ → /θ/	v	v	v	v	v	v	v	v	v	
SI /l, r/ → /j/	v	v	v	v	v	v	v	v	v	v
SI /l, r/ → /l/			v			v	v	v		
Vowel lengthening	v	v	v	v			v		v	v
Fronting process										
Velar fronting	v		v	v	v	v	v	v	v	v
Palatal fronting							v	v	v	
Labialization						v	v		v	
Stopping processes										
Fricatives	v	v	v	v	v	v	v	v	v	v
Affricates	v	v	v	v	v	v	v	v	v	v
Deaffrication							v	v		
Affrication										
Stops					v		v			v
Fricatives				v	v	v	v	v		v
Voicing										
(SIWI and SIWW)	v	v	v	v	v	v	v	v		
Devoicing		v	v	v	v	v	v	v	v	
Backing										
Delabilization		v			v					
Palatalization			v		v	v	v	v	v	
Velarization		v			v		v	v	v	

Unusual processes	1	2	3	4	5	6	7	8	9	10
Syllable reduction	v	v	v	v	v	v	v	v	v	v
Stopping										
/r/	v		v							
/l/	v		v	v		v				v
/j/	v		v							
Denasalization	v	v	v	v			v	v		v
Fricative → /j/	v			v		v				v
/r, l, j,/ → Fricative					v					
Metathesis										
Consonant	v	v	v	v	v	v		v	v	v
Syllable		v					v		v	
Coalescence	v	v	v		v	v	v	v	v	
Nasalization of stops	v	v	v			v				

Table 9.1. *(Cont.)*

Idiosyncratic Processes	1	2	3	4	5	6	7	8	9	10
Metathesis and Migration							v	v		v
Compound simplification										
Noun+Noun	v		v	v	v					
Noun+Verb		v	v							
H-zation										
Substitution	v	v				v	v		v	v
Insertion		v			v					
Assimilation		v								
Nasalization										
Fricatives				v		v	v		v	
Liquids (/r, l/)			v				v	v		
Idiosyncratic velarization			v					v		
(K-zation)								v		
Ejective-zation			v							
Glottalization	v	v	v	v						
Lateralization										
m, b, v → /β/						v	v			
						v	v			

acting processes was reported by Topbaş (1992) in a case study of a child compared to normative data. Fricative gliding was observed in four children. All these patterns are considered non-developmental.

(c) The processes that were not used among normally developing children, or that were found to be very variable, were grouped as idiosyncratic processes (Grunwell 1985). This group also showed a disordered development and the processes were very inconsistent (So and Dodd, 1994). By inconsistency it is meant that the error patterns cannot be explained or interpreted systematically by rules (Table 9.1). Among these processes 'h-zation' was the most frequent one used by six subjects. 'H-zation' used by subject 2 was found to be inconsistent. Although usually the fricatives /s, ʃ, z, f/ were realized as [h], the process was not restricted to these consonants. Both SI and SF 'h-zation' was observed. Within some words, an assimilation process applied after h-zation occurred.

Compound simplification, nasalization of fricatives and glottalization were the next three processes used by four of the ten children. Glottalization usually occurred in SI and SF within word positions. Velarization, used by two children, was considered as a persisting normal process: since velars are acquired early in Turkish, it is assumed that children may have a tendency to use velars in systemic simplifications. However, there was much idiosyncracy in the data. SF velars were fronted which might be accepted as persistent normal, but the velars in other contexts were labialized and fronted, which is unusual for normal children. On the other hand, velarization was observed as occurring very idiosyncratically so that the patterns could not easily be explained by rules. Usually the fricatives were realized as /k/. Analysis of some words showed that after velarization a velar assimilation occurred within the same word. The only prominent note may be that velarization occurred usually, but not always, before front vowels. Ejectivization was observed in only one child.

Discussion

In this study all of the Turkish-speaking children provided examples of persisting normal, unusual, and idiosyncratic processes. None of the children presented a pure phonological delay. Communicative adequacy was highly affected, causing unintelligibility. Although there was evidence for underlying systematic behaviours in the use of some error patterns, there was evidence for inconsistent use as well.

All the children's consonant systems were restricted. Most of the processes considered as persistent normal processes were suppressed at about 3;0 years of age in normal Turkish children's speech. Among these processes, SF deletion of liquids in intervocalic consonant sequences, SF cluster reduction, and liquid deviation are the processes to be suppressed last in normals.

Topbaş (1991) discussed the possibility that the suppression of these processes may continue due to the characteristics of Turkish. However, the use of these processes after the age of five may be an indication of delayed phonological development.

The unusual processes observed are seldom used among normally developing children. A review of the literature shows that such unusual processes are characteristic of an impaired phonological system. Leonard (1985) proposed that children who exhibit unusual phonological behaviour may require considerable clinical attention, as such behaviours signal an impaired system. Similarly, Fey and Stalker (1986) reported that unusual phonological and morphophonological rules are common among phonologically disordered children. In this study, when the children's error patterns were further analysed, there was evidence for systematicity. The systematicity or consistency of these behaviours was also discussed by several authors in the literature (Leonard, 1985; Dodd, 1993; So and Dodd, 1994; Yavaş, 1994). To search for systematicity within an impaired system is particularly important for therapy purposes. Yavaş (1994) reported a case study of a Portuguese-speaking child whose speech error patterns were very different from the ambient language but he found evidence for regularities in these data which is fundamental for assessment and therapy.

In this study, almost all the children exhibited idiosyncratic behaviours. Idiosyncratic behaviours have also been discussed as a characteristic of disordered development (Grunwell, 1985; Dodd, 1993; So and Dodd, 1994). There are controversies as to which behaviours should be accepted as idiosyncratic and whether these idiosyncratic behaviours can be consistent or not. Nevertheless, researchers reported that idiosyncratic behaviours might also be observed among normally developing children. For instance, Menn (1976, 1978), giving examples from assimilation processes, explains that many early rules in child phonology reflect children's self-discovered ways of assimilating target words into preferred forms that can be produced fluently and automatically.

It can thus be inferred that children may create forms in order to be able to communicate. The variability of surface error patterns may cause unintelligibility. However, a detailed analysis may help to find some regularities or consistencies within the system.

In this paper the patterns that were not explained by any regularity and which differ from one child to another were considered as idiosyncratic behaviours. Consequently, the apparent patterns were so inconsistent that it was not easy to make any predictions. Word-by-word analysis gave some indications of what might be helpful therapeutically but such behaviours could not be generalized. Some researchers attribute such inconsistent error patterns to a deficit in motor programming (Dodd, 1993; So and Dodd, 1994). This hypothesis, however, needs further investigation.

In summary, the analysis of this study revealed that the phonological patterns of Turkish phonologically disordered children can be classified not only as *delayed* but as *disordered* as well. Cross-linguistic data from phonologically disordered children can provide important evidence concerning the nature of the disorder (Kopkalli-Yavuz and Topbaş, this volume).

References

Acarlar F (1994) Türkge Kazaniminda sesbilgisel sùregler. PhD dissertation: Hacettepe University, Ankara.

Compton A (1995) Generative studies of children's phonological disorders: a strarergy of therapy. In Singh S (ed.) Measurements in Hearing, Speech and Language. Baltimore: University Park Press.

Dodd BJ (1993) Speech disordered children. In Blanken G, Dittmann J, Grimm H, Marshall J, Wallesch CW (Eds) Linguistic Disorders and Pathologies. Berlin: De Gruyter.

Dodd BJ, Hambly G, Leahy J (1989) Phonological disorders in children: underlying cognitive deficits. British Journal of Developmental Psychology, 7, 55–71.

Fey ME, Stalker CH (1986) A hypothesis-testing approach to treatment of a child with an idiosyncratic (morpho-) phonological system. Journal of Speech and Hearing Disorders 51: 324–36.

Fey M E, Gandour J (1982) Rule discovery in phonological acquisition. Journal of Child Language 9: 71–81.

Fletcher P (1990) The breakdown of language: language pathology and therapy. In Collinge N (ed.) Encyclopedia of Language, London: Routledge.

Grunwell P (1985) Phonological Assessment of Child Speech (PACS). Dorset: NFER-Nelson.

Ingram D (1976) Phonological Disability in Children. London: Edward Arnold.

Ingram D (1981) Procedures for the Phonological Analysis of Children's Language. Baltimore:University Park Press.

Kopkalli-Yavuz H, Topbaş (this volume, Chapter 10) Phonological processes of Turkish phonologically disordered children: Language specific or universal? Proceedings of the 1996 ICPLA Conference, Munich.

Leonard LB (1985) Unusual and subtle phonological behavior in the speech of phonologically disordered children. Journal of Speech and Hearing Disorders 50: 4-13.

Menn L (1976) Pattern, control and contrast in beginning speech: a case study in the development of word form and word function. Unpublished doctoral dissertation, University of Illinois.

Menn L (1978) Phonological units in beginning speech. In Bell A and Bybee J (eds), Syllables and Segments. Amsterdam: North-Holland: 157–71.

So KHL, Dodd BJ (1994) Phonologically disordered Cantonese-speaking children. Clinical Linguistics and Phonetics 8, 3: 235–55.

Topbaş, S (1991) Sesbilgisi Açısındam Dil Edinim Süreci. Paper presented to the Fifth National Linguistics Conference. Turkey, İzmir.

Topbaş, S. (1992) Turkish children's phonological acquisition: implications for phonological disorders. Paper presented to the Sixth International Turkish Linguistics Conference.

Yavaş, M (1994) Extreme regularity in phonological disorder: a case study. Clinical Linguistics and Phonetics 8, 2: 127–39.

Chapter 10
Phonological Processes of Turkish Phonologically Disordered Children: Language Specific or Universal?

HANDAN KOPKALLI-YAVUZ AND SEYHUN TOPBAŞ

Introduction

In recent years the importance of a cross-linguistic approach to language development for impaired children has been emphasized (Fletcher and Grunwell, 1990). Although there are a substantial number of studies describing the nature of language development for impaired children, most of these studies have been with children acquiring Indo-European languages, such as English (Grunwell, 1981, 1985), Swedish (Magnusson, 1983 cited in Beers, 1992), Dutch (Beers, 1992), Italian (Bortolini and Leonard, 1991), and Portuguese (Yavaş, 1994) with the exception of one non-Indo-European language – Cantonese (So and Dodd, 1994). The findings of these studies suggest that phonologically disordered children, like normally developing children, acquire the phonological system of a particular language. As with normally developing children (ND), however, some phonological processes are seen across languages. As the majority of the languages investigated are members of the same language family, strong claims about whether the processes are language-specific or universal cannot be made. This study presents data from phonologically disordered (PD) children acquiring Turkish and compares the findings with those of other languages investigated. Turkish was chosen because it presents data from a non-Indo-European language so that the saliency of the language being acquired and the language specific factors can be determined.

Cross-language comparison

Topbaş and Konrot (this volume, Chapter 9) have investigated the speech of 10 phonologically disordered children (aged between 5 and 7). In this study, the phonological processes observed in PD children were first identified in relation with ND children, and were then categorized as persisting normal, unusual, and idiosyncratic processes as in similar studies in the literature. The 'persisting normal' processes were those observed in ND children. The processes that are seldom used by ND children were classified as 'unusual'. The processes that were not observed in ND children and variable across subjects were categorized as 'idiosyncratic' (see Topbaş and Konrot, this volume, for the details and justification of these classifications). The data presented in Topbaş and Konrot are taken as the basis for Turkish. The Turkish data were compared with six other languages: English, Dutch, Swedish, Italian, Portuguese, and Cantonese. After appropriate categorization of phonological processes the Turkish data were compared with Grunwell (1981, 1985) for English, Magnusson (1983 cited in Beers, 1992) for Swedish, Beers (1992) for Dutch, Bortolini and Leonard (1991) for Italian, Yavaş and Lamprecht (1988) and Yavaş (1994) for Portuguese, and So and Dodd (1994) for Cantonese.

Persisting processes

Persisting processes for Turkish and occurrences in the other languages are presented in Table 10.1.

In Turkish PD children, word-final (WF) cluster reduction, liquid deviation, syllable-final (SF) consonant deletion, velar fronting, and stopping processes were the most frequently used processes. WF cluster reduction was specified as word-final because Turkish does not allow syllable initial (SI) clusters. In Turkish, WF clusters are generally resricted to sonorant + stop sequences. The data indicated that these clusters were reduced by eliminating the sonorant. In other languages, initial cluster reduction is a more common process than final cluster reduction. As a matter of fact, WF cluster reduction is reported only for English.

Liquid deviation is seen across languages and hence appears to be universal. However, the nature of the deviation seems to be different across languages. Liquid deviation patterns of Turkish are different from those of other languages, so this process can be specified as language-specific. The label 'liquid' is used loosely to cover all types of 'r' sounds as well as /l/. Turkish 'r', for example, is a flap /ɾ/ with allophones in complementary distribution. The term liquid was used because Turkish flap behaves like an 'r', and because similar processes

Table 10.1. Persisting normal processes in Turkish and occurrences in other languages.

Persisting Processes	Turkish	English	Dutch	Swedish	Italian	Portuguese	Cantonese
WF Cluster reduction	✓	✓					
Liquid deviation							
SF /l, r/ → /ø/	✓				✓		
SF /l, r/ → /j/	✓			✓		✓	✓ (1subj)
SF /r/ → /l/	✓				✓	✓	
Vowel lengthening	✓						
SF Consonant deletion	✓	✓	✓				✓
Fronting processes							
Velar fronting	✓	✓	✓	✓			✓
Palatal fronting	✓	✓	✓	✓			
Labialization	✓		✓				
Stopping processes		✓		✓	✓		✓
Fricatives	✓		✓				
Affricatives	✓						
SI Consonant deletion	✓		✓	✓			✓
/i/ Deletion	✓						✓
Voicing (SIWI and SIWW)	✓	✓	✓				
Devoicing	✓	✓	✓	✓	✓	✓	
Assimilation Processes		✓	✓	✓	✓	✓	✓
Labial assimilation	✓						
Alveolar assimilation	✓						
Velar assimilation	✓						
Nasal assimilation	✓						
Syllable Deletion	✓	✓	✓	✓	✓	✓	
WI /h/Deletion	✓	✓					✓
Backing							
Delabialization	✓	✓	✓				
Palatalization	✓	✓	✓				
Velarization	✓	✓	✓	✓			✓
Affrication		✓					✓
Stops	✓						
Fricatives	✓						
Reduplication	✓	✓	✓				
Deaffrication	✓	✓			✓		✓

in other languages are reported as such. Turkish liquids were deleted in SF position (both within word (WW) and in WF position) but replaced by /j/ in SIWW position. Italian is the only other language for which liquid deletion is reported but in Italian liquids are deleted both in SI and word-initial (WI) positions. Gliding of liquids (/l, r/ →/j/) is reported for all the other languages except Italian. Depending on the 'r' sound a language uses, 'r' is replaced with /w/ or /j/. In English and

Dutch, for example, 'r' is replaced with /w/, but with /j/ in Swedish and Turkish. (In Table 10.1, the gliding process was restricted to [/l, ɾ/ →/j/] as /w/ was never substituted for liquids in the Turkish data. Thus English and Dutch were not checked for this process.) What 'r' is replaced with seems to depend on the phonetic characteristics of that sound in a language. SI liquid substitution (/ɾ/ →/l/) observed in Turkish was restricted to substitution of /l/ for /ɾ/ . A similar process is also reported in Italian and Portuguese but in these languages either one of the liquids may be substituted with the other. Furthermore, in Italian, substitution of both /ɾ/ and /l/ with /n/ has been observed. Although this seems to be a similar process across languages, the differences in the nature of the deviation suggest that PD children are sensitive to the phonology of the ambient language.

Another common process under liquid deviation was vowel lengthening whereby the vowel preceding the liquid is lengthened as a function of liquid deletion. Vowel lengthening occurred generally in contexts where the liquid was adjacent to another consonant (i.e., SF). Vowel lengthening as a function of liquid deletion is not reported for any other language.[1] This process can thus be classified as language-specific. Although compensatory lengthening has been reported in literature for other languages (e.g. Stemberger, 1992) it is not necessarily a function of liquid deletion.

SF consonant deletion, velar fronting and stopping were processes common both in Turkish and across languages. SF deletion is also reported for English, Dutch, and Cantonese. The most commonly observed fronting process for Turkish was velar fronting. This process has been reported for English, Dutch, Swedish, and Cantonese. Bortolini and Leonard (1991) report that there is a fronting process in Italian but do not specify the nature of the process. None the less, velar fronting seems to be a universal process. Similarly, stopping may also be regarded as a universal process as it is reported for all languages except Portuguese.

Initial consonant deletion in general is a common process among the PD children within a language as well as across languages. However, the type of the consonant and the position of the deletion vary across languages. In Turkish, consonants were deleted in SIWW especially if they were preceded by a consonant. WI consonants, on the other hand, were less likely to be deleted in Turkish. SI consonant deletion has been observed in Dutch, Swedish, and Cantonese but in these languages deletion is not restricted solely to WW. Furthermore, in Cantonese, this process is restricted to fricatives and affricates.

Glide (/j/) deletion was distinguished from other consonant deletions because unlike other consonants, /j/ was mainly deleted SFWW in Turkish. Glide deletion was frequent across Turkish subjects but not across languages. This process is reported only for Cantonese, and was observed in the speech of only one subject. Thus /j/ deletion appears to be specific to Turkish.

Voicing, unusual in Dutch and context-based in English, was restricted to SI position (WW and WI) in Turkish. This is expected as Turkish devoices underlyingly voiced non-continuants (i.e. stops and affricates) in the SF position (Kopkalli, 1993). Application of this process only in SI position suggests that PD children are sensitive to the phonological constraints of the ambient language. In Turkish, devoicing was another frequent process. Devoicing of stops and affricates was again restricted to SI position as voiced stops and affricates cannot occur syllable-finally. Devoicing of fricatives was equally common in both SI and SF positions. Devoicing has been observed in the other languages except for Cantonese.

Assimilation processes were frequently observed in Turkish. Three of the assimilation processes – alveolar, labial, and nasal – were more frequent than velar assimilation. It is difficult to compare individual assimilation processes with those of other languages because assimilation processes have been subdivided differently in different languages. Assimilation is one of the few processes observed in all of the languages investigated.

Other processes have been observed in more than half of the Turkish subjects but less frequently than the processes mentioned above. Syllable deletion has been observed in all languages except Cantonese. In other languages it is the weak syllable that deletes, and/or the position of the syllable may play a role, i.e. pre-tonic, post-tonic. In the Turkish data, syllable deletion does not seem to be a function of stress or position within a word.

WI /h/ deletion was a frequent process in Turkish, although it was not common across languages; only English and Cantonese report having the same process. The /h/ deletion process was identified as a separate process because /h/ behaves differently from other consonants in Turkish. Deletion of /h/ was almost exclusively limited to WI position in Turkish whereas deletion of other consonants (except /j/) were in SI position.

Palatalization, a backing process whereby phonologically [+anterior, +coronal] consonants are substituted by a palatal consonant was frequently observed among Turkish PD children. Palatalization was reported for English and Dutch. Backing process is also reported for Portuguese but in this language backing is to palato-alveolar.

Velarization, another frequent process, refers to the substitution of a non-velar consonant by a velar one. Velar assimilation, on the other hand, refers to the realization of a non-velar consonant as velar due to the presence of other velar(s) within the word. Velar assimilation was not as frequent in Turkish as velarization. Velar sounds, although back sounds and acquired relatively late in other languages, are the earliest sounds acquired in Turkish. Therefore both processes are classified as persisting normal for PD Turkish children. Velar assimilation has not been reported for any other language. Velarization, on the other hand, has been observed in English, Dutch, Swedish and Cantonese but was identified as an unusual process. The difference in the classification of processes is another evidence of the differences across languages; what may be unusual for some languages (English, Dutch, Swedish, and Cantonese) may be usual for others (Turkish).

Affrication of fricatives was more common than affrication of stops in Turkish. Although affrication is a common process in Turkish, it is not so common in other languages (reported for only English and Cantonese).

Less frequent processes were reduplication, deaffrication, palatal fronting, and labialization. Reduplication, a process whereby a syllable is duplicated to form the target word, is reported for English and Dutch. Deaffrication refers to simplification of affricates into fricatives. Velar fronting was the most common fronting process across subjects and across languages (English, Dutch, Swedish, Cantonese). The other two fronting processes were infrequent. Palatal fronting is reported for English and Swedish whereas labialization is reported only for Swedish.

Unusual processes

Unusual processes for Turkish and their occurrences in the other languages are presented in Table 10.2.

Table 10.2. Unusual processes in Turkish and occurrences in other languages.

Unusual Processes	Turkish	English	Dutch	Swedish	Italian	Portuguese	Cantonese
Syllable reduction	✓		✓				
Metathesis		✓	✓	✓	✓		
Consonant	✓						
Syllable	✓						
Coalescence	✓						
Denasalization	✓	✓	✓				
Nasalization of stops	✓			✓	✓		
Stopping							
/r/	✓	✓					
/l/	✓	✓					
/j/	✓	✓					
Fricative → /j/	✓	✓	✓				✓
/r, l, j/ → Fricative	✓	✓	✓				

Some of these processes were frequently observed across Turkish subjects while others were less frequent. Syllable reduction, a frequent
process, refers to partial deletion of a syllable resulting in the change of
the syllable structure (e.g. 'swing' /sʌ-lʉm-dʒʌk/ → [hʌn-ʒʌk]). Syllable
reduction was observed only in Dutch.

Consonant metathesis is a frequent process in Turkish as well as
across languages. In Turkish, consonant metathesis generally occurred
with adjacent consonants. Syllable metathesis (e.g. 'ice cream' /dən-
dʉʂ̌-mʌ/ → [bʉn-də]) was also observed in the Turkish data. This seems
to be specific to Turkish as it has not been specifically reported for any
other language.

Coalescence, two adjacent sounds becoming one, was a common
process among Turkish subjects (e.g. 'truck' [kʌm-jon] → [kʌ-ɲol]).
Coalescence was observed when either a nasal (irrespective of place) or
a liquid occurred next to a glide and resulted in a palatal nasal /ɲ/
which does not occur in the phonetic inventory of Turkish. Such a
process is not reported for any other language and thus appears to be
language-specific.

Denasalization, a process which deletes the feature [+nasal], was
commonly observed in Turkish. This process occurs in English and
Dutch. Nasalization, on the other hand, is a more common process
across languages including Turkish. Nasalization affects different segments in different languages. In Turkish, for example, stops become
nasals while in Portuguese liquids become nasals.

Stopping of liquids and glide /j/ was a rare process among the
languages investigated. In languages other than Turkish, it is only
reported for English and is seen rarely. Similarly, fricative gliding is seen
only in Turkish and English. Liquid and glide frication are observed in
Dutch in addition to Turkish and English.

Idiosyncratic processes

Idiosyncratic processes are presented in Table 10.3. These processes
were not as rare across Turkish subjects as one might predict. H-zation,
for example, has been observed in the speech of seven children. The
majority of these subjects substituted /h/ for another consonant. There
were also examples of /h/ insertion but it was much less frequent.
H-zation is common across languages investigated (Dutch, Swedish,
and Cantonese).

Glottalization, insertion or substitution of a consonant with a glottal
stop, was observed in a number of Turkish subjects as well as in other
languages such as English and Dutch.

Metathesis and migration refers to the interaction of these two
processes (e.g., 'chair' /sʌn-dʌl-jɛ/ → [dʌs-sʌn-ni]). This process appears

Table 10.3. Idiosyncratic processes in Turkish and occurrences in other languages

Idiosyn. Processes	Turkish	English	Dutch	Swedish	Italian	Portuguese	Cantonese
H-zation		✓	✓				✓
Substitution	✓						
Insertion	✓						
Assimilation	✓						
Glottalization	✓	✓	✓				
Metathesis and migration	✓						
Compound simplification							
Noun+noun	✓						
Noun+verb	✓						
Nasalization							
Fricatives	✓						
Liquids (/r, l/)	✓					✓	
Idiosyncratic velarization	✓						
Ejective-zation	✓						
Lateralization	✓	✓	✓	✓			
(m, b, v) → /ß/	✓						

to be specific to Turkish. Although metathesis and migration as separate processes are reported for other languages, it has not been observed as a single process in any other language.

Compound simplification was a process observed for Turkish, but not reported for any other language. Compound simplification refers to the reduction of noun compounds (e.g., 'birthday' /doum # gyny/ → [dʊmdy]) and noun + verb sequences (e.g., '[he is] brushing his teeth' /diʃlerini # fuɯʈʃʌlɯjoɾ̯/ → /diʃlipətə/) to one word. Such a process appears to be specific to Turkish.

Sound changes such as nasalization of fricatives and liquids or idiosyncratic velarization are processes observed in a number of Turkish subjects. Nasalization of fricatives and liquids is also reported in Portuguese. Idiosyncratic velarization (k-zation), substitution of /k/ for a number of different targets in a very idiosyncratic way (e.g. 'bottle' /ʃiʃe/ → [cicæ], 'green'/jeʃil/ → [ɹiɲi]) was not observed in any other language.

Some substitution processes were interesting as the substituted sounds do not occur in the phonetic inventory of Turkish. Although rare, these processes were observed in some of the subjects' speech. Ejective-zation refers to the realization of obstruents (i.e. stops and fricatives) as ejectives (e.g. 'lion' /ʌslʌn/ → [ʌk'cɛn]). Lateralization refers to the substitution of /j, r/ by palatal lateral and alveolar lateral fricative (e.g. '[his] nose' /buɾnʊ/ → [buʎʊ]). Lateralization also occurs in English, Dutch and Swedish. Substitution of voiced bilabial fricative /ß/

for voiced labial sounds /m, b, v/ was observed in Turkish but not in any
other language.

Conclusion

Cross-linguistic comparison of PD children's speech indicates that there
are many universal aspects. However, there are language-specific
aspects too. The comparison of seven languages suggests that vowel
lengthening as a function of liquid deletion, SF /j/ deletion, compound
simplification, idiosyncratic velarization, and ejective-zation are specific
to Turkish. Some processes, such as velarization and velar assimilation,
were observed in other languages but the nature of these processes
appears to be language-specific. Investigation of other languages, especially from different language families, is needed to be conclusive.

There are cross-language differences in terms of processes being
persisting normal, unusual, or idiosyncratic. A process may be, for
example, persisting normal in one language but unusual in another. It
appears that some processes either classified as unusual or idiosyncratic are specific to PD children both across and within languages.
Thus individual differences as well as language specifics need to be considered both in classifications and in therapy.

As Turkish was taken as the basis for the comparison, a number of
processes not occurring in Turkish but reported for the other languages
such as labial lenition (Dutch), /s/ substitution for /h/ (English), initial
cluster reduction (English, Dutch, Swedish), cluster creation (Swedish)
and others reported in case studies, were not included. These also need
to be explored to determine the saliency of the languages.

References

Beers M (1992) Phonological processes in Dutch language impaired children.
    Scandinavian Journal of Logopedics and Phonology 17: 9–16.
Bortolini U and Leonard LB (1991) The speech of phonologically disordered chil-
    dren acquiring Italian. Clinical Linguistics and Phonetics 5: 1–12.
Fletcher P and Grunwell P (1990) A cross-linguistic perspective on child language
    impairment. Clinical Linguistics and Phonetics 4: 25–7.
Grunwell P (1981) The Nature of Phonological Disability in Children. London:
    Academic Press.
Grunwell P (1985) Phonological Assessment of Child Speech (PACS). Windsor:
    NFER-Nelson.
Kopkalli H (1993) A Phonetic and Phonological Analysis of Final Devoicing in
    Turkish. PhD Dissertation: The University of Michigan, Ann Arbor.
Magnusson E (1983) The phonology of language disordered children. Thesis:
    Travaux de l'Institut de Linguistique de Lund.

So L K H and Dodd BJ (1994) Phonologically disordered Cantonese-speaking children. Clinical Linguistics and Phonetics 8: 235–55.

Stemberger J P (1992) A performance constraint on compensatory lengthening in child phonology. Language and Speech 35: 207–18.

Topbaş S and A Konrot (this volume, Chapter 9) Variability in Phonological Disorders: Can we search for systematicity? Evidence from Turkish speaking children. Proceedings of the 1996 ICPLA Conference, Munich.

Yavaş M (1994) Extreme regularity in phonological disorder: a case study. Clinical Linguistics and Phonetics 8: 127–39.

Yavaş M, Lamprecht R (1988) Processes and intelligibility in disordered phonology. Clinical Linguistics and Phonetics 2, 40: 329–45.

Note

1   den Onden (personal communication) states that there is compensatory lengthening after liquid deletion in Dutch. Such a process, however, is not reported in publication (eg Beers, 1992).

Chapter 11
Phonological Awareness and Severe Reading/Writing Delay

NICOLE MÜLLER, ANGELA HURD AND
MARTIN J BALL

Introduction

Phonological awareness and literacy development are generally seen as connected although there is no consensus as to the extent and direction of causality in this connection. However, a widespread assumption, supported by research, is that certain phonological skills precede and support literacy and that, on the other hand, learning to read and spell supports the further development of phonological awareness in children. Much attention in recent years has focused on rhyming and alliteration skills, their relation to other segmentation skills and to the acquisition of literacy (c.f. e.g Bowey and Francis, 1991; Bradley and Bryant, 1983; Bryant, MacLean, Bradley, and Crossland, 1990; Goswami and Bryant, 1990; Huxford, 1995; Mann, 1986; Stackhouse, 1985; Wimmer, Landerl, Linortner, and Hummer, 1991). Huxford (1995, 103) suggests a developmental path of what she calls 'phonemic ability' along the following lines:

1. rhyming.
2. segmenting (hearing) of initial sound in a word.
3. segmenting (hearing) of final sound in a word.
4. segmenting (hearing) of medial sound in a word.

Huxford thus takes rhyming skills as the starting point in phonological skills development. Other studies have shown that both poor readers with no other phonological problems and children with phonological disorders find rhyme and alliteration tasks (as well as other sound awareness tasks) much more difficult than children with age-appropriate reading and spelling skills (c.f. e.g. Bernhardt, Edwards and Rempel, 1995; Magnusson and Nauclér, 1993).

Chris: a case study

The case study presented here concerns 'Chris', a monolingual English speaker, aged 7;10 at the onset of this study. He had received unsuccessful literacy instruction for approximately three years, had virtually no reading, writing or letter-recognition skills, with the exception that he was able to recognize and write a few rote-learned words, such as 'egg' and 'cat'.

Chris's general cognitive ability, hearing and verbal reasoning skills are well within normal limits and he is an active and communicative child. He had experienced speech and language therapy before, having been referred at age 3;0 for language delay, the main problem being delayed phonology. Other aspects dealt with in therapy, and continuing up to the age of 7;10 were auditory memory skills and higher-level concepts (such as time). The one problem remaining in his phonology is that the production of the approximants /l, w, j/ is practically in free variation. However, Chris has no problem discriminating minimal pairs involving approximants, such as 'yes' and 'less'. Chris's metaphonological abilities and phonological skills at the beginning of this study were very limited for a child of his age. He never had any problems repeating words or non-words and could make judgments about minimal pairs (i.e. he could tell whether two words were the same or different) irrespective of the position or the type of the differentiating sound (e.g. initial C, or nucleus V, or final C). He was beginning to acquire knowledge of syllables, i.e. the abilities to clap out the number of syllables in a word. However, he could not make judgments concerning rhyme, alliteration, or individual segments in oddity or naming tasks, and could not play rhyming games. The impression was of a fundamental lack of understanding concerning what the task was about, and an inability to follow patterns provided in examples. Instead, Chris focused on word meaning and semantic fields. For example, when asked for a word that rhymed with 'nose' (such as 'hose' – this was given to him as an example), the response was 'ears'. In a game of 'let's find as many words as we can that sound like "bat", e.g. "fat", "cat" . . .', Chris's contribution was 'kitten'. Oddity tasks were similarly unsuccessful. These were tasks that demanded the identification of the non-alliterating word out of three (e.g. 'fish', 'fun', 'song'), or the non-rhyming word out of three (e.g. 'fish', 'dish', 'song'), Chris would either not answer at all, or guess.

Given the low level of Chris's sound awareness, and the assumed links between literacy and phonological awareness cited above, it is not surprising that literacy instruction tailored for children with age-appropriate metaphonological skills was not successful. A further problem, caused by lack of success over years, was that Chris had become extremely anxious about letters, spelling, reading and writing, and would be greatly distracted by his anxiety. Thus a 'non-spelling' approach was needed.

Establishing segmentation skills: initial results

We decided to focus on segmenting skills with Chris, whereby, at the outset of this stage of his therapy, he was asked to identify sounds in simple CVC nonsense words (with C = fricative, V = long). The segmenting tasks Chris was presented with were very explicit. He was asked to listen to a nonsense word and repeat it. At no stage did he experience problems with repetition. The next instruction was, 'Can you tell me what sound it starts with? Listen again to the word, and say it, and then tell me, what's the first sound you make?'

After a very short time, Chris developed awareness of initial sounds. One side-effect was that he was no longer distracted by word-meaning and he performed well on tasks such as selection tasks (presented with a picture, Chris was asked to choose from three initial consonants), sorting tasks ('Put all the pictures that start with /s/ on one pile'; 'Name all the things in the room that start with /s/') and naming tasks ('what sound does the word start with?' – pointing to a picture). Initially, detection was much easier than production (i.e. producing alliterations, such as 'let's find lots of words beginning with /s/'). However, the definition of 'initial sound' that Chris thus acquired could be described as 'anything in front of the vowel', since he still found it impossible to segment clusters into their component parts and, indeed, found it hard to compare, for example, singleton /s/ with /st/ or /str/, and to identify the common element in these clusters although, again, minimal pairs provided no problems in word-discrimination (e.g. 'are "sing" and "sting" the same or different?') or indeed production. The next step was the identification of final consonants. Again, the definition here was that of a slot in syllable structure, rather than that of a single segment since clusters had clearly the same status as singletons and were not segmented any further.

What proved very difficult indeed for a long time was the identification of vowels. In a task that demanded the identification of the three sounds making up a CVC structure, the identification would typically proceed along the following lines: C1, C2, long hesitation, and then a guess, often returning to C1 or C2. Clearly, the vowel did not count as a 'sound' in Chris's judgment. On the other hand, the distinction of minimal pairs differentiated by a vowel (e.g. 'pot' and 'pit') never caused any problems. However, it soon emerged that this lack of awareness of vowels as segments appeared to be restricted to vowels preceded by a consonantal syllable onset. When confronted with VC structures and asked to identify the sounds they comprised, Chris had no major problems. Although more difficult than in VC structures, the identification of vowels in CV structures was much easier than in CVCs. Only after much effort on Chris's part, explicitly comparing Vs on CVC and VC structures, did vowels acquire the same segmental status in his sound awareness.

Chris acquired the ability to detect and produce rhyme much later than the ability to detect and produce alliterations. This could very well be a direct result of the types of tasks chosen to initiate sound awareness: since Chris found it impossible to cope with rhyme or deletion, very explicit identification tasks were devised, which may have led to a strong focus of attention on one slot in syllable structure.

Questions

Several questions arise from the path of Chris's progress. For example:

(a) What is the relation between rhyme and alliteration and how do both relate to other segmentation skills – i.e. what skills do they presuppose?
(b) What was Chris's (meta)phonological representation of the syllable when he began to acquire sound awareness, especially with regard to the commonly proposed basic division into onset and rhyme unit, and with regard to the vowel as syllabic nucleus?

Alliterations and rhymes

There is a body of literature that treats onset and rhyme tasks as being of equal difficulty for children with normally developing phonological/metaphonological skills (e.g. Bowey and Frances, 1991), although 'equal difficulty', however measured, does not mean that the same skills and processes are involved in the two types of tasks. Other studies have found differences between alliteration and rhyming tasks, with rhyming being easier (e.g. Bernhardt et al., 1995). Work with children suffering from severe phonological disorders has shown that rhyming and alliteration skills do not necessarily develop at the same time; some children find it easier to produce rhymes than alliterations, whereas others who are able to alliterate cannot produce rhymes.

There may be several reasons why some children find it easier to produce rhymes than alliterations. One may be that many children are conditioned from a very early age to be sensitive to rhyming through listening to nursery rhymes or songs, whereas alliteration tends to be introduced through literacy training (i.e. words beginning with the same letter, rather than sound). Another, phonological, reason that has been suggested[1] is that if a child is able to divide a word into onset and rhyme unit, then the child can produce a rhyme by maintaining the stronger phonological unit, i.e. the rhyme unit, which is acoustically more prominent, while replacing the acoustically less prominent onset. On the other hand, alliteration requires that the onset is maintained while the vowel (the acoustic prime of the syllable) and the coda are changed.

This reasoning, however, presupposes that alliteration starts with an onset-rhyme division. But is this division, i.e. a segmentation, actually necessary to match alliterating pairs of words? In other words, is it possible to identify the first 'sound' in a word, without segmenting that 'sound' from the rest of the word? If we define alliteration as 'identify the first "sound", and call up another word that starts with the same sound', then whatever comes after that first sound can be disregarded. It might be possible that all that is required is a partial segmentation, i.e. the identification of certain characteristics of a string of sounds, namely the characteristics which are present at the very beginning of that string. One need only scan as far as is necessary to match another string of sounds with the first one. Much the same may be true for the identification of beginning sounds. In a task such as 'what sound does /fi:t/ start with', what the child needs to do first of all is to start saying the word. The question is where to stop. This boundary may be signalled by a change in articulatory and/or acoustic characteristics, in the case of the above example, from fricative to vowel. In Chris's case, this 'boundary effect' may indeed have been crucial in the acquisition of segment-awareness. We may see how this could have happened if we consider again the great difficulties he had in recognizing vowels as segments and the fact that, for a long time, clusters were treated in the same way as singleton consonants. In other words, what may have happened in the course of Chris's work on identifying sounds was that he identified beginnings and ends, and if there was more than a beginning and an end, as in a CVC structure, the vowel represented the boundary between the two.

Syllable structure

We may thus profitably turn to the question of what Chris's problems tell us about the type of syllable structure that he uses in his attempts to spell, read and identify sounds metaphonologically.[2] In modern phonological theories (see, for example, Carr, 1993) it is generally accepted that the syllable has a hierarchical structure, which can be represented as in Figure 11.1. Here, the syllable is divided first into an onset and rhyme, and the rhyme is divided into a nucleus and a coda. While the nucleus is a required part of any syllable, both onsets and codas can be unfilled in English. Onsets and codas in English can be complex, i.e. further divided, and this accounts for syllable initial and final consonant clusters.

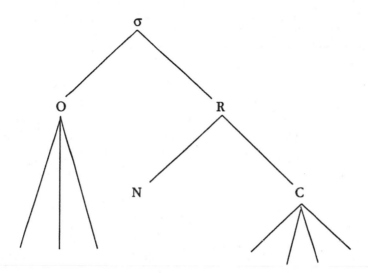

Figure 11.1. *Syllable structure.*
σ: syllable; O: onset; R: rhyme; N: nucleus; C: coda

The literature referred to earlier (e.g. Huxford, 1995) suggests clearly that in normal phonological development, abilities to rhyme and then to alliterate are acquired earlier, whereas the ability to distinguish final and medial sounds comes later. We also know from the production side that abilities with consonant clusters develop late. This suggests that the model given in Figure 11.1 can also be used to summarize the normally developing child's development of syllable awareness. Working down the tree, we see an initial ability with the 'onset' and 'rhyme' units (that rhyming precedes alliteration is possibly due to the greater acoustic prominence of the rhyme unit as noted earlier) and only later an ability to separate the nucleus and coda and then to deal with complex onsets and codas.

However, Chris's syllable structure (in terms of metaphonological abilities) does not resemble the one in Figure 11.1, or even a reduced version of Figure 11.1. His different behaviour in terms of vowel recognition (i.e. metaphonological recognition; not perception) depending on vowel position demonstrates that he does not have an established nucleus unit. His lack of ability with rhyming tasks shows that he does not even have an undivided rhyme unit although his more accurate alliterative skills suggest that some kind of syllable initial unit does exist. This, coupled with his abilities with final consonant recognition, suggests that Chris has a syllable initial unit and a syllable final unit, but nothing in between. Therefore, if vowels are in this initial slot they are recognized but, if a consonant precedes the vowel, it is moved out of the initial slot and, assuming a final consonant is present, is now outside of Chris's possible syllable structure and so is ignored. Chris does not allow complex initial or final slots, so is unable to deal with consonant clusters. We can show Chris's syllable structure in Figure 11.2. We would suggest that such a syllable structure for metaphonological abilities is not simply a delayed version of normal development but represents an atypical situation. This would help explain why there has been, until recently, such a lack of improvement in Chris's recognition and spelling skills, as attempts to move him down a normal developmental pathway are hampered by the fact that he was not yet even at the beginning.

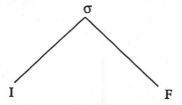

Figure 11.2. Chris's metaphonological syllable structure.
σ: syllable; I: initial unit; F: final unit

We must remember, however, that Chris's production abilities and perception abilities (e.g. in recognizing that minimal pairs are different, if not how they are different) suggest that he is using a normal syllable structure at the speech production/perception level. His problem clearly lies in the lack of linkage between the phonological domain and the metaphonological one.

As noted above, it may well be that these 'units' that we posit for Chris might not be of traditional segment length. It may be that the extra demands on Chris caused by a request to perform a metaphonological operation (such as identifying segments or rhymes, or reading or spelling) result in him being able to recognize syllables initially and finally those acoustic cues that allow him to make a match with his stored phonological units. Everything else is ignored, or possibly treated as boundary information.

Recent improvements in the recognition of Vs in CVC structures suggest a trend towards a syllable structure more like Figure 11.1 than Figure 11.2 – in other words a bringing together of phonological and metaphonological syllable structures. However, continuing problems with the recognition and spelling of consonant clusters would lead us to believe that advances in this direction must await the firm establishment of an onset–rhyme, and nucleus–coda syllable hierarchy in Chris's metaphonological domain.

References

Bernhardt B, Edwards S, Rempel R (1995) Metaphonological skills of typically developing three-year-olds and children with phonological disorders. In: Powell TW (Ed) Pathologies of Speech and Language: Contributions of Clinical Phonetics and Linguistics. New Orleans: ICPLA, pp 135–42.

Bowey JA, Francis J (1991) Phonological analysis as a function of age and exposure to reading instruction. Applied Psycholinguistics 22: 91–121.

Bradley L, Bryant PE (1983) Categorising sounds and learning to read - a causal connection. Nature 301: 419–21.

Bryant PE, MacLean M, Bradley LL, Crossland J (1990) Rhyme and alliteration, phoneme detection, and learning to read. Developmental Psychology 26: 429–38.

Carr P (1993) Phonology. London: Longman.

Goswami U, Bryant PE (1990) Phonological skills and learning to read. Hove: Lawrence Erlbaum Associates.

Huxford L (1995) Teaching a phonemic strategy for reading: implications for research. Dyslexia 1: 96–107.

Magnusson E, Nauclér K (1993) The development of linguistic awareness in language-disordered children. First Language 13: 93–111.

Mann VA (1986) Phonological awareness: the role of reading experience. Cognition 24: 64–92.

Stackhouse J (1985). Segmentation, speech difficulties and spelling difficulties. In: Snowling M (Ed) Children's Written Language Difficulties. Windsor: NFER-Nelson.

Wimmer H, Landerl K, Linortner R and Hummer P (1991) The relationship of phonemic awareness and reading acquisition: more consequence than precondition but still important. Cognition 40: 219–49.

Notes

1 We are grateful to Eva Major for her most helpful contribution to this discussion.

2 We will use the term 'metaphonological' to refer to Chris's abilities in these areas, as opposed to production and perception abilities.

Chapter 12
Homonyms in Children's Productions of Consonant Clusters

SHARYNNE McLEOD, JAN VAN DOORN AND
VICKI A. REED

Introduction

Consonant clusters are among the last aspects of phonology to be mastered both by children who have normally developing speech (Smit, Hand, Freilinger, Bernthal and Bird, 1990) and by those who have impaired speech (Shriberg and Kwiatkowski, 1980). Children often produce homonyms in their attempts to produce consonant clusters (e.g. Scobbie, Hardcastle, Fletcher and Gibbon, 1995) particularly as a result of cluster reduction. For example, when many young children attempt to say 'bread', they say a word which sounds like 'bed'.

Homonymy has attracted attention in the literature for two major reasons: the reason for homonymy is unresolved and the assumptions about homonymy in children's underlying representations are being reconsidered. Firstly, there has been debate regarding the reason for homonymy in child phonology. Some researchers have argued that children create homonyms to increase the number of items in their lexicon ('homonym strategy') (Lleo, 1990; Stoel-Gammon and Cooper, 1984; Vihman, 1981) whereas others have argued that children try to avoid the occurrence of homonyms in their speech (Ingram, 1975; 1985; Leonard, Schwartz, Allen, Swanson and Loeb, 1989). Further systematic longitudinal studies are required to add information to this debate.

The second issue regards the assumptions behind underlying representations of homonyms. Speech-language pathologists have targeted the reduction of homonymy in intervention (c.f. Ingram, 1981) and have employed techniques such as minimal pairs therapy to establish contrastive productions between homonymous forms (e.g., Gierut, 1991; Saben and Costello-Ingham, 1991). The assumption behind this intervention approach is that children do not have different underlying representations of the homonymous forms. An alternative view is that homonyms may occur because children are unable to make perceivable phonetic distinctions rather than because they. lack phonological knowledge between the two forms (Priestly, 1980; Scobbie, Gibbon, Hardcastle and Fletcher, 1996). This may occur as a result of children's developing speech motor control systems (Scobbie et al. 1996). It is thus suggested that these children do have different underlying representations of the homonymous forms and intervention based on minimal pairs may not be the most appropriate. The term 'covert contrast' (Hewlett, 1988; Scobbie et al., 1995) has been used to describe these differences between seemingly homonymous forms that are not perceived by a listener. Detection of covert contrasts has occurred using acoustic measures (e.g. Macken and Barton, 1980; Maxwell and Weismer, 1982; McLeod and Isaac, 1995; Scobbie et al., 1995; Tyler, 1995) and other instrumental analyses such as electropalatography (Gibbon, 1990) (see Gibbon and Scobbie, 1997, for a review).

Systematic research is required to further explore unresolved issues surrounding the existence, nature and purpose of homonyms. Consonant clusters provide a unique opportunity to examine homonymy in children's speech acquisition and underlying phonological representations. Experiments can be constructed using a potentially homonym-rich environment due to the wide occurrence of consonant clusters in English, the number of potential homonyms that can be created as a result of cluster reduction and the late age at which children acquire clusters. Such experiments are not possible for many of the other sound classes as children acquire mastery at an early age and potential homonyms are beyond the vocabulary level of the children. There is limited information regarding the nature and occurrence of homonymy in children's productions of consonant clusters. The impact of factors such as dependence on cluster type or age of subjects on the resulting number and type of homonyms has not been explored. It has also been assumed that when children produce a homonym in their attempt to produce a consonant cluster that it is as a result of cluster reduction. It is possible that children create other unique forms when producing clusters. Finally, underlying representations of consonant clusters can be examined by studying acoustic distinctions between the production of potential homonyms containing consonant clusters and their singleton counterparts. The purpose of this study was thus to conduct a systematic longitudinal examination of the nature and frequency of homonymy in normally developing young children and to describe the dependence of homonymy on cluster type and age.

Method

Sixteen normally developing Australian children with a cross-section of ages from 2;0 to 2;11 years (mean 2;6) participated in the study. Each subject was found to have normal hearing, cognition (Griffiths, 1984), phonology (phonological repertoires were compared to Dodd, 1995; Dyson, 1988; Stoel-Gammon, 1987), expressive language (mean length of utterance, Miller, 1981), receptive language (Reynell and Huntley, 1985) and oromusculature (Robbins and Klee, 1987) during an assessment by a speech pathologist, an audiologist, and a psychologist.

Longitudinal speech data for each child was recorded on to audio cassettes at monthly intervals for six months. Each month the subjects produced twelve sets of three words based on the target clusters /br, dr, gr, kl, st, sk, sn, sw/. Each set of words contained a word with one of the target clusters in word-initial position, and two of its potential homonyms (e.g., ski, sea and key). Word production was elicited by presenting computer graphic pictures of the 36 words in a sequence that did not place potentially homonymous words together.

Identification of homonyms

Homonyms were identified from phonetic transcription of all words in the speech corpus (16 x 6 x 36 words). At the time of each recording, the subjects' responses were transcribed on-line using narrow transcription, and then were checked against the audio tape recordings following data collection. The reliability of the transcription was established by having a second judge carry out exactly the same procedure for 10 per cent of the data. The phoneme-by-phoneme agreement between judges for broad transcription was 0.92 and narrow transcription was 0.85.

Homonyms were judged at three levels: via broad transcription, narrow transcription and acoustic measures. For example, ski produced as [kʰi] was considered to be a homonym with key produced as [ki:] at the level of broad transcription whereas every diacritic had to be the same to be considered homonymous via narrow transcription. Results from the narrow transcription generally showed similar trends to the broad transcription so were not documented in the present investigation.

Acoustic analyses were conducted on a subset of homonyms to determine whether the subjects were signifying a covert contrast between the cluster and singleton words in the homonyms. The homonyms chosen for acoustic analysis were those generated by cluster reduction of /sk/ to /k/ and /st/ to /t/. Voice onset time (VOT) for the word-initial stop was measured from the digitised waveforms (20 kHz), using a Kay CSL 4300B. The accuracy of the VOT measurements was one pitch period (approximately 5 ms for children's speech). Other measures (reported in McLeod, van Doorn and Reed, 1996) included relative energy for aspiration of the stops /k/ and /t/, duration and spectral distribution for fricative /s/ and VOT for /k/.

Results

The homonyms judged from broad phonetic transcription were investigated according to their frequency of occurrence, type of realization,
dependence on cluster type, and variation with children's ages. The
data allowed these features to be examined from both cross-sectional
and longitudinal perspectives.

Frequency of occurrence and realizations of homonyms

All children in the study produced homonyms on at least one occasion
for at least one cluster type. Over all six sessions for all children, an
average of 19.5% of the word sets contained homonyms, ranging from
2.8% to 50.0% across subjects.

There were three realizations of homonyms. The majority (88.3%) of
homonyms were produced as a result of cluster reduction. Four-fifths
of those were created between the cluster and the first element of the
cluster (e.g. *bread* and *bed*, and the remaining fifth were with the second element (e.g. *bread* and *red*). Examples of first and second element reduction were found for all cluster types. Homonyms due to
cluster reduction occurred for 13 subjects across all target cluster types.

Secondly, 7.6% of homonyms occurred due to the addition of a
phoneme to a non-cluster word creating a homonym with the clustered
word (e.g. *sweet* and *wheat* were both realized as [swit]). Homonyms
due to cluster creation occurred for 10 subjects across three cluster
types (/br, sn, sw/).

The remaining 4.0% of homonyms were created between the non-
cluster words. For example, the eldest subject realised both sail and
nail as [seɪʊ]; whereas she produced snail as [sneɪʊ]. This type of
homonym occurred for six subjects across four different cluster contexts (/br, sn, st, kl/).

Occurrence of homonyms in different consonant clusters

The occurrence of homonyms varied according to cluster type. For all
subjects, across all six measurements, the consonant clusters that had a
high occurrence of homonyms were /br/ (29%), /st/ (24%), and /sn/
(23%). The consonant cluster that had the lowest occurrence of
homonyms was /sw/ (10%). It is interesting to note that only half of that
10% were produced by cluster reduction. This is a far lower proportion
than the overall average of 88% of homonyms resulting from cluster
reduction.

Table 12.1 shows the number of children who demonstrated
homonym production for each cluster type, and homonym realization
category. For all target clusters, there were realizations of homonym by

cluster reduction. The three /Cr/ cluster types showed the greatest number of children using cluster reduction, while /sw/ showed the least number of children using cluster reduction. However, /sw/ had the greatest number of children using either cluster creation or non-cluster homonym realizations.

Table 12.1. Number of children exhibiting homonym production for each target cluster type, showing the categories of realization that occurred for the homonyms

Realization	/br/	/dr/	/gr/	/kl/	/st/	/sk/	/sn/	/sw/
Cluster reduction only	9	10	8	7	6	7	5	3
Other homonyms	2						3	6
Both categories (on different occasions)	3			1	1		2	1
Total number	14	10	8	8	7	7	10	10

Relationship between the incidence of homonymy and age

There was a reduction in the number of homonyms produced by the subjects for both the cross-sectional measurements and also for the longitudinal measurements for subjects in each age group. Table 12.2 shows the proportion of word sets containing homonyms for each age group and each session. Where there was more than one child for a particular age group, the data were averaged across children. The reduction of homonym production across children of increasing ages can be seen from the columns in Table 12.2. The same trend can be seen (to a lesser degree) from the rows in Table 12.2, which contain the longitudinal data. Children tended to produce homonyms as a result of cluster reduction when they were younger and cluster creation as they grew older.

Acoustic measures

There were 12 token pairs where subjects produced [ki] for both ski and key; or [tɪk] for both stick and tick. The mean VOT of the plosives in the target words that contained consonant clusters (mean = 26.31 ms; SD = 18.52 ms) was significantly shorter (p<0.0001) than that of plosives in the singleton target words (mean = 80.18 ms; SD = 40.45 ms), using a paired two-sample t-test. Statistical significance was not reached for the other acoustic measures: relative energy for aspiration of stops /k/ and /t/, duration and spectral distribution for fricative /s/ and VOT for /k/ (see McLeod, van Doorn and Reed, 1996 for further details).

Table 12.2. Percentage of word sets containing homonyms for each measurement occasion, and each represented starting age. The number of children at that age is shown in brackets.

Age yr;m at first session (# subjects)	% word sets containing homonyms at each measurement session					
	Session 1	Session 2	Session 3	Session 4	Session 5	Session 6
2;0 (2)	41.7	70.8	37.5	20.8	16.7	33.3
2;1 (1)	57.1	83.3	75.0	50.0	58.3	0.0
2;2 (1)	33.3	50.0	27.3	41.7	58.3	41.7
2;3 (1)	41.7	25.0	50.0	33.3	41.7	25.0
2;6 (1)	0.0	0.0	0.0	25.0	8.3	0.0
2;7 (3)	11.1	13.9	2.7	2.7	8.3	5.5
2;8 (2)	20.8	16.7	16.7	12.5	16.7	4.2
2;9 (1)	33.3	91.7	33.3	33.3	16.7	0.0
2;10 (3)	2.8	11.1	0.0	2.8	5.6	8.3
2;11 (1)	0.0	0.0	8.3	0.0	8.3	0.0

Discussion

Homonyms were found to be present in approximately one-fifth of the word sets. This figure could be indicative of the maximum number of homonyms present in normal young children's productions of consonant clusters in a homonym-rich environment. This finding can be compared with Leinonen-Davies' (1988) who hypothesized that the mean functional loss (FLOSS) (number of homonymous pairs) as a result of word-initial cluster reduction was low compared to other processes. The different findings may be due to the fact that Leinonen-Davies' results were hypothesized on the basis of the correct production of words in the common vocabulary of children aged 5;11–6;11 whereas the present research reports actual productions of words in a homonym-rich environment by children aged 2;0–3;4. Furthermore, Leinonen-Davies' hypothesized productions may be an underestimation of the extent of homonymy from cluster reduction since not all potentialities of homonyms were included. For example, Leinonen-Davies included only instances of homonymy between words commencing with /sn/ and /n/, whereas the present study found a similar extent of homonymy between words commencing with /sn/ and /n/, and /sn and /s/. The actual extent of homonymy in young children's spontaneous speech is likely to be found somewhere between the figure from the present investigation and the result of Leinonen-Davies.

There was a reduction in homonymy as the subjects grew older, with few occasions of homonymy after the subjects' third birthdays. This finding occurred cross-sectionally as well as longitudinally for individual subjects across visits; although the longitudinal result occurred to a lesser extent. Homonymy has been described as a developmental stage through which children pass in their acquisition of adult-like phonology (Macken and Barton, 1980). For example, Lleo (1990) found four stages of increase and decline in the extent of homonymous types in her daughter's speech between the ages of 1;7 and 2;11. Lleo suggested that the stages were a result of the interaction between number of homonymous types, lexical growth and syllabic development.

Three realizations of homonyms occurred in the present investigation: homonyms created by cluster reduction, cluster creation and changes in the non-clustered words. The majority of homonyms were created by cluster reduction. Only the occurrence of homonyms as a result of cluster reduction is usually reported (e.g. Scobbie et al., 1995; Tyler, 1995). This is not surprising as cluster reduction is one of the most common phonological processes affecting consonant clusters (Shriberg and Kwiatkowski, 1980). However, rare examples of cluster creation have been reported in the literature in speech-impaired children (Leonard et al., 1989). The present investigation suggests that homonymy as a result of cluster creation may not be as rare as expected, since 10 of the 16 subjects demonstrated at least one example of cluster creation. In the present investigation the type of homonymy interacted with the age of the subject. Younger subjects were more likely to demonstrate homonymy as a result of cluster reduction, older subjects were more likely to have instances of homonymy as a result of cluster creation.

Homonyms were more likely to be created with the retention of the first element of the consonant cluster. This finding is similar to the findings regarding cluster reduction in a non-homonymy context by normally developing children (Smit, 1993) and children with phonological impairment (Chin and Dinnsen, 1992; McLeod, van Doorn and Reed, 1997).

Only one acoustic measurement showed systematic and significant differences between singleton and clustered contexts. Word-initial /s/ + stop clusters which had been reduced to a stop had significantly less aspiration duration for the stop in the cluster target word than that for the singleton target word. This finding may suggest a covert contrast between the subjects' productions of the words (c.f. Scobbie et al., 1995) and is consistent with findings by other researchers who have considered children's development of VOT (e.g. Catts and Kamhi, 1984). No other time or spectral measures reached statistical significance as there was a high degree of inter- and intra- subject variability. The findings for the other measures do not rule out the notion of covert contrasts (indeed there was typically a difference for each token pair) but suggest that the covert contrasts were individualized for specific subjects and specific words or clusters.

Consonant clusters provide a unique opportunity to study homonym production in young children. The present investigation provides systematic longitudinal and cross-sectional data on 2-to-3-year-old children's productions of consonant clusters in a homonym-rich environment. Their nature, frequency, and dependence on cluster type and the child's age were described. Preliminary acoustic investigations suggest the presence of covert contrasts in children's productions of consonant clusters, thus providing insight into underlying representations. These data can be used to further unravel the reality of children's productions of homonyms so that discussion can continue on the purpose and nature of homonymy in children's development.

References

Catts H, Kamhi A (1984) Simplification of /s/ + stop consonant clusters: a developmental perspective. Journal of Speech and Hearing Research 27: 556–61.

Chin SB, Dinnsen DA (1992) Consonant clusters in disordered speech: constraints and correspondence patterns. Journal of Child Language 19: 259–85.

Dodd B (1995) Children's acquisition of phonology. In B Dodd (Ed) Differential Diagnosis and Treatment of Speech Disordered Children. London: Whurr, pp 21–48.

Dyson AT (1988) Phonetic inventories of 2- and 3-year old children. Journal of Speech and Hearing Disorders 53: 89–93.

Gibbon F (1990) Lingual activity in two speech-disordered children's attempts to produce velar and alveolar stop consonants: Evidence from electropalatographic (EPG) data. British Journal of Disorders of Communication 25: 329–40.

Gibbon, F and Scobbie, JM (1997) Covert contrasts in children with phonological disorder. Australian Communication Quarterly. Autumn, 13–16.

Gierut JA (1991) Homonymy in phonological change. Clinical Linguistics and Phonetics 5: 119–37.

Griffiths R (1984) Griffiths Mental Development Scales. Amersham: Association for Research in Infant and Child Development.

Hewlett N (1988) Acoustic properties of /k/ and /t/ in normal and phonologically disordered speech. Clinical Linguistics and Phonetics 2: 29–45.

Ingram D (1975) Surface contrast in children's speech. Journal of Child Language 2: 287–92.

Ingram D (1981) Procedures for the phonological analysis of children's language. Baltimore: University Park Press.

Ingram D (1985) On children's homonyms. Journal of Child Language 12: 671–80.

Leinonen-Davies E (1988) Assessing the functional adequacy of children's phonological systems. Clinical Linguistics and Phonetics 2: 257–70.

Leonard LB, Schwartz RG, Allen GD, Swanson LA, Loeb DF (1989) Unusual phonological behaviour and the avoidance of homonymy in children. Journal of Speech and Hearing Research 32: 583–90.

Lleo C (1990) Homonymy and reduplication: on the extended availability of two strategies in phonological acquisition. Journal of Child Language 17: 267–78.

Macken MA, Barton D (1980) The acquisition of the voicing contrast in English: a study of voice onset time in word-initial stop consonants. Journal of Child Language 7: 41–74.

Maxwell EM, Weismer G (1982) The contribution of phonological acoustic, and perceptual techniques to the characterization of a misarticulating child's voice contrast for stops. Applied Psycholinguistics 3: 29–43.

McLeod S, Isaac K (1995) Use of spectrographic analyses to evaluate the efficacy of phonological intervention. Clinical Linguistics and Phonetics 9: 229–34.

McLeod S, van Doorn J, Reed VA (1996) Homonyms and cluster reduction in the normal development of children's speech. In P McCormack, A Russell (Eds) Proceedings of the Australian International Conference on Speech Science and Technology, Canberra: Australian Speech Science and Technology Association pp 331–6.

McLeod S, van Doorn J, Reed VA (1997) Realizations of consonant clusters by children with phonological impairment. Clinical Linguistics and Phonetics. 2: 85–113

Miller JF (1981) Assessing language production in children: Experimental procedures. Austin TX: Pro-Ed.

Priestly TMS (1980) Homonymy in child phonology. Journal of Child Language 7: 413–27.

Reynell J, Huntley M (1985) Reynell Developmental Language Scales. Windsor: NFER-Nelson.

Robbins J, Klee T (1987) Clinical assessment of oropharyngeal motor development in young children. Journal of Speech and Hearing Disorders 52: 271–7.

Saben CB, Costello-Ingham J (1991) The effects of minimal pairs treatment on the speech-sound production of two children with phonologic disorders. Journal of Speech and Hearing Research 34: 1023–40.

Scobbie JM, Hardcastle WJ, Fletcher P, Gibbon F (1995) Consonant clusters in disordered L1 acquisition: A longitudinal acoustic study. In Proceedings of the XIIIth International Congress of the Phonetic Sciences, Stockholm pp 706–9.

Scobbie JM, Gibbon F, Hardcastle WJ Fletcher, P (1996) Covert contrast as a stage in the acquisition of phonetics and phonology. In Scobbie JM (Ed.) QMC working papers in speech and language sciences 1: 43–62.

Shriberg L, Kwiatkowski J (1980) Natural Process Analysis. New York: John Wiley.

Smit AB (1993) Phonologic error distributions in the Iowa-Nebraska articulation norms project: Word-initial consonant clusters. Journal of Speech and Hearing Research, 36, 931–47.

Smit AB, Hand L, Freilinger JJ, Bernthal JE, Bird A (1990) The Iowa articulation norms project and its Nebraska replication. Journal of Speech and Hearing Disorders 55: 779–98.

Stoel-Gammon C (1987) Phonological skills of 2-year-olds. Language, Speech, and Hearing Services in Schools 18: 323–9.

Stoel-Gammon C, Cooper JA (1984) Patterns of early lexical and phonological development. Journal of Child Language 11: 247–71.

Tyler AA (1995) Durational analysis of stridency errors in children with phonological impairment. Clinical Linguistics and Phonetics 9: 211–28.

Vihman MM (1981) Phonology and the development of the lexicon: evidence from children's errors. Journal of Child Language 8: 239–64.

Chapter 13
A Phonetically-Based Feature Geometry for the Analysis and Classification of Disordered Pronunciation

BARRY HESELWOOD

Introduction

The componential nature of realizations of phonemes (i.e. allophones) offers a basis for phonetically detailed comparisons between normal and disordered pronunciation and can provide a framework for classifying instances of disordered pronunciation into types according to how the componential structure of an allophone deviates from the norm. The following assumptions provide the framework:

1. Phones are componential – that is, they can be analysed into phonetic features. Phonetic features are not systematic in that we cannot state them as a finite set, nor should they necessarily be considered as simple atomic elements. For example, [voiced] could be said to consist of both pitch and amplitude, either of which might be manipulated phonologically by a speaker in place of some other phonetic parameter (Leonard, 1985).
2. The phonetic features of a phone form a structure of dependency relations. The concept of dependency is central to non-linear approaches to phonology (McCarthy, 1988) and is one with important applications to disordered speech. Examples of speakers whose phones contain normal phonetic features but in deviant dependency relations are given below.
3. Phonetic features have the potential for distinctive function. In any realization of a phoneme certain phonetic features will be realiza-

tions of distinctive features while others will be phonologically
redundant; distinctive features themselves are entities at the same
level of abstraction as phonemes and do not enter into dependency
relations (see Figure 13.1). An example of a speaker transferring distinctive function from one feature to another feature which never
normally has it in English is given below.

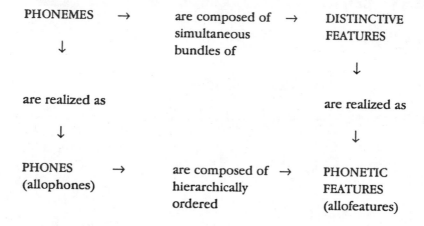

Figure 13.1. Componential and realizational relations between phonetic and
phonological entities.

4. Dependencies are grounded in properties of the speech production
   system and to that extent are universal.
5. The governing feature for any phone is always an airstream feature.
   This is motivated by the fact that all audible speech is dependent on
   a source of aerodynamic energy. An example of a speaker splitting
   dependent features between two different airstream features is discussed at length in Heselwood (1997) and more briefly below.

Figure 13.1 partially represents the relationship between phonetic and
phonological entities that forms part of the theoretical background
underpinning the approach, but the usefulness of the classificatory
scheme does not depend crucially on adhering to this view.

Structural and functional deviance

A pronunciation error may be classified as either structurally or functionally deviant according to the following definitions:

Structural deviance: a phone is structurally deviant if its feature structure exhibits a dependency relation not normally found in the language
being spoken.

Functional deviance: a phone is functionally deviant if a component feature has distinctive function that does not normally have distinctive function in the language being spoken.

Structural deviance

As an example of structural deviance we can take [h͡n̥] as a realization of /s/, a common realization in children with cleft palate even after repair and after velo-pharyngeal sufficiency has been established – the so-called 'habit factor' (Hardcastle, Morgan Barry and Nunn, 1989; for a discussion of phonetic symbols for this and similar realizations in cleft palate speech see Harding and Grunwell, 1996). Both [h͡n̥] and the normal realization [s] involve voicelessness, alveolar articulation and friction but while the friction is produced in the oral chamber for [s] it is produced in the nasal chamber for [h͡n̥]. This difference can be represented as a difference in the dependency relation of the feature [fricative] as shown in Figure 13.2.

/s/ > [h͡n̥]

Feature structure for [s]:   Feature structure for [h͡n̥]:

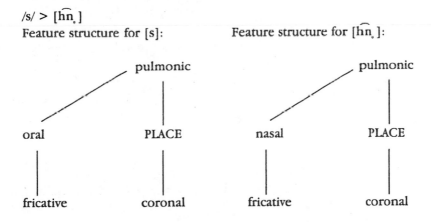

Figure 13.2. Feature dependency of [fricative] in [s] and [h͡n̥]. LARYNX node not included.

Functional deviance

An example of functional deviance is provided by a case of a child of 6;7 realizing /t/ as [tʰ], and /k/ as [tˢ] in initial stressed syllable position, as in *tap* and *cap*. The locus of the opposition has shifted from the hold to the release phase so that the opposition is between [aspirated] and [affricated] instead of [coronal] and [dorsal]; the feature structures for the normal and the deviant realizations are represented in Figure 13.3. Following a suggestion by Steriade (1991, cited in Kenstowicz (1994)) the two phases have separate feature structures.

/t/ > [tʰ],   /k/ > [tˢ]

Feature structure for the normal realizations [tʰ] and [kʰ]:

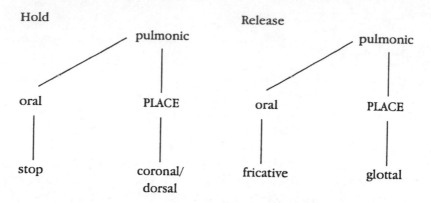

Feature structure for the deviant realizations [tʰ] and [tˢ]:

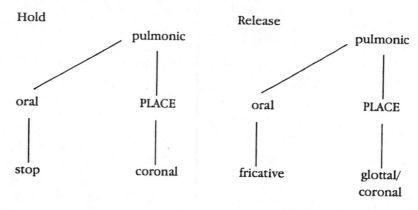

Figure 13.3. Feature structures showing the normal coronal–dorsal opposition in the hold phase and the child's deviant glottal–coronal (aspirated–affricated) opposition in the release phase. LARYNX node not included.

The deviance of [tˢ] as a realization of /k/ is of course quite obvious without considering the functional status of the [ˢ] component but the distinctive use of affrication, when it is not used distinctively in the ambient language, is a different kind of deviance. By the same criterion the aspiration of the child's [tʰ], although normal as a redundant feature, is being used distinctively and therefore deviantly: it has distinctive function in the child's system but not in the ambient language. Functional deviance, then, involves a deviant opposition, not just a deviant realization, and one of the terms of the opposition may, as here, be realized quite normally when considered from a purely phonetic perspective.

Feature disjunction and feature adjunction

These two kinds of deviance can be defined as follows:

Feature disjunction: There is feature disjunction when features that normally occur in the same feature structure occur in different feature structures. Structures resulting from disjunction may associate to the same slot in syllable structure, as in the example given below, or to different slots.

Feature adjunction: There is feature adjunction when features that normally occur in different feature structures occur in the same feature structure.

Feature disjunction

An example of feature disjunction is the use of the nasal click [ŋ͡ǂ] for [j], observed repeatedly in the speech of an adult with Down's syndrome in dysfluent contexts (see Heselwood, 1997, for a study of this speaker's use of clicks). This deviant realization contains some of the same features as [j] but distributed across two structures rather than one, each being governed by a different airstream feature. Figure 13.4 compares these realizations.

The features [sonorant], [coronal] and [oral] have distinctive function in [j] (to distinguish it from realizations of, for example, /d/, /w/ and /n/ respectively) and these features are present in the deviant realization. The nasal component provides [sonorant], the click component provides [coronal], and all clicks are [oral] by definition. The presence of the features [nasal] and [dorsal] can be attributed to the speaker's pathology: it seems that one of the symptoms of his dysfluency is an involuntary dorsovelar closure and his solution to the problem of producing a [j] in this condition is to generate [sonorant] in the part of the vocal tract comprising the larynx, pharynx and nasal chamber, and to carry out the [coronal] articulation in the form of a click using the dorsovelar closure to generate a velaric ingressive airstream. The vocal tract is behaving as two independent systems with the click superimposed on the nasal. The products of each of these systems, the [ŋ] and the [ǂ], associate to the same syllable slot, the one that would norm-ally accommodate the target [j] (note that the [ǂ] component is also a case of structural deviance because no phoneme in normal English has an allophone governed by [velaric]). In some cases speakers may repackage a target singleton as a cluster, for example /f/ > [ps] (Bates and Watson, 1996) where the disjunction associates to different syllable slots.

[ŋ͡ːɬ] for [j]
Feature structure [j]:

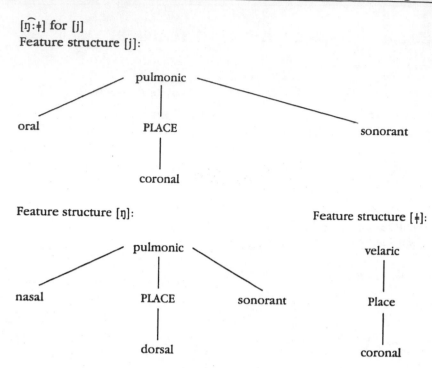

Feature structure [ŋ]:   Feature structure [ɬ]:

Figure 13.4. Feature structures for [j] and the [ŋ] and [ɬ] components of [ŋ͡ːɬ] showing feature disjunction. LARYNX node not included.

Feature adjunction

Cases where a feature from one segment is anticipated in an earlier segment, or perseverates into a later segment, are instances of feature adjunction. In non-linear phonology these assimilatory phenomena are described as 'feature spreading' (Kenstowicz, 1994). For cases where two or more target segments fuse into a single segment clinical phonologists have used the term 'feature synthesis', for example [m̥] as a disordered realization of the /sm-/ cluster (Grunwell, 1987). This is feature adjunction in its most extreme form. A less extreme example is provided by JP, a boy of 4;2, diagnosed as phonologically disordered. JP was found by the present author to neutralize [labial]–[coronal] oppositions in the context of a following rounded vowel, pronouncing *toy* as [pʷɔɪ], *do* as [bʷu], *sun* (northern English /sʊn/) as [pʷʊn], etc. It is quite normal to anticipate the labialization of the vowel by adjoining the labialization feature [prolabial] (Watson, 1993), together with its governing feature [labial], to the release phase structure of the preceding consonant, but JP also adjoins it to the hold phase structure (i.e. he spreads the feature too far to the left). If the hold phase structure has the feature [stop], as do all of this speaker's obstruents, then [labial] and [stop] will co-occur and result in [b] or [p]. The structures are given in Figure 13.5.

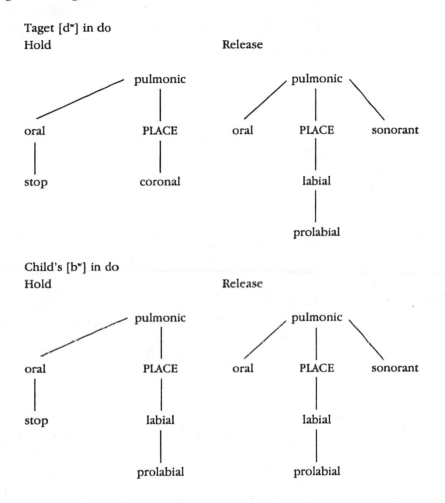

Figure 13.5. The adjunction of [prolabial] and its governing feature [labial] to the feature structure of the hold phase of a target coronal plosive. LARYNX node not included.

Conclusion

By focusing on the componential structure of phones it is possible to compare disordered realizations of distinctive features with normal realizations and to demonstrate the ways in which they differ. The notion of distinctive function, and therefore the notion of phonological opposition, is crucial and the category of functional deviance enables oppositions, not just their terms, to be identified as deviant. There is scope to apply this category to the so-called 'subphonemic' distinctions uncovered by Macken and Barton (1980), while feature adjunction and feature disjunction may be useful general categories for investigating the kinds of syntagmatic interactions that have been observed in developmental disorders, e.g. between consonants and vowels (Bates and Watson, 1996).

References

Bates S, Watson J (1996) Consonant vowel interactions in developmental phonological disorder. In Caring to Communicate: Proceedings of the Golden Jubilee Conference of the Royal College of Speech and Language Therapists, York, October 1995. London: Royal College of Speech and Language Therapists, 274–9.

Grunwell P (1987) Clinical Phonology. 2nd edn. London: Croom Helm.

Hardcastle W, Morgan Barry R and Nunn M (1989) Instrumental articulatory phonetics in assessment and remediation: case studies with the electropalatograph. In Stengelhofen J (Ed) Cleft Palate. Edinburgh: Churchill Livingstone.

Harding A, Grunwell P (1996) Characteristics of cleft palate speech. European Journal of Disorders of Communication 31, 4: 331–57.

Heselwood B (1997) A case of nasal clicks for target sonorants: a feature geometry account. Clinical Linguistics and Phonetics 11(1): 43–61.

Kenstowicz M (1994) Phonology in Generative Grammar. Oxford: Blackwell.

Leonard LB (1985) Unusual and subtle phonological behaviour in the speech of phonologically disordered children. Journal of Speech and Hearing Disorders 50: 4–13.

McCarthy J (1988) Feature geometry and dependency: a review. Phonetica 43: 84–108.

Macken MA and Barton D (1980) The acquisition of the voicing contrast in English: a study of voice onset time in word initial stop consonants. Journal of Child Language 7: 41–74.

Steriade D (1991) Aperture positions and syllable structure. Paper presented at the Organization of Phonology conference, University of Illinois.

Watson J (1993) Aspects of verb morphology in a Yemeni k-dialect. Working Papers in Language and Linguistics No.16, Dept of Modern Languages, University of Salford.

Chapter 14
A Paradox in
Process-Based Analysis[1]

ISAO UEDA, TOMOHIKO ITO AND TOMOHIKO SHIRAHATA

Introduction

It has been pointed out in descriptive studies that the Japanese /ɾ/ is acquired in the latest stage of phonological development (Ishikawa, 1930; Sakauchi, 1967; Takagi and Yasuda, 1967; Yasuda, 1969; Nakanishi, Owada and Fujita 1972). It is also an oft-cited fact that the Japanese /ɾ/ is one of the segments that is most likely to undergo misarticulation, whether it is functional or organic (Fukusako, Sawashima and Abe, 1976; Matsushita, 1981; Nagafuchi, 1985; Nagayama, 1985). In both cases, the misproduction of /ɾ/ is generally referred to as 'rhotacism'. A detailed study reported in Murata (1970) recognizes two types of rhotacism. In one type, the word-initial target /ɾ/ is replaced by [d], while the word-medial target /d/ is replaced by /ɾ/. In the other type, however, the target /ɾ/ is replaced by [d] irrespective of the place where it appears. It is further suggested in Murata (1970) and Nakanishi, Owada, and Fujita (1972) that the first type (hereafter type A) is developmentally more primitive and clinically more serious than the second type (hereafter type B). Thus far no explicit explanation whatsoever has been provided on rhotacism itself, nor on the relationship between the two types of rhotacism.

The purpose of this paper, then, is to provide an account of rhotacism. We first show that currently dominant process-based analysis fails to give a plausible explanation for rhotacism and then we analyse the data within the framework of 'underspecification'. We claim that in the underlying representation of type A the feature [flap] is underspecified, but that in that of type B, the default value of [flap], minus, is actually specified. As a result of this, we further suggest that in the earliest stage of phonological development at least some features should be non-specified or underspecified, that in the next stage the child should learn to utilize the default value and that, finally, the child should learn the maximal contrasts between the phonemes.

Rhotacism type A

Let us observe the data for type A reported by Murata (1970) in Table 14.1. In the word-initial position, the target /r/ is misproduced as [d], but the target /d/ is correctly produced as [d]. In the word-medial position, however, the target /r/ is correctly produced as [ɾ], but the target /d/, in its turn, is misproduced as [ɾ].

Table 14.1 Rhotacism Type A

Word-initial position

(Target /r/ is misproduced as [d])

Phonetic forms	Target forms	Gloss
dappa	ɾappa	trumpet
doosokɯ	ɾoosokɯ	candle
demoŋ	ɾemoŋ	lemon
disɯ	ɾisɯ	squirrel

(Target /d/ is correctly produced as [d])

Phonetic forms	Target forms	Gloss
daɾuma	daɾuma	tumbler
doobɯtsɯeŋ	doobɯtsɯeŋ	zoo
denʃa	denʃa	tram

Word-medial position

(Target /r/ is correctly produced as [ɾ])

Phonetic forms	Target forms	Gloss
paɾaʃɯɯto	paɾaʃɯɯto	parachute
gɯɾoobɯ	gɯɾoobɯ	glove
teɾebi	teɾebi	TV
soɾa	soɾa	sky

(Target /d/ is misproduced as [ɾ])

Phonetic forms	Target forms	Gloss
sɯbeɾiɾai	sɯbeɾidai	slide
dʒiɾooʃa	dʒidooʃa	car
namiɾa	namida	tear
bwɾoo	bɯdoo	grape

Natural process analysis and traditional generative analysis

In this section, we examine the data from type A rhotacism in Table 14.1 under two earlier frameworks that are still dominant in the clinical field. First, let us examine natural process analysis or phonological process analysis, proposed by, among others, Hodson (1980), Ingram (1976), Shriberg and Kwiatkowski (1980), Weiner (1979). Based on natural phonology (Stampe, 1973), natural process analysis claims that misarticulation is triggered by various processes that are 'innately' natural. This analysis would posit one process as in (1) for the misarticulation of target /ɾ/ in the word-initial position and another process as in (2) for the misarticulation of target /d/ in the word-medial position.

(1) ɾ → d (Stopping)
(2) d → ɾ (Rhotation)

This, however, results in two conflicting processes existing in one phonological system. It is self-evident that two processes that are supposed to be innately natural cannot go together in one single system.

Let us turn to traditional generative analysis (Dinnsen, 1984; Dinnsen, Elbert and Weismer, 1980; Maxwell, 1984) which is based on the feature system as developed in Chomsky and Halle (1968). Given that Japanese /ɾ/ and /d/ are different from each other in distinctive features in that /ɾ/ is specified as [+flap] and /d/ as [−flap], this analysis would postulate a phonological rule as in (3).

(3) [+consonantal, -nasal, +voiced] → [−flap] / #___

This particular formalization states that the underlying representation of the surface [d] is /ɾ/, and rule (3) operates in the word-initial position, yielding the misproduction of [d]. However, this rule is also insufficient in that the selection of the underlying representation is arbitrary. Equally possible is the postulation of the underlying /d/ and of the phonological rule (4) which converts the underlying /d/ into the surface [ɾ] in the word-medial intervocalic position.

(4) [+consonantal, −nasal, +voiced] → [+flap] / [+syllabic] ___ [+syllabic]

Analysis of type A

Noting the theory of underspecification (Archangeli, 1984, 1988) we claim that both /ɾ/ and [d] are underspecified or underlyingly non-specified in terms of the feature [flap], and posit the following underlying representation for /ɾ/ and [d] as in Figure 14.1.

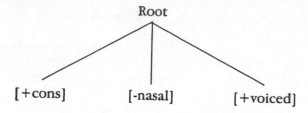

Figure 14.1. Underlying representation for [d] and [ɾ].

We further propose that the default value of [flap] be negative given the wider distribution of [d] in type B discussed below. The default value is specified later in derivation. The realization of [ɾ] is a lenition process with the spreading of [+sonorant] from the preceding vowel, which results in [+flap]. Japanese has no other segment that is specified as [+consonantal, -nasal, +voiced, +sonorant] than /ɾ/.

Rhotacism type B

In this type the target /ɾ/ is produced as [d] without regard to the position where it occurs. The target /d/, on the other hand, is correctly produced as [d] in all positions. Let us examine the data in Table 14.2 below.

Table 14.2 Rhotacism Type B

Word-initial position

(Target /ɾ/ is misproduced as [d])

Phonetic forms	Target forms	Gloss
dappa	ɾappa	trumpet
doosokɯ	roosokɯ	candle
demoŋ	remoŋ	lemon
disɯ	risɯ	squirrel

(Target /d/ is correctly produced as [d])

Phonetic forms	Target forms	Gloss
daɾɯma	daɾɯma	tumbler
doobɯtsɯeŋ	doobɯtsɯeŋ	zoo
denʃa	denʃa	tram

Word-medial position

(Target /ɾ/ is misproduced as [d])

Phonetic forms	Target forms	Gloss
padaʃɯɯto	paraʃɯɯto	parachute
gɯdoobɯ	gɯroobɯ	glove
tedebi	terebi	TV
soda	sora	sky

(Target /d/ is correctly produced as [d])

Phonetic forms	Target forms	Gloss
suubedidai	suuberidai	slide
ʤidooʃa	ʤidooʃa	car
namida	namida	tear
bwdoo	buudoo	grape

Type B rhotacism is developmentally less primitive and clinically less serious.

Analysis of type B

Let us embark on the analysis of the phonological system of type B. First we begin with the underlying represention of [d] produced for the target /d/ because the determination is somewhat straightforward. The representation of [d] for /d/ is in Figure 14.2, which is the same as the one in Figure 14.1, with the feature [flap] underspecified. The coronal stop [d] is the 'default' with respect to the feature [flap] and the default value is filled in the later stage of derivation.

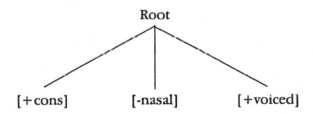

Figure 14.2. Underlying representation of [d] for /d/.

The determination of the underlying representation for [d] produced for the target /r/ is rather a complicated matter. Given that the child perceptually distinguishes [d] and /r/ from each other, we need to posit two different underlying representations for the two d's, namely [d] for /d/ and [d] for /r/. Here, let us introduce the concept of 'shadow-specification' (Dinnsen, 1993; Dinnsen and Chin, 1995; Ueda, 1996a, 1996b). The shadow-specification is a modified version of radical underspecification wherein a sound may actually be specified for the default value when the child can distinguish two sounds in perception but cannot in production. In this particular case, then, the default value is [-flap], which is actually (and therefore wrongly) specified in the child's underlying representation of [d] for /r/ as in Figure 14.3.

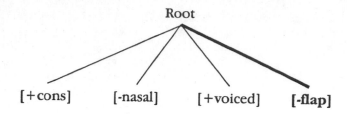

Figure 14.3. Underlying representation for [d] for /ɾ/.

Thus the shadow-specification enables the representation of '[d] for /ɾ/' to be differentiated from that of '[d] for /d/'. Moreover, the phonetic evidence for misproduction follows directly from the specification; it is [d] that is misproduced.

Conclusion

In this paper we have discussed two types of rhotacism. In the more primitive type A, the feature [flap] is underspecified both for the target /d/ and /ɾ/. However, in the more developed type B, the feature is underspecified for the target /d/, but is actually specified (shadow-specifed) as [-flap] for the target /ɾ/, hence the misproduction of the surface [d]. We have emphasized the fact that type A is developmentally more primitive and clinically more serious. In fact, Murata (1970) reports that the phonological system of a type B subject changed to become an adult-like phonological system in terms of the target /ɾ/ after seven months, while that of type A subjects did not. This evidence leads us to suggest that the child's specification changes from 'underspecified' to 'shadow-specified', then to 'fully specified' in the course of phonological acquisition. Further study is necessary to determine whether or not this developmental process holds for other phenomena in phonological acquisition.

References

Archangeli D (1984) Underspecification and Yawelmani phonology and morphology. MIT dissertation.

Archangeli D (1988) Aspects of underspecification theory. Phonology 5: 183–2.

Chomsky N, Halle M (1968) The Sound Pattern of English. New York: Harper and Row.

Dinnsen D (1984) Methods and empirical issues in analyzing functional misarticulation. In Elbert M, Dinnsen D, Weismer G (Eds) Phonological Theory and the Misarticulating Child. ASHA Monograph 22: 5–17.

Dinnsen D (1993) Underspecification and phonological disorders. In Eid M, Iverson G (Eds) Principles and Prediction: The Analysis of Natural Language. Philadelphia: John Benjamins.

Dinnsen D, Chin S (1995) On the natural domain of phonological disorders. In Archibald, J (Ed) Phonological Acquisition and Phonological Theory. New Jersey: Lawrence Erlbaum.

Dinnsen D, Elbert M, Weismer G (1980) Some typological properties of functional misarticulation systems. In Dressler, W (ed.) Phonologica 1980. Innsbruck: Innsbrucker Beiträge zur Sprachwissenschaft.

Fukusako Y, Sawashima M, Abe M (1976) Shoni ni mirareru koon no ayamari (iwayuru kinoteki koon shogai) ni tsuite: sono rinsho keiken. Onsei Gengo Igaku 17: 60–71.

Hodson B (1980) The Assessment of Phonological Processes. Danville: The Interstate.

Ingram D (1976) Phonological Disability in Children. London: Edward Arnold.

Ishikawa S (1930) Hatsuon hattatsu no bunsekiteki kenkyu. Aichiken Jido-Kenkyusyo Kiyo 5: 115–33.

Matsushita K (1981) Shogaiji no gengo keisei katei: koon no kakutoku ni tsuite. Hattatsu Shogai Kenkyu 3: 28–36.

Maxwell E (1984) On determining underlying phonological representation in children: a critique of the current theories. In Elbert M, Dinnsen D, Weismer G (Eds) Phonological Theory and the Misarticulating Child. ASHA Monograph 22: 59–68.

Murata K (1970) Yoji no Kotoba to Hatsuon: Sono Hattatsu to Hattatsu Shogai. Tokyo: Baifukan.

Nagafuchi M (1985) Gengo Shogai Gaisetsu. Tokyo: Taishukan.

Nagayama K (1985) Shindan to chiryo. In Kumae T, Nishikawa M, Tomita N (Eds) Gengo shogai no Chiryo to Shindan. Kyoto: Nakanishiya.

Nakanishi Y, Owada K, Fujita N (1972) Koonkensa to sono kekkani kansuru kousatsu. Bulletin of the Research Institute for the Education of Exceptional Children: Tokyo Gakugei University 1.

Sakauchi T (1967) Kodomono koon noryoku ni tuite. Gengoshogai Kenkyu 68: 13–26.

Shriberg L, Kwiatkowski J (1980) Natural Process Analysis: A Procedure for Phonological Analysis of Continuous Speech Samples. New York: Wiley.

Stampe D (1973) A dissertation of natural phonology. University of Chicago dissertation.

Takagi S, Yasuda A (1967) Seijo yoji (3-6 sai) no koon noryoku. Shonihoken Kenkyu 25: 23–8.

Ueda I (1996a) On the phonology of Japanese 'kappacism'. In Powell T (Ed) Pathologies of Speech and Language: Contributions of Clinical Phonetics and Linguistics. New Orleans: The International Clinical Phonetics and Linguistics Association.

Ueda I (1996b) Segmental acquisition and feature specification in Japanese. In Bernhardt B, Gilbert J, Ingram D (Eds) Proceedings of The University of British Columbia International Conference on Phonological Acquisition Somerville, Mass: Cascadilla Press.

Yasuda A (1969) Articulatory skills in three-year-old children. Studia Phonologica 5: 52–71.

Weiner F (1979) Phonological Process Analysis. Baltimore: University Park Press.

Note

1   We are grateful to the following people for their comments and suggestions on earlier versions of this paper: Itsue Kawagoe, Haruo Kubozono, Armin Mester, Ichiro Miura, Toshiyuki Tabata and Shin'ichi Tanaka. This work was supported in part by a grant-in-aid from the Japanese Ministry of Education for the specially promoted project entitled Emergence of Cognition and Language.

Chapter 15
Phonological Encoding Processes in Children with Developmental Apraxia of Speech[1]

INGE BOERS, BEN MAASSEN AND
SJOEKE VAN DER MEULEN

Introduction

This paper presents the first results of a longitudinal study comparing the development of speech planning in children who have developmental apraxia of speech (DAS) to children who speak normally. It reports acoustic characteristics of coarticulation produced within and between syllables for three children with DAS and three children who speak normally.

Children with DAS are characterized by speech that is often unintelligible due to many sound substitutions and omissions. According to Hall, Jordan and Robin (1993) and Thoonen, Maassen, Wit, Gabreëls and Schreuder (1996) the most salient speech characteristics of children with DAS at about 5 years of age are: largely unintelligible speech, high consonant error rates, many context-related substitutions, groping, and inconsistency of errors.

The experiments on coarticulation reported in this paper are based on a series of studies by Susan Nittrouer and her colleagues (Nittrouer, 1993, 1996; Nittrouer, Studdert-Kennedy and McGowan, 1989). These studies revealed that, in children with normal speech development, coarticulation of gestures between syllables matures earlier than coarticulation within syllables. By the age of 3, children who speak normally mastered an adult level of intersyllabic coarticulation, but articulatory gestures for the coproduction of segments within the syllable continued to be refined until at least the age of 7. Moreover, control of jaw movements matured at a faster rate than that of tongue movements.

In the present study we addressed the question of whether children with DAS follow the same developmental trends as those found by Nittrouer in children who speak normally. Thus, the question was: do 5-year-old children with DAS show the same coarticulation processes in perceptually correct speech as normal-speaking 5-year-old children?

Method

Subjects

The cases presented here are clear examples of DAS. They were referred and selected according to clinical criteria described in Hall et al. (1993) and Thoonen et al. (1996). Furthermore, the following exclusion criteria were applied: no hearing problems, no problems with language comprehension, no organic disorders in the orofacial area, no gross motor disturbances, no dysarthria and normal intelligence. It was not easy to find such clear cases. Of the 70 children in the age group 4;6 to 6;6 who were referred with the diagnosis DAS, only 30 were selected as clear cases. Of these 30 children, 10 had additional language comprehension difficulties. 'Clear developmental dyspraxia' does not, therefore, seem to be a very common phenomenon.

The three children with DAS were: RL (age 5;0 yrs), PM (5;10 yrs) and KB (5;11 yrs). The normal children were: JD (age 5;0 yrs), TS (5;6 yrs) and RV (5;11 yrs). They were all boys, and passed the selection criteria, in particular normal hearing and a receptive language score higher than 80, according to a standardized Dutch language comprehension test.

Speech samples

The stimulus-set consisted of nonsense syllables of the schwa-fricative-vowel type. The following combinations were used: /əxa əxi əxu/ and /əsa əsi əsu/ . Instead of the alveolar – palatal distinction /s/ - /ʃ/ used by Nittrouer, the alveolar–velar distinction /s/ - /x/ was used in this study. The articulatory positions of these consonants are further apart. The velar fricative /x/ is very common in Dutch.

All items were repeated six times and were spoken in a carrier phrase. The children were encouraged to imitate the experimenter's speaking rate and intonation. The recordings were made at the child's school in a quiet room using a portable DAT recorder and a headset microphone.

Acoustic analysis

Speech samples were digitized at 25 kHz and relevant sections (i.e. schwa-fricative-vowel segments) were spliced out. The second formant trajectory was used as a measure of the amount of coarticulation. To do this, a pitch synchronous LPC analysis was applied, overlaid on the spectrogram of the utterance. These analyses were executed by means of a Kay Elemetrics Computerized Speech Lab model 4300.

F2 was measured at six points through the utterance: at schwa midpoint and end, in the fricative portion of the signal 30 ms before vowel onset, at the vowel transition onset and end, and at vowel midpoint (see Figure 15.1). The automatic formant trajectory measurements were post-processed by means of a smoothing procedure developed at our speech laboratory.

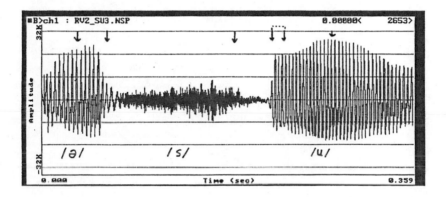

Figure 15.1. Example of speech sample: oscillogram and spectrum. With arrows the moments are indicated at which F2 was determined.

The F2-traces shown in Figure 15.2 and the following figures are all mean F2 trajectories over six tokens that were all produced perceptually correctly (except for the schwa of one dyspraxic child, PM). The x-axis represents time (not absolute); the y-axis represents the mean frequency of the second formant over six tokens.

Results

Coarticulation between syllables

As the three children who speak normally performed very similarly, data from only one child are used to describe the pattern (see Figure 15.2). Differences in F2 of schwa due to upcoming vowel are very small in context /_s_/, and slightly larger in context /_x_/. As expected, schwa F2 is highest when followed by the vowel /i/ and lowest when followed by the /u/.

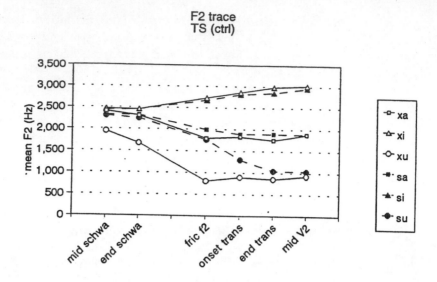

Figure 15.2. F2-traces (means of six tokens) for all utterances spoken by the normally speaking child TS, who is representative of the three children who speak normally.

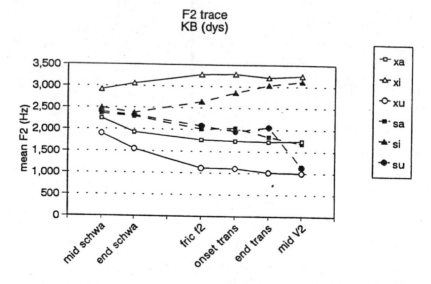

Figure 15.3. F2-traces (means of 6 tokens) for all utterances spoken by the child with DAS called KB.

The dyspraxic child KB, presented in Figure 15.3, shows the same pattern as the normal child when schwa is followed by an /s/; in that context schwa production is fairly constant. However, in context /_x_/ the schwa production differs much more as a function of the upcoming vowel.

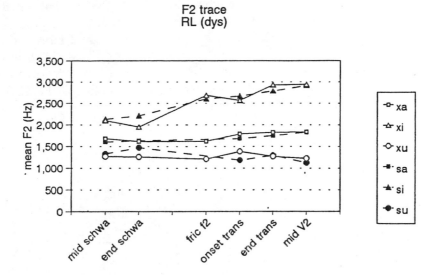

F2 trace
RL (dys)

Figure 15.4. F2-traces (means of six tokens) for all utterances spoken by the child with DAS called RL.

In the dyspraxic child RL, presented in Figure 15.4, strong coarticulation effects are found between syllables. Moreover, the size of the effect is as large in context /_s_/ as it is in context /_x_/.

No coarticulation between syllables could be observed in dyspraxic child PM due to the high overall level of F2. These schwas sounded like /i/.

To summarize, the F2 values for the normal children in this study corroborate Nittrouer's (1996) data. At 5 years of age, children who speak normally master intersyllabic coarticulation at an adult level. In the context of the velar fricative /_x_/ the children who speak normally experience a larger upcoming vowel effect on the schwa than in the context of /_s_/. Much larger upcoming vowel effects on the schwa were found for the children with DAS, showing immature articulation. For both groups coarticulation effects were stronger in the context of /_x_/. Apparently, body movement for /x/ allows 'penetration' of the upcoming vowel to a larger extent than tongue-tip movements for /s/.

Coarticulation within syllables

For the control child TS, presented in Figure 15.2, there is already evidence of the upcoming steady state F2 value of the vowel 30 ms before its onset. The F2 traces gradually move towards the steady state F2 value. This effect is stronger in context /_x_/ than in context /_s_/.

The dyspraxic child KB, presented in Figure 15.3, shows a different pattern in context /_s_/ 30 ms before vowel onset. At this point in the utterance /a/ and /u/ are not distinguished whereas /i/ is. The case of /su/ is interesting in this regard because there is no gradual F2 movement towards the steady state as was apparent for the normal child. In contrast to the weak coarticulation effect in context /_s_/, a very strong coarticulation effect is found in context /_x_/, similar to the children who speak normally.

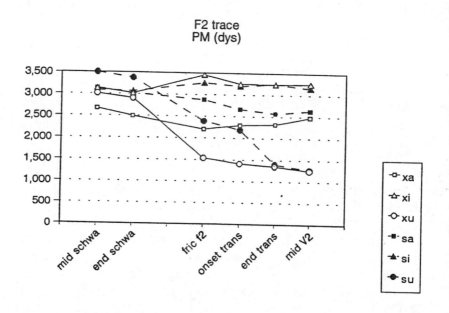

F2 trace
PM (dys)

Figure 15.5. F2-traces (means of six tokens) for all utterances spoken by the child with DAS called PM.

The dyspraxic child PM, presented in Figure 15.5, who shows a very odd between-syllable coarticulation pattern, shows evidence of the upcoming vowel 30 ms before its onset, but for this child, too, the /su/ trace differs from that of the normally speaking child. The F2 value of the steady state is reached at a later point in time.

The dyspraxic boy RL, presented in Figure 15.4, did not show any measurable effect with the upcoming vowels /a/ and /u/ 30 ms before the onset of the vowel in the context /_s_/. He did show an effect, however, in the velar fricative stimuli.

To summarize: the upcoming vowel was reflected 30 ms before vowel onset for both the normal and the dyspraxic children. This coarticulation effect is stronger in the context of velar fricatives than in the context of alveolar fricatives. All three children with DAS showed slow F2 transitions in /su/, indicating delayed anticipatory coarticulation (see also Ziegler, 1989; Ziegler and von Cramon, 1986).

Discussion and conclusion

The children with DAS show a stronger influence of the upcoming vowel on the schwa than the children who speak normally. This indicates a stronger coarticulation between syllables, which, according to Nittrouer, reflects a less well-syllabified utterance.

Within the syllable the children with DAS show a smaller effect of the vowel on the preceding alveolar fricative than children who speak normally, indicating a weaker coarticulation within the syllable. This effect was not found for the velar fricative. It would be interesting to compare these child data with adult velar fricative data. The choice of /s/ and /x/ in the present study offers greater opportunity for differential effects related to place-of-articulation than the study by Nittrouer (1996) in which /s/ and /ʃ/ were examined.

Both the between- and within-syllables effects depend on the fricative that is being produced. The difference seems to be related to the articulators involved, in this case tongue body for the velar fricative /x/ versus the tip of the tongue for the alveolar fricative /s/. Thus, the coproduction of schwa, j/x/ and vowel is considered homorganic (only tongue body involved) and the coproduction of schwa, /s/ and vowel heterorganic (tongue body and tongue tip involved). The three children with DAS seem to operate according to the 'everything moves at once' principle in the homorganic productions – more so than the children who speak normally. In the heterorganic productions, schwa-vowel (tongue-body) and fricative (tongue-tip) movements seem less well integrated in children with DAS, resulting in slow transitions.

The following quotation from Nittrouer (1996) seems to apply:

> one aspect of speech development may very well involve gaining greater independence among gestures that use articulators of increasingly closer anatomical proximity. (p.388)

References

Hall PK, Jordan LS, Robin DA (1993) Developmental Apraxia of Speech. Austin, TX: Proed.

Nittrouer S, Studdert Kennedy M, McGowan RS (1989) The emergence of phonetic segments: evidence from the spectral structure of fricative vowel syllables spoken by children and adults. Journal of Speech and Hearing Research 32: 120-32.

Nittrouer S (1993) The emergence of mature gestural patterns is not uniform: Evidence from an acoustic study. Journal of Speech and Hearing Research 36: 959-72.

Nittrouer, S (1996) How children learn to organize their speech gestures: further evidence from fricative vowel syllables. Journal of Speech and Hearing Research 39: 379–89.

Thoonen G, Maassen B, Wit J, Gabreëls F, Schreuder R (1996) The integrated use of maximum performance tasks in differential diagnostic evaluations among children with motor speech disorders. Clinical Linguistics and Phonetics 10: 311–36.

Ziegler W, Von Cramon D (1986) Disturbed coarticulation in apraxia of speech: acoustic evidence. Brain and Language 29: 34-47.

Ziegler W (1989) Anticipatory coarticulation in aphasia: more methodology: a reply to Sussman et al. (1988) and Katz (1988). Brain and Language 37: 172-6.

Note

1   The Netherlands Organization for Scientific Research (NWO) is gratefully acknowledged for funding this project. This research was conducted while the first author was supported by a grant from the Foundation and Educational Sciences of this organization (575-56-084) awarded to the second and third authors.

ARTICULATION

Chapter 16
Acoustic Analysis of Infant CV Protosyllables

CREIGHTON J. MILLER, JAMES R. PIROLLI,
MARSHA ZLATIN-LAUFER AND RAY DANILOFF

Introduction

Several recent investigations have refocused attention upon the acoustic and phonetic patterns produced by very young children as a way to relate early preverbal behaviours to the emergence of communicative competence (e.g. Davis and MacNeilage, 1990; de Boysson-Bardies and Vihman, 1991; Halle and Vihman, 1991; Goodell and Studdert-Kennedy, 1993). These studies generally focused on specific acoustic features thought to be relevant in adult speech. This study investigated a variety of acoustic features in the vocalizations of very young children, with the goal of determining which features share characteristics with more mature forms and how developmental changes reflect the paired emergence of communicative awareness and speech motor organization in very young children. Stop-CV-like tokens were the focus for the study because they are prevalent in early vocalizations, they provide easily-measured acoustic indicators of consonantal and vocalic articulation and they are generally held to reflect maximal coproductive encoding in speech (Lieberman and Mattingly, 1985).

Method

Monosyllabic CV-like protosyllables were collected from the vocalizations of three normally developing first-born infants as they progressed from 6 months to 14 months in chronological age. The data were obtained from archival recordings of bimonthly assessments in a longitudinal study of discourse development in young children (Zlatin, 1976). These recordings took place in a sound-attenuated chamber, fitted as a playroom, while the infants (two females, one male) interacted with their parents. A collection of 680 candidate CV utterances was selected from a much larger set of infant utterances that were either (a) multisyllabic or (b) non-stop-CV-like in apparent phonetic identity. From these 680 candidates, 180 stop-CV-like protosyllables were selected and digitized for acoustic analyses. About 80% of the selections (144 items) were scored in the original study as being produced by the child in question with clear communicative intent (Zlatin, 1976). The criteria for selecting individual syllables for analysis required that: (a) the signal-to-noise ratio in the audio recording was sufficient that the acoustic analyses could be accomplished, (b) each token was consistently transcribed by three trained phoneticians, and (c) F1 and F2 trajectories could be clearly identified throughout the utterance.

Tokens selected for analyses were prefiltered at 150 Hz to 10 kHz and subjected to 12-bit digitization at a 20 kHz sampling rate on a PC-based laboratory system for acoustic signal capture and analysis (Miller, 1991; Miller, Roussel, Daniloff and Hoffman, 1991). All acoustic measurements accomplished with this system were based upon digitally generated time/amplitude displays and 2048-point DFT spectra calculated at critical temporal positions. The DFT analyses were performed upon 10 ms samples that were preconditioned with a 200-point symmetric Hanning window. The use of this system and the associated strategies for the analysis of child and infant vocalizations are described in Miller (1991).

Spectral measures

DFT spectra were generated at 15 ms intervals along each syllable beginning at the point of articulatory release. F1 and F2 frequencies at these locations were determined by identifying the appropriate peaks in the DFT spectra (the analysis software automatically provides a cursor-based frequency readout). These values were used to determine each syllable's formant profiles and to determine transition onset- and offset-frequencies, transition durations and transition rates for the consonantal intervals. The 15 ms separation between successive DFT spectra was reduced when necessary to ensure at least four measurement points across the consonantal transition interval.

Amplitude measures

The amplitude envelope was estimated from the magnitude of the time-amplitude wave form in a manner similar to that described for the formant measures, beginning at articulatory release and progressing at 10 ms intervals. In addition to the syllabic amplitude profile, onset- and offset-amplitudes for the consonantal interval and time-to-peak syllable amplitude were derived from these measures. A separate peak-picking routine calculated an amplitude shimmer contour for each syllable on the basis of strategies outlined by Ramig et al. (1988, 1990).

The acoustic measures were (a) evaluated as profiles for the consonant-to vowel interval, and (b) assessed for mean and standard deviation, and compared to adult norms. Where published data were available, comparisons were made with those adult norms. Other assessments of the relation between measures of the infant protosyllables and adult forms were based upon CV data produced by the second author (JP) for the English stop-CV syllables in the carrier phrase, 'Say CV again', produced at a moderate tempo with stress on the CV (C=/b, d, g, p, t, k/, V=/i, ɪ, e, ɛ, ae, ɑ, ɔ, o, ʊ, u/). In the profile analyses each syllable was also evaluated for (a) CV amplitude envelope regularity; (b) total number of peaks in the CV amplitude envelope; (c) the presence or absence of aspiration noise in the syllable, and (d) number of burst-release transients at articulatory release.

Results and discussion

All temporal and spectral measures were initially divided into six age categories (5–6, 7–8, 9–10, 11–12, 13–14, and 15–16 months, respectively) and evaluated for developmental trends. Inspection of the syllable profiles, and the central tendency and variability measures, did not reveal any notable age trends; accordingly, all subsequent analyses were based upon the grouped data.

Of the 680 initial candidate protosyllables, 370 were classified by the scorers as stop-CV items and 190 of these, slightly over half the identified data set, were excluded from further analysis because they were not consistently identified in phonetic analysis. Of the 180 total protosyllables that were analysed, one-third (58 syllables) was judged to have aberrant transitions. Most of these transition aberrancies were cases where F2 transition onset frequencies differed by more than 20% from expected values, given the apparent phonetic labels assigned to them, a criterion taken from Rabiner (1968). Since judges consistently identified these tokens despite highly atypical transition cues it must be assumed that a third of the tokens were identified with respect to acoustic cues not typically used in adult speech. A number of additional exemplars showed 'transition overshoot', where formant values progressed well beyond typical steady-state values and then fell back to those values. It should be noted, however, that transitions in the protosyllables showed adult-like monotonicity in transition rate, thus indicating smooth, co-ordinated articulatory movements during the bulk of the transition.

Average syllable durations for the infant protosyllables were 364 ms, as compared to 234 ms for the adult CVs. This finding compares well with 350 ms durations reported for the first element in infant trisyllable utterances by Levitt and Aydelott-Uttman (1992) and Vihman (1996). Stop-like CV syllable durations for very young children are considerably longer than comparable adult productions. Figure 16.1 compares the dispersion of average durations for the infant protosyllables with the adult CVs produced by JD, where it is clear that both the central tendency and the range is greater in the infants' productions.

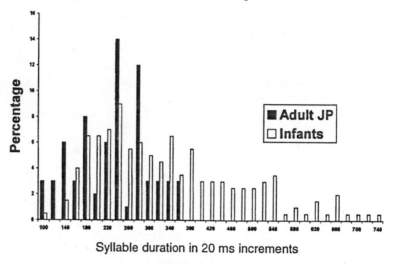

Syllable duration in 20 ms increments

Figure 16.1. Syllable duration frequency histogram comparing infant and adult magnitudes.

Measures of amplitude onset duration, from articulatory release to the point of maximum envelope amplitude, averaged 48 ms for the infants and 54 ms for the adult, an 11% disparity. Transition duration (the interval from first appearance of F1 or F2 to F2 steady-state) measures for infants averaged 43 ms, while the adult value was only 35 ms – a 22% disparity. Interestingly, the interval from articulatory release to peak velocity of amplitude change, a critical factor in both consonant and vowel articulation according to Furuii (1986), is considerably longer for the infant protosyllables (37 ms) than for the adult CVs (11 ms). As might be expected, however, the vocalic element is greatly prolonged for the infant utterances (257 ms versus 144 ms). In contrast to these modest durational disparities between adult and child mean values, variances for the adult and child measures were of comparable magnitude in all but a few cases.

The findings in this study make it clear that, even though infants' articulatory gestures tend to be longer (slower) than those of adult speakers, temporal patterning is nevertheless more precise and less variable than is spatial precision *per se*. The self-organizing perspective on dynamic perceptual-motor planning of infant speech (Thelen, 1991) suggests that complex interactions of biological growth, social/sensory experience and sensorimotor predilections lead to the emergence of articulatory competence (Vihman, 1996). Our results suggest surprisingly little change in protosyllable temporal forms and spatial accuracy for stop-vowel-like combinations over the period of this study. Is it possible that the protosyllables initially attained are sufficiently adult-like for about six months, so that refinement/mastery can be diverted to other phonetic and grammatical matters such as acquiring trains of multisyllabic utterances replete with prosodic forms as well as acquisition of additional sounds? Subsequent pressure for increased articulatory precision might only arise somewhat later, in response to the eventual need to keep initial sets of spoken words distinct from one another. It would be most interesting to enlarge the study to include children aged 2-to-3 months (at Oller's 'gooing' stage; Oller 1980). At that stage such factors as nasality and articulatory imprecision would render the analyses difficult but the results might eliminate the temporo-spatial pattern for the earliest biologically determined protosyllabic forms.

References

Boysson-Bardies B de, Vihman MM (1991) Adaptation to language: evidence from babbling and first words in four languages. Language 67: 297–319.

Davis B, MacNeilage PF (1990) Acquisition of correct vowel production: a quantitative case study. Journal of Speech and Hearing Disorders 33: 16–27.

Furuii S (1986) On the role of spectral transitions for speech perception. Journal of the Acoustical Society of America 80: 1016–25.

Goodell E, Studdert-Kennedy M (1993) Acoustic evidence for the development of gestural coordination in the speech of 2-year-olds: a longitudinal study. Journal of Speech and Hearing Research 36: 707–27.

Halle P, Vihman MM (1991) Beginnings of prosodic organization: Intonation and duration patterns of disyllables produced by Japanese and French infants. Language and Speech 34: 299–318.

Levitt AG, Aydelotte-Utman JG (1992) From Babbling towards the Sound Systems of English and French: a longitudinal two-case study. Journal of Child Language 19: 19–49

Lieberman A, Mattingly I (1985) The motor theory of speech perception revised. Cognition 21: 1–36.

Miller CJ (1991) WavEdit: General purpose program for waveform capture/manipulation/analysis. Users' Manual. Baton Rouge: Creighton J. Miller.

Miller CJ, Roussel N, Daniloff R, Hoffman P (1991) Estimates of formant frequency in synthetic infant CV tokens. Clinical Linguistics and Phonetics 5: 283–96.

Oller DK (1980) The emergence of the sounds of speech in infancy. In G Yeni Komshian, J Kavanagh and C Ferguson (Eds) Child Phonology, 1: Production. New York: Academic Press.

Rabiner L (1968) Speech synthesis by rule: an acoustic domain approach. Bell Systems Technical Journal 47: 17–37.

Ramig L, Scherer R, Titze I, Ringel R (1988) Acoustic analysis of voices of patients with neurological disease: a rationale and preliminary data. Annals of Otology, Rhinology and Laryngology 97: 164–72.

Ramig L, Scherer R, Klasner E, Titze I, Horii Y (1990) Acoustic analysis of voice in amyotropic lateral sclerosis: A longitudinal study. Journal of Speech and Hearing Research 55: 2–14.

Thelen E (1991) Motor aspects of emergent speech; a dynamic approach. In N Krasnegor, D Rumbaugh, R Schieffelbusch, M Studdert-Kennedy (Eds) Biological and Behavioral Determinants of Language Development. Hillsdale, NJ: Earlbaum Associates.

Vihman M (1996) Phonological Development: The Origins of Language in the Child. Cambridge, MA: Blackwell.

Zlatin MA (1976) Final report, National Institutes of Education. Project No. 3-4014, Grant No. NE-G-00-3-001. Resume in Resources in Education.

Chapter 17
Covert Contrast and the Acquisition of Phonetics and Phonology[1]

JAMES M SCOBBIE, FIONA GIBBON, WILLIAM J
HARDCASTLE AND PAUL FLETCHER

Phonetic and phonological development

The speech and language therapist relies on impressionistic transcriptions of speech as the major source of information about speakers' abilities and the nature of any disorders. This is necessary because the intention of the speaker should be perceived and understood correctly, but transcription and other forms of listener-oriented analysis are not sufficient as there may be important aspects of speech that are clinically relevant but are simply not heard (and may be unperceivable).

For example, in the analysis of early speech, transcription shows extensive neutralization of phonological contrasts, with a corresponding range of homophony far in excess of the target language. It is obvious that, as the child matures, it is able to successfully convey an increasing number of non-homophonous categories. It is also obvious, however, that the child does not articulate contrasts in an adult-like way at first. In consequence, the point at which the child starts to articulate a detectable contrast and the point at which the child's contrastive behaviour is perceived by a transcriber need not be synchronous. There can be a delay between the production of contrast and the perception of that contrast by others. This is the stage of 'covert contrast':[2] impressionistic homophones are acoustically or articulatorily different (Figure 17.1, Stage 2). Figure 1 recognizes the fact that children's phonetic systems are acquired and develop over a period of years. Gradual changes in the phonetic characteristics of a child's speech precede and follow the emergence of phonological contrast.

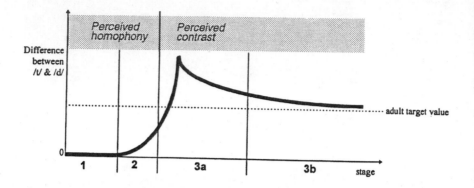

Figure 17.1. Schematic model of the acquisition/maturation of a cue to the contrast between /t/ and /d/. The y-axis represents any instrumentally measured value, e.g. a difference in VOT. Stage 1 = articulatory homophony, 2 = covert contrast, 3a = immature contrast, 3b = mature contrast. The curve shows a relatively rapid differentiation to an immature maximum followed by a more gradual asymptotic approximation to the adult target.

The clinical relevance of covert contrast stems from the fact that one of the common developmental speech disorders, 'functional articulation' or 'phonological' disorder (Ingram, 1981; Grunwell, 1981) is defined at least in part in terms of categorial neutralization of contrast (Gibbon and Scobbie, in press). There is a critical difference between a contrast simply being absent from a child's system and a contrast not being readily perceptible in their speech. Moreover, it has been shown that the remediation of phonological disorders is related to children's knowledge of their phonological system (e.g. Rockman, 1983). The judgement of 'knowledge' is based on transcription. In the case of covert contrast, however, the child has greater phonological knowledge than a transcription can ever reveal.

In summary, the acquisition of perceivable phonological contrast logically necessitates the acquisition and mastery of the numerous interacting phonetic cues that convey a contrast to the listener. A logical possibility for which there is mounting empirical evidence is that phonological contrasts may be unperceivable due to developmental errors in the acquisition of phonetic skills. Moreover, phonetic development is known to continue for years after a perceivable phonological contrast is produced. Yet very little is known about how these aspects of linguistic development interact. We feel therefore that the instrumental study of phonetic cues and parallel study of phonological contrasts is essential (Weismer, 1984; Gibbon, 1990). In the early stages of such work it is necessary to carry out longitudinal studies of cue maturation before and after a contrast is 'acquired' in the traditional phonological sense.

In the rest of the paper we present a case of covert contrast in its clinical context from the longitudinal MRC Cluster Acquisition Project at Queen Margaret College, Edinburgh (Scobbie, Gibbon, Hardcastle and Fletcher, in press; Scobbie, Hardcastle, Fletcher and Gibbon, 1995).

Methodology

In this longitudinal acoustic study of cluster acquisition in Scottish English, a heterogeneous group of nine children, diagnosed as having phonological disorders, were recorded six times at intervals of approximately four months. We elicited multiple instances of sentences of the form 'Give me spear please' in a series of 10 games, all of which involved the child being given the appropriate picture for the elicited sentence. The dialogue was thus relatively relaxed and naturalistic. No game involved rhyming or alliterating words. 'Spear' is one of 28 targets designed primarily to probe the acquisition of /s/+stop clusters. In this paper we discuss durational results for /sp/, /st/ and /sk/, plus the singletons /t/ and /d/, in three rime environments: /ir/, /or/, /ae/. The lexical items were *tie, dye, sty, spy, sky; tear, deer, steer, spear, skier; tore, door, store, score.* (We also collected tokens of *spot, speak* and *skate,* but these short rimes are not discussed here.) Six tokens of each were digitised. A variety of durational events such as consonantal closure, VOT and fricative duration were analysed on a KAY CSL. In this paper we focus on VOT. See Scobbie et al. (in press) for further details.

Covert contrast in subject DB

In this section we report a case of covert contrast in DB, a boy aged 4;01, diagnosed as having a phonological disorder (the initial referral was at 3;05 years of age). See Appendix for a case history and Scobbie et al. (in press) for further discussion and details. We present materials from his Session 1.

Impressionistic analysis

DB's phonological/phonetic system was analysed impressionistically (Tables 17.1, 17.2, 17.3). DB was largely unintelligible and in his speech, minimal triples such as *tie, dye* and *sty* were therefore transcribed as homophonous: [ta:]. A phonological analysis would attribute the homophony to processes of voicing neutralization and cluster reduction.

Table 17.1 Some of DB's developmentally normal and idiosyncratic process

Typical processes	Unusual processes
voicing neutralization	long-distance liquid metathesis
cluster reduction	labial cluster preference
de-rhoticization	vowel devoicing
	diphthong reduction

Table 17.2. Broad transcriptions indicative of DB's processes

Examples of processes	Broad transcriptions
voicing neutralisation	tear & deer = variably [tia] & [tʰia], tie & dye = [ta:]
cluster reduction	sty = [ta:], string = [flɪç]
long distance liquid metathesis	pencil = [flɛn?ɔx], wool = [wlu]
labial cluster preference	train = [flix], glove = [flif], string = [flɪç]
vowel devoicing	peak & beak & speak = variably [pikh:] & [pi̥kh:]
diphthong reduction	tie & die = variably [ta:] & [ta?a]

Table 17.3. DB's initial consonant inventory (session 1). His only initial cluster was [fl] ~ [pl]

p	t	k
f	s ʃ ɬ	x
m	n	
w	l j	

Durational analysis

Durational analysis of DB's speech revealed why no voicing contrast for initial stops had been transcribed. Mean VOT for /t/ was 36ms and for /d/, 35ms. Moreover, /st/ was realized as a stop with 33ms of aspiration. (Standard deviations were 16ms, 20ms and 13ms respectively.) Together, these coronal stops are realized as voiceless with a mean VOT of 34.6ms. This average sits on or above the boundary of the short-lag range of about 0–20ms (e.g. Zlatin and Koenigsknecht, 1976). According to Macken and Barton (1980: 42) the developmental acquisition literature is in 'overwhelming agreement' with Jakobson that prior to the acquisition of a VOT-cued /voice/ contrast, all stops are voiceless and unaspirated. Twenty eight per cent of DB's VOT values are long-lag, i.e. greater than 40ms, shared between /t/, /d/ and /st/. Perhaps this is an indication that DB's homophony does not result simply from a default or 'pre-contrastive' neutralized system.

Moreover, the distribution of VOT is both highly structured and influenced by the adult phonological system. Figure 17.2 shows that the identity of the following vowel has an adult-like, but highly exaggerated effect on DB's VOT. Two-way ANOVA confirms the effect of rime on VOT, $F(2,2) = 17.25$, $p = 0.011$. (Onsets are not distinguished: $F(2,2) = 0.26$, $p = 0.78$). In adult speech, VOT is affected by the height of the following vowel. Klatt (1975: 691) reports that the average VOT of voiceless (i.e. aspirated) stops before /i, u/ is about 15% greater than before /ɛ, æ/. Note the much greater effect in Figure 17.2. DB is able phonetically to time phonation onset but not to cue the appropriate contrast.

We do not know whether such a large effect of vowel height on VOT is normal for young children. Perhaps DB is in Stage 3a because this cue to vowel height, and indeed Stage 3a behaviour of 'secondary' cues to a contrast has been noted occasionally before (exaggerated vowel duration differences conditioned by final obstruents were observed by Krause, 1982).

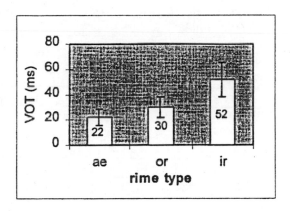

Figure 17.2. Mean VOT (± 1 sd) for coronal onsets before low, mid and high vowels.

Spectral analysis

The size of the glottal aperture during stop closures is a component of the contrast between voiced and voiceless stops: /t/ has glottal abduction in preparation for the high airflow required for aspiration at stop release. Modal voicing may consequently be achieved more slowly at the onset of voicing after /t/, with the first few glottal cycles having 'breathy' or murmured phonation. We performed spectral analysis on these early cycles, looking for possible covert differences in phonation type. The measurement we used is a robust local measure of phonemic breathiness: spectral tilt as localized in the difference of amplitude of the first two harmonics in the spectrum (Ladefoged and Antoñanzas-Barroso, 1984). We call this 'H1p', for 'first harmonic prominence'

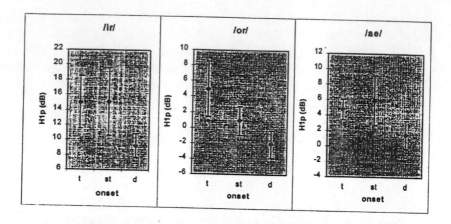

Figure 17.3. H1p means (±1 sd) for DB, organized by rimes.

(Scobbie et al. in press). Analysis revealed a steeper spectral tilt in 'tear' in the relationship of the first and second harmonics. This was true for all three vowel heights (which have a large influence on the absolute value of H1p), as indicated in Figure 17.3.

A two-factor ANOVA indicated that the contrastive effect of the rimes was highly significant $F(2,2) = 52.38$, $p = 0.0014$. In addition to the large absolute difference in H1p that the rime makes, these results show a relative difference between /d/ and either /t/ or /st/. This difference proves that DB has a covert contrast in this system. The covert contrast in onsets was significant $F(2,2) = 11.11$, $p = 0.023$.

Longitudinal analysis

This analysis is at an early stage (Scobbie et al., 1995), but some preliminary findings are relevant here. Impressionistically, the homophony between initial /t/, /d/ and /st/ resolved within four months (by Session 2). Phonological acquisition of these three syllable onsets was thus complete and would attract no further clinical intervention, nor would there be any indication of further development from transcriptions of DB's speech, yet we would clearly expect further phonetic development.

DB's VOT is of interest here. Taking just the values for /t/ from the high rimed 'tear' and the low rimed 'tie', in session 1 (4;01), with DB in Stage 2 for VOT, the means are approximately 50ms and 20ms respectively. In Session 2 (4;05), when DB has acquired onset-determined VOT and thus can convey the contrast between /t/ and /d/ overtly, the means increase to approximately 140ms and 90ms respectively. These values are too high for adult English and are examples of the target overshoot in Figure 17.1 (Stage 3a). Note, too, that the vowel height effect is maintained in Stage 3a: in Session 1, /t/'s VOT before /ir/ is about 30ms or 150% greater than /t/'s VOT before /ae/; in Session 2, the high vowel conditions an increase in VOT of about 50ms, or 60%.

Over the subsequent sessions, which do not accompany any change in the systematic phonological relationship between /t/, /d/ and /st/, we might expect the motoric development to cause the duration of VOT to fall and its standard deviation to decrease. This is the case in general but there is no simple linear progression. For example, in Session 5 (5;06), a year after Session 2, VOT for *tear* is approximately 130ms, and 90ms for *tie* and the variability is much greater than for Session 2. Overall, VOT does fall back towards a shorter value by Session 6 (5;10) but not by much (to approximately 95ms for *tear* and 80ms for *tie*). So approximately one year and five months after aspiration has been achieved, DB is still firmly in Stage 3a, demonstrating the very slow phonetic approximation to adult norms.

The effect of the rime on /t/'s VOT diminishes across the sessions, however, until in Session 6, the VOT of *tear* is only approximately 15% longer than the VOT of *tie*, so that for this aspect of his system, DB has reached Stage 3b.

Different aspects of DB's VOT are at different developmental stages at different times. Figure 17.1 is therefore not a model of the acquisition of a phonemic contrast in all its phonetic complexity: different but related cues to a contrast may be expected to follow their own developmental route. Phonetic maturity is reached only when the entire constellation of motorically based cues transmitting the contrast have reached adult values, each in their own time.

Summary

DB displays a clear case of impressionistic homophony between /t/, /d/ and /st/ backed up by quantitative durational analysis. To this extent DB appears to have no contrast for initial stop /voice/. Durational analysis explains why /t/, /d/ and /st/ are perceived as homophones, but has revealed the surprising fact that DB has acquired some of the aspects of VOT and can vary the duration of aspiration by over 100% from 22ms to 52ms in a linguistically relevant way (based on the rime). Spectral analysis revealed that DB did, however, have a covert contrast between initial /t/ and /d/. This was possibly due to his having acquired an appropriate glottal configuration for aspiration without having applied his timing abilities to the onset.

References

Gibbon, F (1990) Lingual activity in two speech-disordered children's attempts to produce velar and alveolar stop consonants: evidence from electropalatographic (EPG) data. British Journal of Disorders of Communication 25: 329–40.

Gibbon, F, Scobbie JM (in press) Covert contrasts in children with phonological disorder. Australian Communication Quarterly.

Gibbon F, Scobbie JM, Hardcastle WJ and Fletcher P (1996) Covert contrast as a stage in the acquisition of phonetics and phonology. Poster presented at ICPLA München.

Grunwell P (1981) The Nature of Phonological Disability in Children. London: Academic Press.

Hewlett, N (1988) Acoustic properties of /k/ and /t/ in normal and phonologically disordered speech. Clinical Linguistics and Phonetics 2: 29–45.

Ingram, D (1981) Procedures for the Phonological Analysis of Children's Language. Baltimore, MD: University Park Press.

Krause, SE (1982) Developmental use of vowel duration as a cue to postvocalic consonant voicing. Journal of Speech and Hearing Research 25: 388–93.

Ladefoged P, Antoñanzas-Barroso N (1984) Computer measures of breathy voice quality. UCLA Working Papers in Phonetics 61: 79–86.

Macken MA, Barton D (1980) The acquisition of the voicing contrast in English: a study of voice onset time in word-initial stop consonants. Journal of Child Language 7: 41–74.

Rockman BK (1983) An experimental investigation of generalization and individual differences in phonological training. PhD dissertation, Indiana University, USA.

Scobbie JM, Hardcastle WJ, Fletcher P, Gibbon F (1995) Consonant clusters in disordered L1 acquisition: a longitudinal acoustic study. Proceedings of the XIIIth International Congress of the Phonetic Sciences 706–9. Stockholm.

Scobbie JM, Gibbon F, Hardcastle WJ, Fletcher P (in press) Covert contrast as a stage in the acquisition of phonetics and phonology. In Michael Broe and Janet Pierrehumbert (Eds) Papers in Laboratory Phonology V. Cambridge: Cambridge University Press.

Weismer G (1984) Acoustic analysis strategies for the refinement of phonological analysis. In Elbert M, Dinnsen DDA, Weismer G (Eds) Phonological Theory and the Misarticulating Child. ASHA Monographs 22: 30–52. Rockville MD: ASHA.

Zlatin MA, Koenigsknecht RA (1976) Development of the voicing contrast: a comparison of voice onset time in stop perception and production. Journal of Speech and Hearing Research 19: 93–111.

Notes

1   This research was supported by MRC grant #G9117453: 'An instrumental investigation of consonant cluster acquisition in phonologically disordered and normally developing children.' Thanks to: DB and M, and all our MRC subjects and families for their participation; Alison Sinclair, the speech and language therapist responsible for DB's treatment; audiences at Labphon, the Manchester Phonology Meeting, ICPLA München, and others. This paper is based on the poster presented at ICPLA (Gibbon et al., 1996) 'Covert Contrast as a Stage in the Acquisition of Phonetics and Phonology', and on the oral presentation at Labphon 5. Copies of the poster are available from the authors at Queen Margaret College, and the written version of the Labphon 5 presentation is forthcoming (Scobbie et al., in press).

2   The term 'covert contrast' is from Hewlett (1988: 31). The earliest comprehensive study was Macken and Barton (1980), on whose work Figure 17.1 is based.

Appendix - DB's case history

0 years

DB had acute perinatal asphyxia at birth, with subsequent hypoxic encephalopathy. During the first five days of life he experienced seizures and transient acute tubular necrosis with mild renal failure. He was ventilated during this period. The seizures were treated with medication for the first year. There were no recurrences of seizures following this. No further medication was prescribed. The health visitor has monitored DB's development during pre-school years in all areas (e.g. motor, cognitive, social skills) and, apart from speech, this has been unremarkable. His hearing has been tested regularly and has always been found to be normal.

3;5 years

DB was referred for speech/language assessment. Receptive language, expressive syntax and lexical development were found to be in advance of age level. Speech was unintelligible, characterized by some normal phonological processes and some unusual or idiosyncratic features (see Table 17.1). DB was found to be a shy boy, lacking in confidence.

3;9–4;0 years

DB started regular, weekly therapy. His speech was mostly unintelligible. An orofacial examination showed that structure and function were normal and sound imitation was good, except for velars and post-alveolar consonants, which were produced as alveolars. His discrimination of sounds that were not in inventory was good. In therapy, DB was co-operative but shy. Therapy during this period focused on achieving an alveolar/velar contrast in word initial position. After several therapy sessions, velar sound imitation was achieved. Velar production progressed quickly over this period and, at the end of this time, velars were being produced correctly in all contexts except in polysyllabic and word-final position.

4;0–4;3 years

Velar production continued to progress well and speech became intelligible. Therapy focused on the idiosyncratic production of obstruent production in word final position, also the voicing contrast /t d/, affricates, clusters /tr/ and /kr/, and one session on the [fl] clusters arising from long-distance metathesis of /l/.

4;3–4;9 years

Review period (no regular therapy). At 4;9 years, DB's sound system was considered to be appropriate for his age, with only minor sound immaturities. Speech intelligibility at this stage was good, even in sentences where the context was not known. He was given no further therapy.

Chapter 18
A Perceptual and Electropalatographic Case Study of Pierre Robin Sequence

SARA HOWARD

Introduction

This case study examines the speech production of a young boy, Danny, with Pierre Robin Sequence (Shprintzen, 1992). A perceptual analysis at the age of 6 and a perceptual and electropalatographic (EPG) analysis at 13 are compared and reveal many features typically associated with the condition or its ensuing medical treatment. EPG analysis illustrates Danny's articulatory difficulties particularly effectively.

Pierre Robin Sequence

Pierre Robin Sequence (PRS), which is most often found accompanying other craniofacial syndromes such as Treacher Collins, Stickler or velo-cardiofacial syndrome, is a comparatively rare condition that has received little attention from clinical linguists. Because of difficulties establishing clear criteria for diagnosis, estimations of its incidence vary, ranging from 1 in 50 000 to 1 in 2000 (Sadewitz, 1992). Pierre Robin Sequence is traditionally associated with a distinctive triad of symptoms: micrognathia (mandibular hypoplasia), cleft palate and upper airway obstruction (Shprintzen, 1992). It is believed that the symptoms have a developmentally sequential relationship: the small lower jaw is the primary anomaly and is then the causative factor in both the cleft palate and the airway obstruction. Upper airway obstruction in PRS is often, although not always, the product of glossoptosis: the tongue, which is posteriorly positioned in a relatively small oral cavity, tends to fall back into the pharyngeal space making contact with the rear pharyngeal wall and thus blocking the airway (Sher, 1992). This in turn causes the serious respiratory difficulties typically encountered in PRS. As these problems are life-threatening to the infant or neonate in many cases, surgical intervention is often necessary to facilitate respiration, either in the form of a glossopexy, where the tip of the tongue is sutured to the lower lip, or tracheostomy (Sadewitz, 1992).

Literature on speech development in PRS is sparse and typically lacking in phonetic or phonological detail but there seems to be evidence that the individual's speech production will be significantly affected by the type of surgery he or she has received. Stuffins (1989) and Argamaso (1992) suggest that glossopexy has a relatively minor and temporary effect on speech development in PRS. Alveolar targets may tend to be produced as blade articulations and may be dentalized, but Argamaso comments that, for most children with PRS who receive a glossopexy, speech development will be essentially normal. For children with PRS who undergo tracheostomy, however, particularly those with long-term tracheostomies that may remain in place for several months or even for years, the prognosis for speech development is less good. These children show the typical effects of tracheostomy on speech development: abnormal babbling and early motor and articulatory development; abnormal phonation; a tendency to produce posterior consonantal articulations; abnormal vowel production. They may also be at risk of receptive and expressive language development (Bleile, 1993). Many children with PRS also show features of speech production linked to cleft palate, most markedly abnormalities of resonance leading to hypernasality and audible nasal emission. Some also show significant cognitive impairments that may necessitate special education.

Case history

Danny was born prematurely, by breech delivery, at 31 weeks gestation. He had a low birth weight and was diagnosed as having a central cleft of the soft palate and an abnormally small mandible. These factors, together with serious respiratory difficulties and a failure to thrive suggested a diagnosis of Pierre Robin sequence. At 0;4 Danny's respiratory difficulties necessitated a tracheostomy, which remained in place until 1;9. His cleft palate was repaired at 2;0. Danny had a history of feeding difficulties, transient moderate conductive hearing impairment, moderate learning difficulties and a degree of general hypotonicity. His general development, including that of speech and language, was delayed and in time a moderate learning disability was also identified.

Danny at 6: a perceptual analysis

At 6;1 Danny had received speech and language therapy for three years, focusing on his expressive and receptive language, but had no intervention aimed at articulatory or phonological abilities despite the fact that a high level of unintelligibility had been noted on several occasions in his medical and speech and language therapy notes.

A perceptual analysis of Danny's speech production at 6;1 was undertaken, based on a corpus of 443 words, combining single word elicitation and spontaneous speech. Live transcription proved particularly difficult and live observation was combined with a narrow phonetic consensus transcription made from a high-quality video recording and carried out by two clinical linguists.

Danny's speech production at 5;1 showed features consistent with PRS and subsequent treatment by tracheostomy. It is illuminating to examine his speech in relation to the subsystems of resonance, phonation and articulation. Whilst general resonance and signalling of oral/nasal contrasts were remarkably well-preserved, given his history of cleft palate, phonatory activity was markedly perceptually abnormal, resulting in a hoarse, aperiodic voice quality, although appropriate contrasts between voiced and voiceless targets were generally maintained.

Many of Danny's problems hinged around difficulties in achieving specific articulatory movements, particularly those involving the tongue. These affected both place and manner of articulation. In general Danny was successful in producing appropriate sound segments according to the broad classes of plosive, fricative and approximant. This suggests that he had internalized these contrasts at the level of phonological representation and also that he was successful in manipulating the degrees of approximation of active and passive articulators that form the articulatory underpinning of the phonological organization. There were only very occasional examples where realisations cross sound classes (e.g./f/ → [b͡β], /ð/ → [d], /s/ →[ɹ], /v/→[ʔp].). Contrasts between plosives and affricates and between fricatives and affricates were less successfully realized: affricates were sometimes realized as plosives and sometimes as fricatives. There were too few tokens of affricates in the data to make confident explanatory statements: the overlap between affricates and other sound classes could suggest that Danny had not yet established a clear category at a phonological level of organization or it might imply an articulatory timing difficulty in the co-ordination of the complex closure and release phases of target affricates. Even in normally developing phonology, of course, affricates are late to be incorporated successfully into the sound system (Gibbon, 1994). Although Danny made a clear distinction between approximants and other sound classes it is striking that no examples of lateral approximants occurred anywhere in the data. The range of approximants that Danny produced all had a central airstream.

Danny achieved an accurate place of articulation for bilabial and velar targets and in doing so contrasted them clearly and successfully with other target segments. He was much less successful in maintaining appropriate place contrasts for alveolar and post-alveolar targets and examination of his difficulties in this area of his speech production helps to explain a significant amount of his reduced intelligibility and the perceptual impression of a severely disordered and atypical sound system.

That Danny would have difficulties with tip and blade articulations might be predicted from the combined influences of Pierre Robin anatomy and physiology, cleft palate and tracheostomy. These difficulties are well illustrated by the target fricative data. Various targets were produced at unusual places of articulation so that, for example, target /s/ was realized variably as /ɸ/, /ç/, and /x/. There was also a significant degree of overlap between other fricative labiodental, dental, alveolar and post-alveolar targets: all were produced on some occasions as palatal or velar fricatives. The dental and labiodental fricatives, however, also overlapped on occasions in realizations as bilabial fricatives. It is striking that the labiodental fricatives appear to have two characteristic and articulatory dissimilar variants: bilabial and palatal/velar fricatives, not only perceptually different but also produced by two different articulator systems, the lips and the tongue dorsum. Alveolar place of articulation was also problematic for Danny in his production of approximants. Whereas /w/ and /j/ were generally realized appropriately, the approximants produced with the tip and blade of the tongue, /l/ and /r/, were variably produced, but never at the correct alveolar or post-alveolar location. In summary, at 6;1, whilst there is evidence of some phonological organizational impairment, Danny's speech disorder can be largely characterized in terms of articulatory constraints related to the symptoms and surgery for PRS.

Danny at 13: a perceptual and electropalatographic analysis

At 13;10 Danny had received several years of special educational support and speech and language therapy for language and literacy but had still not received any speech and language therapy intervention aimed at articulation or phonology. Perceptual analysis of Danny's speech at 13;10, based on a similar corpus to that collected at 6;1, revealed a similar picture in many ways to his speech at 5;0. Resonance remained normal and, whereas phonation remained hoarse and aperiodic, contrasts between voiced and voiceless targets were typically clearly marked. Apart from his abnormal voice quality, Danny's major problem remained that of the accurate realization of alveolar and post-alveolar consonantal segments. Although the bilabial fricative realisations of target sibilant fricatives noted at 5;1 had now disappeared, his system showed an avoidance of alveolar and post-alveolar places of articulation and a tendency to produce many alveolar and post-alveolar targets more posteriorly in the oral cavity, typically realizing them variably as palatals or velars. It is also noteworthy that the other target consonants produced in normal speech with the tongue tip, the dental fricatives /θ/ and /ð/, were produced by Danny as /f/ and /v/. Whilst this is an acceptable variant for the regional accent which Danny speaks (an urban variety of northern British English), it is significant that this was not a variant used by the rest of his family. The lateral approximant /l/ and the post-alveolar median approximant /r/ were also produced at places of articulation that do not involve tongue-tip activity. Thus Danny's system of realisations of tip/blade consonants was as follows:

/t/ → [t, t̪, c] /d/ → [d, d̪, ɟ]

/θ/ → [f]   /ð/ → [v]   /s/ → [ç, x]   /z/ → [j, ɤ]   /ʃ/ → [ç, x]   /ʒ/ → [j, ɤ]

/tʃ/ → [t͡ɕ, tʃ, c͡ç]   /dʒ/ → [d͡ʑ, dʒ, ɟ͡ʝ]

/n/ → [n, ɲ, ŋ]

/l/ → [j, ʊ, (lj)]   /r/ → [w, ʊ, ɥ]

Simultaneous EPG recordings of the single word data from the perceptual corpus had been made using the Reading EPG3 (Hardcastle, Gibbon and Jones, 1991). These data gave a clear picture of lingual-palatal contact activity during speech production, which proved particularly useful for examining Danny's realizations of target alveolar and post-alveolar consonants. Although EPG cannot identify which part of the tongue is making contact with the palate, it gives very detailed information about certain aspects of lingual gestures over time and about lingual activity that may not be auditorily perceptible (see e.g. Hardcastle and Edwards, 1992; Howard and Varley, 1995).

Figure 18.1 shows a composite representation of lingualpalatal contact patterns for a selection of alveolar and post-alveolar consonant targets over a number of productions and in a number of contexts. This is based on a technique devised by Gibbon, (1990). Each item shows the frame of maximum lingualpalatal contact for each of six alveolar or post-alveolar targets using a percentage scale.

The most consistent patterns, revealing little inter-token variability, are those for target /s/ and /ʃ/. Perceptually realised as voiceless fricatives on the borders of the palatal/velar continuum, the EPG patterns confirm a consistent pattern of backing. The patterns for the two targets are very similar with only a suggestion of a slightly more anterior tendency towards /ʃ/.

A comparison of the contact patterns for /s/ and /t/ reveal some interesting differences. Fletcher (1989) suggests that /s/ emerges developmentally as a suppression of the closure phase of /t/ and that we would

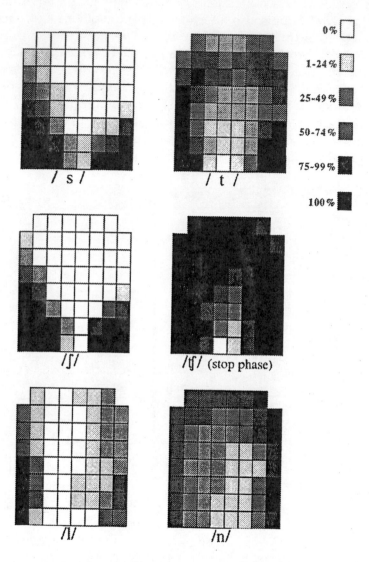

Figure 18.1. Lingual-palatal contact patterns for alveolar and post-alveolar consonant targets.

thus expect a very similar place of articulation for the two segments in any one individual's speech. For Danny, however, contact patterns for /t/ revealed a much more anterior articulation than for /s/, although, significantly, still with consistent narrowing in the region of the border of the hard and soft palates, echoing the contact patterns in this region for /s/ and /ʃ/. The fact that only one of the electrodes in the anterior region of the palate was contacted for 100% of the tokens could, from this method of representation, suggest that Danny never achieved the complete anterior closures necessary for plosive articulations. However, inspection of inter-token differences suggests an alternative explanation: Danny always made a complete closure for /t/ but the location and the width of closure varies markedly both between words and between multiple realizations of the same word.

Lingual palatal contact patterns for the frame of maximum contact in the stop phase of the target affricate /tʃ/ were very different from those for /t/ and identify quite consistently broad patterns of contact that extend more posteriorly over the palate, in anticipation of the velar fricative with which Danny realized the /ʃ/portion of the affricate. These patterns echo those found by Gibbon, (1994), illustrating the articulatory conflict which results for affricates for speakers who have markedly different places of articulation for targets /t/ and /ʃ/.

The target nasal /n/, like /t/, had very variable contact patterns. It was sometimes realized with an alveolar or post-alveolar closure but in postvocalic syllable final position the perceptual impression of an alveolar nasal sometimes appeared to consist of a heavily nasalized vocal element with very little evidence of lingual palatal contact.

The target alveolar lateral approximant /l/ was never judged as perceptually normal in the data and the EPG patterns confirm that this target was never articulated normally. Whereas /l/ is normally realized by contact between the tip or blade of the tongue and the alveolar ridge with some significant lowering of one or both sides of the tongue, in Danny's EPG data there were no examples where he achieved central alveolar contact and the most frequent contacts were made between the sides of the tongue and the lateral margins of the palate: Danny appeared to be doing the opposite of what is required for the successful articulation of this target. Subsequent EPG investigation of Danny's speech and also of non-speech oral movements revealed that, in trials over several weeks, Danny was never able to make a lingual contact at the alveolar ridge unless the sides of the tongue were elevated at the same time to make contact with the sides of the palate.

Discussion

Danny's problems in producing /l/ encapsulate the specific articulatory basis of his speech disorder at 13;10. He had particular difficulty with tip and blade target consonants which, taking his attempts at the articulation of /l/ into account, appeared to be linked not only to a habitual retracted setting of the tongue, but to specific anatomical or neuromuscular lingual impairment. It is significant that in the early literature ankyloglossia (tongue-tie) has been associated with Pierre Robin, although assessment of the full range of Danny's apical lingual movements did not immediately suggest this as a clear cut explanation for his specific articulatory deficit. The residual phonological impairment present at 6;1 had resolved, leaving a sound system where specific articulatory constraints undermined Danny's attempts to signal phonological contrasts. The specific nature of these articulatory deficits is being investigated further at the time of writing.

References

Argamaso RV (1992) Glossopexy for upper airway obstruction in Robin Sequence. Cleft Palate Craniofacial Journal 29: 232–38.

Bleile K (1993) Children with long-term tracheostomies. In Bleile K (Ed) The Care of Children with Long-term Tracheostomies. San Diego: Singular.

Fletcher SG (1989) Palatometric specification of stop, affricate and sibilant sounds. Journal of Speech and Hearing Research 32: 736–48.

Gibbon F (1990) Lingual activity in two speech disordered children's attempts to produce velar and alveolar stop consonants: evidence from electropalatographic (EPG) data. British Journal of Disorders of Communication 25: 1–14.

Gibbon F (1994) A description of affricate production in a group of speech-disordered children using electropalatography. Third Congress of the International Clinical Linguistics and Phonetics Association, Helsinki, Publications of the Department of Phonetics, University of Helsinki, pp 35–42.

Hardcastle WJ, Edwards S (1992) EPG-based descriptions of apraxic speech errors. In Kent R (Ed) Intelligibility in Speech Disorders: Theory, Measurement and Management. Philadelphia: John Benjamins, pp 287–328.

Hardcastle WJ, Gibbon F, Jones W (1991) Visual display of tongue-palate contact: electropalatography in the assessment and remediation of speech disorders. British Journal of Disorders of Communication 26: 41–74.

Howard SJ, Varley RA (1995) Acquired speech disorder: differential diagnosis using perceptual and instrumental analysis. In Perkins MR, Howard SJ (Eds) Case Studies in Clinical Linguistics. London: Whurr.

Sadewitz V (1992) Robin Sequence: changes in thinking leading to changes in patient care. Cleft Palate – Craniofacial Journal 29: 246–53.

Sher A (1992) Mechanisms of airway obstruction in Robin sequence: implications for treatment. Cleft Palate – Craniofacial Journal 29: 224–31.

Shprintzen RJ (1992) The implications of the diagnosis of Robin sequence. Cleft Palate – Craniofacial Journal 29: 205–9.

Stuffins GM (1989) The use of appliances in the treatment of speech problems in cleft palate. In Stengelhofen J (Ed) Cleft Palate: The Nature and Remediation of Communication Problems. London: Churchill Livingstone, pp 111–35.

Chapter 19
Cross-Language (Cantonese/English) Study of Articulatory Error Patterns in Cleft Palate Speech using Electropalatography (EPG)[1]

FIONA GIBBON, TARA L WHITEHILL, WILLIAM J HARDCASTLE, STEPHANIE F STOKES, AND MORAY NAIRN

Introduction

Cross-language studies of cleft palate speech are of particular interest since they provide unique evidence of the relative influence of biomechanical as opposed to linguistic features on the development of speech. Phonetic errors that arise as a direct consequence of the structural abnormality are predicted to occur in all languages. For example, one consequence of velopharyngeal dysfunction could be nasal realizations of obstruent targets. However, other types of speech errors could develop during the speech acquisition period due to the child actively compensating for a structural defect in order to produce maximally intelligible speech. The Eurocleft Speech Group (1994) state that such compensatory articulations 'do not result directly from the structural deficit: they result from strategies adopted by the speech production system to overcome or minimize the effects of this deficit' (p. 113). It is possible that a child acquiring one language could adopt quite different compensatory articulations from a child acquiring another language, depending on the phonology of the language being acquired, so giving rise to language-specific speech error patterns. These compensatory gestures can become habitual, and persist not only after the normal speech acquisition period but also after any earlier physiological or structural anomalies have been corrected – by surgery for example. It might be predicted that the physical constraints imposed by the oro-facial abnormality involved in cleft palate would override any language-specific differences. This has been the overall finding of studies that have investigated phonetic characteristics of cleft speech in a number of European languages (for example, the Eurocleft Speech Group, 1994). Studies investigating cleft-type speech errors in languages where the phonological systems are as different as Cantonese and English are par-ticularly valuable in identifying language-specific error patterns (e.g. Stokes and Whitehill, 1996)

Cantonese and English phonology

Cantonese is a Chinese dialect spoken by the majority of people in Hong Kong and neighbouring provinces. The Cantonese phonological system differs from English on a number of important dimensions. For example, in terms of contrastive segments in syllable initial position, there are fewer segments than in English (17 in Cantonese as opposed to 24 in English). All Cantonese oral stops are unvoiced, with aspirated and unaspirated cognates occurring in syllable initial position. There are three fricatives (one lingual) in Cantonese, constituting a smaller system than in English which has eight fricatives with four contrasting places of articulation, with voiced/voiceless cognates. Syllable structure is simpler in Cantonese than in English, with two clusters (kw and k^hw), although most people now view these as coarticulated (velar/bilabial) unit phonemes (Cheung, 1986). The languages differ in the distribu-tion of phonemes in syllable structure – for example, fricatives and affricates do not occur in syllable final position in Cantonese. The phonotactic structure of syllables in Cantonese is (C)V(V)(C) where parentheses indicate optional elements. This is simple, compared to English where it is possible to have sequences of up to three conson-ants in syllable initial and four in final position. Cantonese is a tone lan-guage. In other words tone operates lexically to change meaning. Historically the number of tones is controversial but six contrastive tones are generally accepted today (Cheung, 1986).

Perceptual characteristics of cleft-palate speech

Previous work on the phonetic characteristics of English cleft-palate speech, based largely on perceptual analyses, has revealed a number of speech abnormalities commonly found in these speakers. These abnor-malities include weakened obstruent sounds, a tendency for place of articulation to be retracted (particularly for plosive and fricative sounds) the occurrence of double articulations, secondary articulations (especially velarization and glottalization) and the presence of nasal emission during the production of obstruent sounds (Stengelhofen, 1989; and see Harding and Grunwell, 1996, for a recent review). In a perceptual study of seven Cantonese-speaking children with cleft palate (Stokes and Whitehill, 1996) abnormalities were identified that have not typically been noted for English-speakers. Specifically, three children deleted initial consonants and two children produced bilabial fricatives for /s/ targets. Deletion of initial consonants has also been found by Dodd and So (1994) in Cantonese children with hearing impairment. Both studies have hypothesized that the functional load of tones in Cantonese permits speakers to maintain contrast by relying on tone rather than on initial consonants in certain contexts.

EPG characteristics of cleft-palate speech

A variety of EPG error patterns has been found to be typical of cleft-palate speech (see Hardcastle and Gibbon, 1997, for a review). In particular, spatial distortions have been reported extensively, which involve both excessive and more posterior tongue palate contact than that found in normal speakers. A number of general categories emerge (see Suzuki, Yamashita, Michi and Ueno, 1981; Yamashita and Michi, 1991; Yamashita, Michi, Imai, Suzuki and Yoshida, 1992) including lateralized articulations, palatal/velar place of articulation and nasopharyngeal articulations (Hardcastle and Gibbon, 1997, give a description of the EPG patterns that typically accompany these categories). Although double articulations have long been recognized as being characteristic of cleft-palate speech, EPG has revealed a specific type (Gibbon and Hardcastle, 1989; Dent, Gibbon and Hardcastle, 1992) involving complete velar constriction. These types of double articulations are not obvious from a perceptual analysis. In a study by Whitehill, Stokes, Hardcastle and Gibbon (1995) simultaneous alveolar/velar lingual contact during production of velar targets was noted in two Cantonese-speaking children who had residual alveolar clefts that were unobturated at the time of the recording. These authors hypothesized that the tongue tip/blade was being raised in an attempt to 'block' the alveolar cleft.

Method

The aim of this study was to extend the work of Stokes and Whitehill (1996) by examining EPG data from two groups of speakers (Cantonese and English) with speech disorders associated with cleft palate. For this study EPG recordings were made of 10 subjects from each language (mean age for Cantonese speakers – 11 years; mean age for English speakers – 13 years). The Reading EPG3 system was used (Hardcastle, Gibbon and Jones, 1991). The subjects were consecutive referrals to the respective centres in Hong Kong and UK, and were referred for EPG therapy because of significant ongoing speech problems, which were not resolving. They were not controlled for age, medical history, type of cleft or the presence or extent of velopharyngeal dysfunction (see Table 19.1 for subject details). One normal control was used in each group. Segments (target sounds) that were common to both languages were selected from a large corpus of speech data for the purpose of this study (/p, pʰ, t, tʰ, s, n, k, kʰ, l/ in Cantonese and /p, b, t, d, s, n, k, g, l/ in English – see the Appendix to this chapter).

Table 19.1 Subject details. Key: CA - chronological age; REPAIR - age (in months) at primary repair; N/A - not applicable (non-cleft speakers); UCLP(r) - right unilateral cleft lip and palate; UCLP(l) - left unilateral cleft lip and palate; BCLP - bilateral cleft lip and palate; CVPD - congenital velopharyngeal disproportion; CP - cleft palate only; WNL - within normal limits; HI - hearing impairment; VPI - velopharyngeal insufficiency; HxVPI - history of velopharyngeal incompetence, now resolved; M - male; F - female; PriorTx - history of prior speech therapy.

SUBJECTS	CA	REPAIR	TYPECLEFT	HEARING	VPI	M/F	OCCLUSION	PRIOR TX
Cantonese								
WHK	11	N/A	N/A	WNL	WNL	M	Normal	No
CSY	7	36	UCLP(r)	WNL	Hx VPI	F	Class III	Yes
CYK	8	36	BCLP	HI	WNL	M	Class III	Yes
LWK	11	16	UCLP(1)	WNL	WNL	M	Class III	Yes
LHZ	9	18	BCLP	WNL	VPI	M	Class III	Yes
KYM	4	22	UCLP(r)	WNL	WNL	M	Class III	No
LKF	17	168	BCLP	WNL	VPI	F	Normal	No
LWY	13	18	BCLP	WNL	VPI	M	Class III	Yes
HMC	5	12	UCLP(l)	HI	VPI	M	Class III	No
ICC	20	12	UCLP(l)	WNL	VPI	M	Class III	Yes
SHW	7	24	UCLP(r)	HI	VPI	F	Class III	Yes
English								
AW	12;04	N/A	N/A	WNL	WNL	M	Normal	No
BY	12;0	18	UCLP(l)	WNL	Hx VPI	M	Class III	Yes
CB	8;08	58	CVPD	WNL	Hx VPI	F	Normal	Yes
ED	10;0	20	CP	WNL	Hx VPI	F	Normal	Yes
GR	11;01	36	UCLP(r)	WNL	Hx VPI	M	Normal	Yes
GB	8;06	50	CVPD	WNL	Hx VPI	M	Normal	Yes
PB	9;07	36	UCLP(l)	HI	VPI	M	Class III	Yes
SH	8;02	13	CP	WNL	Hx VPI	M	Normal	Yes
TG	8;11	73	CVPD	HI	Hx VPI	M	Normal	Yes
RM	20;07	36	UCLP (l)	WNL	Hx VPI	M	Class III	Yes
DS	36;00	18	UCLP (l)	WNL	Hx VPI	M	Class III	Yes

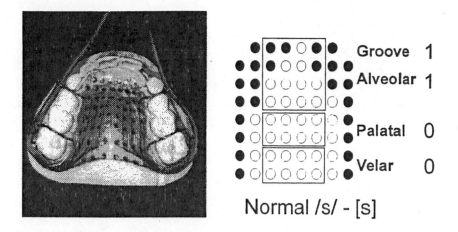

Figure 19.1. A photograph of an EPG palate is shown on the left, and an individual EPG palatogram illustrating the profiling scheme shown on the right (see text for details).

EPG classification scheme

A profiling scheme was developed to characterize the articulatory features of each subject. The rationale for the EPG profiling scheme was that it should be quick and easy to use, that it should include phonetic and clinically meaningful parameters and that it should enable comparison between normal and abnormal EPG patterns. The profiling procedure involved firstly selecting the EPG frame of maximum constriction from the full EPG printout for the target sounds. Each frame extracted was then classified according to the following binary scheme:

Constriction in the alveolar zone: 1 = yes; 0 = no;
Constriction in the palatal zone: 1 = yes; 0 = no;
Constriction in the velar zone: 1 = yes; 0 = no;
Presence of a groove: 1 = yes; 0 = no;

The classification was based on tongue/palate contact made in three regions (alveolar, palatal, velar) of the central zone (the central four electrodes in any of the eight rows) of the artificial palate (see Figure 19.1). Constriction was defined as involving a minimum of two electrodes contacted in the central zone in any row. The presence of a groove was indicated by a channel of uncontacted electrodes, which could exist in the posterior region or extend into the anterior region of the palate. In the posterior region, the channel had to be 1 to 2 uncontacted electrodes in width in rows 5–8, and in the anterior region, the channel had to be 1 to 3 uncontacted electrodes wide in rows 1–4 of the palate.

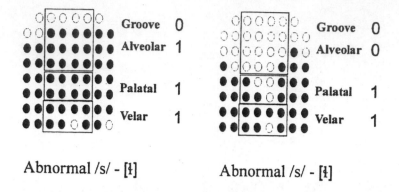

Abnormal /s/ - [ɬ]   Abnormal /s/ - [ɬ]

Figure 19.2. Examples of two abnormal EPG patterns from different English speakers to illustrate the classification system. Both productions were transcribed as alveolar lateral fricatives. The different EPG characteristics are captured by the binary classification shown to the right of each palatogram.

	Groove	Anterior	Palatal	Velar	IPA
p	0	0	0	0	p
b	0	0	0	0	b
t	0	0	1	1	t
d	0	1	1	1	ɟ
s	0	1	1	1	ɬ
n	0	1	1	1	n
k	0	1	1	1	k
g	0	1	1	1	g
l	0	0	0	0	l

Figure 19.3. Profile of EPG error patterns for one English cleft speaker (DS), based on the classification system described (see text for details). Shaded boxes indicate abnormality.

Two examples of abnormal productions of /s/ targets, with the appropriate EPG classifications are shown in Figure 19.2. Both of these productions were heard as alveolar lateral fricatives. It can be seen from the EPG palatograms that neither has a central groove and both have abnormal palatal and velar contact. One obvious difference between the two EPG patterns is that the left-hand one has contact that extends into the alveolar region. This difference is reflected in the error classifications. Figure 19.3 shows the EPG profile of one English cleft speaker (DS), where shading indicates abnormal EPG or perceptual classification (IPA symbol). For this speaker, there was abnormal velar/palatal EPG contact for alveolar obstruents although these were not heard as abnormal. There was also abnormal anterior contact for velar targets. Bilabials had no lingual contact and were heard as acceptable productions (i.e. normal) and from this it is possible to conclude that bilabials presented no problems for this speaker.

Results

EPG/perceptual features found in both languages

The EPG patterns were examined statistically for cross-language differences. None of the phoneme-by-zone-by-group data were significant. Although there were some differences between English and Cantonese in EPG contact patterns, these differences were not significant. For example, more of the English speakers had maximum constriction in the velar zone for /s/ (six out of 10) than the Cantonese-speakers (two out of 10) but the difference was not statistically significant ($V = 3.17$, $p > 0.05$, chi-square $= 0.17$). Similarly, although more of the English speakers had maximum constriction in the alveolar zone for /d/, (eight out of 10) than did the Cantonese speakers (five out of nine – there was one missing datum), this difference was also not statistically significant ($V = 1.24$, $p > 0.05$, chi-square $= 0.07$).

Thus, a number of error patterns were found in both the Cantonese and English cleft-palate speakers (see Table 19.2). Over half of the Cantonese and English subjects produced anterior targets (/b, p, t, d, l, n, s/) with excessive contact in the posterior regions of the EPG palate, in other words in the palatal/velar regions. The remaining group produced all lingual targets (/t, d, k, g, l, n, s/) with minimal EPG contact. For these sounds the site of constriction was inferred from the perceptual analysis. This auditory-based analysis suggested that speakers were producing these sounds either further back than the most posterior row of EPG electrodes, for example in the pharyngeal or glottal regions, or further forward than the most anterior row of EPG electrodes, for example in the dental or labial regions. In addition, in both languages /s/ targets were produced by many of the subjects with complete constriction across the palate, in other words with no groove present. These productions were variously realized as lateralized or nasal fricatives.

Table 19.2 EPG/perceptual features found in both languages

	Cantonese %	English %
Complete constriction across the palate for /s/	40	60
EPG contact in posterior regions for anterior targets	60	70
Minimal tongue palate contact for lingual targets	40	30

EPG/perceptual language-specific features

Some features were evident in the Cantonese data only (see Table 19.3). Alternations of n/l were found in Cantonese, but not in the English data. This is not a cleft-type error pattern, and can be directly attributable to a sound change that is currently occurring in the language, where /n/ usage in syllable initial position in the younger generation is in decline (Cheung, 1986). There were, however, some differences between the languages in the realization of /s/, with bilabial fricatives occurring only in the Cantonese data set. Some features were evident only in the English data. For example, double labial-velar articulations for bilabial targets were found in two of the 10 speakers. Two of the English speakers had nasal escape of air during production of /s/ targets (and complete velar constriction during their production) but a central airstream for /ʃ/ targets.

Table 19.3 EPG/perceptual features found in either Cantonese or English

	Cantonese %	English %
n/l alternations	60	0
bilabial fricatives for /s/ targets	20	0
anterior EPG contact plus velar constriction for /k, kʰ/ targets	20	0
labial/velar double articulations for /p, b/	0	20
complete EPG constriction plus nasal friction for /s/ targets	0	20

Phonemes most likely to show error patterns

In order to quantify which phonemes were most susceptible to error, data derived from the EPG classification were subjected to statistical analysis (chi-square). This analysis revealed (for groups collapsed together) the following overall pattern of vulnerability to disruption (with /t/ being the most vulnerable):

$$/t/ \rightarrow /s/ \rightarrow /d/ \rightarrow /k/ \rightarrow /g/ \rightarrow /n/ \rightarrow /l/ \rightarrow /b/ + /p/$$

The order of susceptibility of phonemes for Cantonese and English was essentially the same in the sense that lingual obstruents were the most vulnerable, followed by liquids with bilabial stops the least likely to be produced as errors. The order for each language was as follows:

Cantonese: /t/ → /k/ → /s/ → /d/ → /g/ → /n/ → /l/ → /b/+/p/

English: /s/ → /d/ → /t/ → /k/ → /g/ → /n+l/ → /b/+/p/

The difference in ordering of the first four phonemes may be indicative of a sampling artefact (small sample size). Table 19.4 shows the percentage of accuracy (in terms of EPG patterns) of each phoneme for Cantonese and English cleft speakers.

Table 19.4 The percentage of accurate EPG patterns for each phoneme in Cantonese and English

Target phoneme	Cantonese % Correct	English % Correct
/t/	10	30
/k/	20	50
/s/	40	10
/d/	40	20
/g/	40	60
/n/	70	60
/l/	80	60
/b/	100	80
/p/	100	80

Discussion

The data from the classification system revealed several error patterns that were common to both languages, most obviously retracted place of articulation. Retracted articulations were also found in the Eurocleft Speech Group (1994) study and may be a language-universal feature of cleft-palate speech. A number of possible factors may be related to this widespread finding. For example, the need to build up oral pressure for lingual and labial obstruent targets in the presence of velopharyngeal dysfunction might result in the development of compensatory pharyngeal and glottal articulations since these are the only available regions of the vocal tract where air pressure build-up is possible. A similar phenomenon might occur where an oral fistula is present, resulting in palatal or velar articulations. As expected the cleft speakers from both languages had the greatest difficulty with lingual obstruents, followed by liquids, with bilabials being the least vulnerable to disruption. Target /s/ was realized as a lateralized fricative by some speakers in both languages. Lateralized articulations are usually produced with increased

EPG tongue contact and this increased contact may be related to a lack of tactile feedback in the alveolar region. Another possible factor is the presence of abnormal palate shape, dental anomalies or malocclusion, although the relationship between these factors and speech error patterns has not been investigated systematically to date.

Some features were noted in the Cantonese speakers that have not been reported as occurring frequently in English speakers. For example, there were some differences in the realization of /s/ targets in the two languages. As in the previous work by Stokes and Whitehill (1996), bilabial fricatives were found to occur only in the Cantonese data set. This has not been found widely in English cleft speech either in this study or in other studies that have used perceptual analysis (Harding and Grunwell, 1996). The phenomenon of initial consonant deletion, reported by Stokes and Whitehill (1996) as occurring in some Cantonese cleft speakers, was not recorded in this study. Finally, two of the English speakers produced nasal fricatives for /s/ targets, but produced a central airstream for /ʃ/ targets, resulting in a distinction between these two phonemes which could be identified easily by listeners. It is possible that these speakers were attempting to produce a clear contrast for these targets, a requirement for English but not for Cantonese.

The results of this study support previous findings that language-specific error patterns do occur, at least for cleft speakers of languages that are as different as Cantonese and English (Stokes and Whitehill, 1996). There is clearly a need for more studies of this type to look more closely at the effects of the target phonology on compensatory articulations. In particular, more cross-linguistic studies of other languages such as Putonghua, which has a large number of fricative contrasts, are needed to investigate the effect of the size of the fricative inventory on compensatory strategies.

Extracting phonetically useful information quickly from EPG recordings is a practical problem, particularly in the clinical setting, and the classification system described in this paper does appear to be useful for this purpose. However, a relatively small amount of speech data was analysed in this study, so verification is needed with larger numbers of subjects and greater amounts of speech data. A preliminary attempt to establish the reliability of the profiling system was encouraging, although this will need to be investigated in a more systematic way in future studies.

References

Cheung, KL (1986) The phonology of present day Cantonese. Unpublished doctoral dissertation: University College, London.

Dodd BJ, So LKH (1994) The phonological abilities of Cantonese-speaking children with hearing loss. Journal of Speech and Hearing Research 37: 671–79.

Dent H, Gibbon F, Hardcastle WJ (1992) Inhibiting an abnormal lingual pattern in a cleft palate child using electropalatography (EPG). In: Leahy MM, Kallen JL (Eds) Interdisciplinary Perspectives in Speech and Language Pathology. University of Dublin, Trinity College, Eire. 211–21.

Eurocleft Speech Group: Brondsted K, Grunwell P, Henningsson G, Jansonius K, Karling J, Meijer M, Ording U, Sell D, Vermeij-Zieverink E, Wyatt R (1994) A phonetic framework for the cross-linguistic analysis of cleft palate speech. Clinical Linguistics and Phonetics 8: 109–25.

Gibbon F, Hardcastle WJ (1989) Deviant articulation in a cleft palate child following late repair of the hard palate: a description and remediation procedure using Electropalatography (EPG). Clinical Linguistics and Phonetics 3: 93–110.

Hardcastle WJ, Gibbon F (1997) Electropalatography and its clinical applications. In: Ball MJ, Code C (Eds) Instrumental Clinical Phonetics (2nd edition). Whurr Publishers: London. 149–93.

Hardcastle WJ, Gibbon FE, Jones W (1991) Visual display of tongue-palate contact: Electropalatography in the assessment and remediation of speech disorders. British Journal of Disorders of Communication 26: 41–74.

Harding A, Grunwell P (1996) Characteristics of cleft palate speech. European Journal of Disorders of Communication 31: 331–57.

Stengelhofen J (1989) The nature and causes of communication problems in cleft palate. In: Stengelhofen J (Ed) Cleft Palate. Edinburgh: Churchill Livingstone.

Stokes SF, Whitehill TL (1996) Speech error patterns in Cantonese speaking children with cleft palate. European Journal of Disorders of Communication 31: 45–64.

Suzuki N, Yamashita Y, Michi K, Ueno T (1981) Changes of the palatolingual contact during articulation therapy in the cleft palate patients: Observation by use of dynamic palatography. Paper presented at the 4th International Congress of Cleft Palate and Related Craniofacial Abnormalities, Acapulco, Mexico, May 1981.

Whitehill T, Stokes S, Hardcastle W, Gibbon F (1995) Electropalatographic and perceptual analysis of the speech of Cantonese children with cleft palate. European Journal of Disorders of Communication 30: 193–202.

Yamashita Y, Michi K (1991) Misarticulation caused by abnormal lingual-palatal contact in patients with cleft palate with adequate velopharyngeal function. Cleft Palate-Craniofacial Journal 28: 360–6.

Yamashita Y, Michi K, Imai S, Suzuki N, Yoshida H (1992) Electropalatographic investigation of abnormal lingual-palatal contact patterns in cleft palate patients. Clinical Linguistics and Phonetics 6: 210–17.

Note

1 This research was supported by grants from the British Council/HK Research Grants Council (JRS 92/48), the Simon KY Lee Research Fund (Grant no. 375/050/7216) and CRCG (Grant no. 337/050/0007) from the University of Hong Kong. Thanks are due to Hilary Dent and Wilf Jones for their assistance and to all the subjects and families for their participation.

Appendix: speech material.

	Cantonese	English
Target phonemes	/p, pʰ, t, tʰ, s, n, k, kʰ, l/	/p, b, t, d, s, n, k, g, l/
Examples of words	/t/-dek, /tʰ/-tek, /s/-sek,	/p/-puddle, /s/-circus,
	/k/-geng, /kʰ/-kek, /l/-lin.	/k/-castle, /g/-gold, /n/-nose.

Chapter 20
Phonetic Development in Children with Cochlear Implants Trained Using the Auditory-Verbal Philosophy

LINDA DANIEL, M HENOCH, MARTIS OKON, RAY DANILOFF, TRACEY M. JONES, KARRIE SURBER

Introduction

The benefits received from a cochlear implant during the post-implant period depend upon the age of onset of hearing loss and language level at onset, hearing level, age of subject at implantation, type and individual's use of implant fitted, integrity of cognitive/neuromuscular systems, and the type and intensity of habilitation-rehabilitation (Tyler, 1993). To date most research on speech production in implanted children reports on training that involves total communication or classroom-based oral communication (Hasenstab and Tobey, 1991; Tobey, Angelette, and Marchison, 1991; Tobey, Pancamo, Steller, Brimacombe, and Beiter, 1991; Tyler, 1991; Tye-Murray, Spencer, and Woodworth, 1995). Systematic use of intensive auditory-verbal (AV) has recently been reported (Bertram, 1995; Rice, Gibki, Marciano, Shakes, and Bissaker, 1995 Grogan, Barker, Dettman and Blamey, 1995; Daniel, 1996, 1997). The AV-rehabilitation philosophy (Pollack, 1985) has been applied by Daniel, (1990, 1996) to children with cochlear implants. The AV method used by Daniel typically involves two 60-minute intensive training sessions per week with the child, the therapist and at least one parent in attendance. Parents observe and participate in each therapy session and are programmed to provide AV instruction to the child seven days per week throughout their daily communicative routines. The AV philosophy focuses upon redirecting the child's selective attention from visual input to auditory input. The initial months of AV training include use of gesture, toys and props to train children to react to combinations of gestures and simple and complex non-speech, nonsense speech, and simple words so that auditory attention, identification, searching, discrimination, recall, association, etc can be acquired before therapist and parent become dyadic partners in early verbal interchange with the child. The lessons partake of whole language methods and procedures (Norris and Hoffman 1993) as the instruction and learning become sufficiently complex to sustain mainstreaming some children into an all-hearing classroom. To date, the first author has succeeded in mainstreaming 12/24 implanted children throughout the country with another 14 in training. The present study reports growth of phonetic production in three children enrolled in her training programme. The data were phonetically transcribed, using Tait (1993) and Tait and Lutman's (1994) protocols, from video tapes made of each formal training session over a specified post-implantation period. The speech produced underestimates the length and complexity of utterance somewhat since much of the discourse is didactic rather than more relaxed play or family-interaction scenes of discourse (Okon, 1995).

Subjects

Table 20.1 lists essential characteristics of the three very different children reported herein. The youngest, child 'A', commenced AV therapy at 16 months. Initially she wore binaural hearing aids (HAs) with FM inconsistently for four months and at 20 months wore a TRANSONIC transposition aid more successfully for two months before implantation with a NUCLEUS 22 prosthesis. At the period of implantation, she generally uttered to her parent a few meaningless, monosyllabic vocalizations with flat pitch and 'nasalization'. After 5 months of AV training her utterances became contingent on therapist utterances (turn-taking); and nasality and mono-pitch declined rapidly (Okon, 1995).

At the onset of training, with 40-50 dB HL across the speech frequencies, she silently 'mouthed' simple labial CV syllables in response to speech directed at her. Her MLU remained at 1.0 throughout (Figure 20.2). Her utterance productivity rose from 11 at the first post-implant session to a peak of 53 at two months (Figure 20.7). Use of diverse syllable types rose from 2 to 7-9, but no consonant clusters (Figure 20.3) ever emerged. Vowel diversity (Figure 20.1) rose from 1 to 8; canonical syllable strings and slightly later, variegated syllable string (Figures 20.5, 20.8) emerged during training. Over five months, this child, who initially used groans, screams, and occasional monosyllables progressed through babbling and began to reply to speech directed at her with oral

monosyllables with substantial vocalic, consonantal, and syllable structure diversity (Figures 20.1 to 20.8). For five months she recapitulated
elements of her earlier babbling and was poised on the verge of producing her first meaningful words during training. Parental report indicated in the fifth month of training that she had uttered her first words at
home, so these data probably underestimate her phonetic competence.
Therapy was discontinued on 30 August 1995 when the family situation
changed.

Table 20.1. Subject Characteristics From: Caseload of Linda A. Daniel, M.A. CCC-A,
M.S. Comm. Dis.

	Child A	Child B	Child C
Age at loss: Etiology:	birth CMV infection	birth 'KIDS' syndrome	birth unknown
Physical disability:	mild cerebral palsy in lower extremities	—	—
Age at implant:	24 months	90 months	33 months
Non-verbal intelligence:	developmentally 'normal' MacArthur, DOCS tests	normal (clinical impression); Symptoms of mild learning disability	normal (clinical impression)
Therapy prior to implant:	auditory verbal (8 months)	total communication (60 months)	auditory verbal (15 months)
Implant:	NUCLEUS 22	NUCLEUS 22	NUCLEUS 22
HA use:	TRANSONIC HA, 60dB HL @ the low frequencies	bilateral HA, 45–70dB HL, sloping across speech frequencies	bilateral HA, with FM; HL @ 45–75 dB HL, sloping across speech frequencies
Prosthesis use:	40–50dB HL across speech-frequencies with NUCLEUS	40–45dB HL across speech-frequencies with NUCLEUS	35–45dB HL across speech- frequencies with NUCLEUS

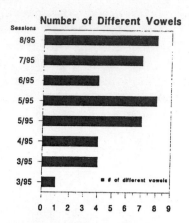

Figure 20.1. Number of different vowels for child A

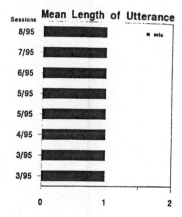

Figure 20.2. Mean utterance length for child A

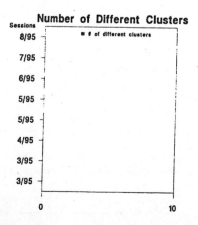

Figure 20.3. Number of different clusters for child A

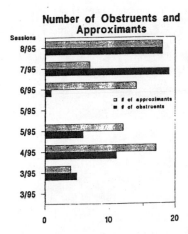

Figure 20.4. Number of obstruents and approximants for child A

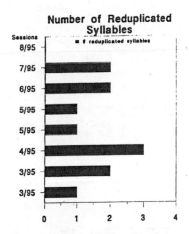

Figure 20.5. Number of reduplicated syllables for child A

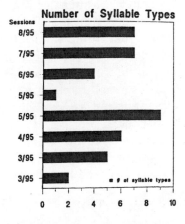

Figure 20.6. Number of syllable types for child A

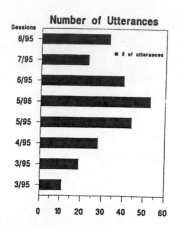

Figure 20.7. Number of utterances for child A

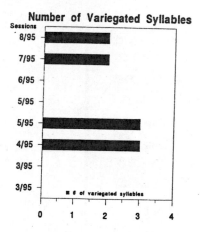

Figure 20.8. Number of variegated syllables for child A

Child 'B' entered therapy at age 7;6 after five years of total communication training using bilateral hearing aids. Selected samples, covering 1½ years of child B's extensive recordings made during therapy, were analysed. This female child exhibited 'KIDS' genetic syndrome, and manifested mild to moderate learning disabilities, with a clinical impression of otherwise age-normal intellectual development. She received a NUCLEUS 22 implant at age 7;6 and achieved 40—45 dB HL throughout the speech frequencies. She continued to sign spontaneously during therapy for months after implantation. Her rated intelligibility rose from 0 to four (on an eight-point scale) and nasality was minimal at the last session reported. The first author, familiar with her speech, said that it was 60 to 70% intelligible during her last reported therapy session and two years later (1997) is nearly 80% intelligible to familiar listeners.

Child 'B''s relatively diverse phonetic repertoire, at the start, matched that of a normal 2½ year old (Vihman, 1996). In 1½ years of AV training, her MLU (Figure 20.15) tripled (2.65 to 6.43), utterance productivity (Figure 20.12) soared (in the last session) from 153 to 830, the number of clusters (Figure 20.11) produced rose from 46 to 89 and diversity of cluster types (Figure 20.9) roughly doubled from 10 to 21. The number of approximants (Figure 20.13) used in a session increased almost fivefold (148-624), while obstruents (Figure 20.16) (most stops) nearly doubled (418-755). The predominant initial CV syllable structure declined from 75% to 55% of utterances. Use of different syllable structures (Figure 20.9) did not increase in number. In 18 months, this child rose from the developmental level of a 2½-year-old to that of a 4-year-old. Her vocal quality and intelligibility rose well, and with the exception of syllable types and diversity, her utterances reflected swift development of oral competence.

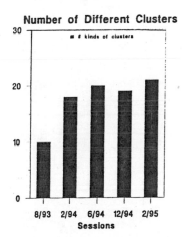

Figure 20.9. Number of different clusters for child B

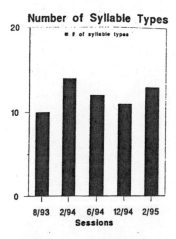

Figure 20.10. Number of syllable types for child B

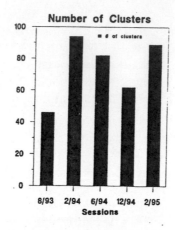

Figure 20.11. Number of clusters for child B

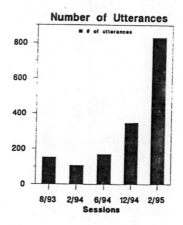

Figure 20.12. Number of utterances for child B

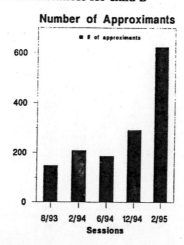

Figure 20.13. Number of approximants for child B

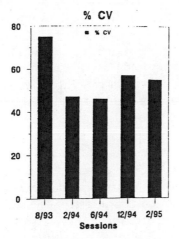

Figure 20.14. Percentage of CV-syllables for child B

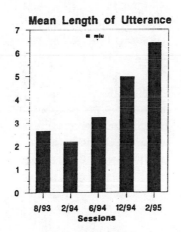

Figure 20.15. Mean utterance length for child B

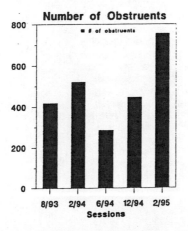

Figure 20.16. Number of obstruents for child B

Child 'C' suffered congenital deafness. He received binaural hearing aids at 17 months and 14 months later, a NUCLEUS 22 implant at 31 months. He had 15 months of pre-implant AV therapy with an effective HL of 95 dB. He had acquired 76 different monosyllabic words by the time of implantation. He was in training from 17 months to the present (1997), and was mainstreamed into his neighbourhood hearing classroom. His developmental path is especially well-detailed (48 months).

Implant thresholds were obtained from 35-45 dB across the speech frequency range. While his MLU during post-implant training rose only to 4.54 at the last session, it must be cautioned that one- and two-word utterances suffice for much of the activities used in each training session. Anecdotal parental reports indicate near age-normal conversational MLU, use of the telephone, out-of-sight verbal communication, and so forth.

Over the 54-month AV training period, his MLU for lessons nearly tripled (1.21 to 4.54). The MLU at the first lesson post-implant was 1.84. Total utterances (Figure 20.24) were up sixfold (51 to 375), syllable productivity (Figure 20.24) increased nineteenfold (94-1704), obstruent consonants (Figure 20.19) nearly tripled and cluster usage (Figure 20.21) increased almost 25 times (from six to 169). This child's development was more smoothly synchronous, probably because of early and lengthy auditory verbal training, and lack of mild neurological complications characteristic of child 'B'. This child's acquisition resembled that of normal peers, except that it was somewhat slower overall. His rated intelligibility score increased from 3.5 to 9.0, suggesting near normal intelligibility, which complemented his high phonetic quality.

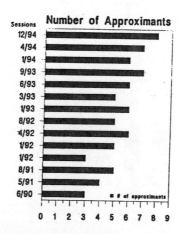

Figure 20.17. Number of approximants for child C

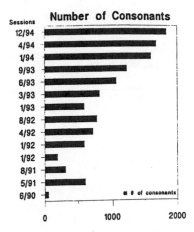

Figure 20.18. Number of consonants for child C

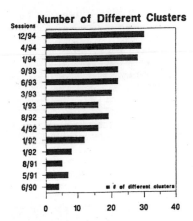

Figure 20.19. Number of different clusters for child C

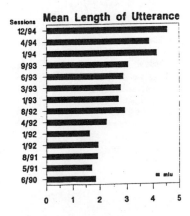

Figure 20.20. Mean length of utterances for child C

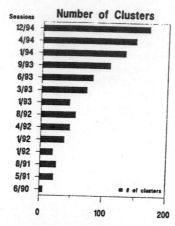

Figure 20.21. Number of clusters for child C

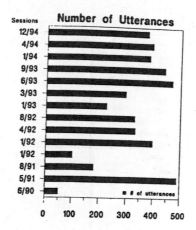

Figure 20.22. Number of utterances for child C

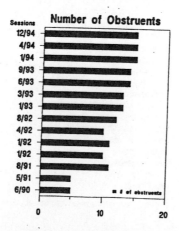

Figure 20.23. Number of obstruents for child C

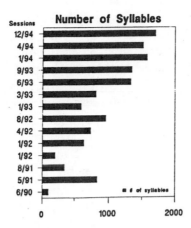

Figure 20.24. Number of syllables for child C

Discussion

For child 'A', eight months of AV therapy (five months post-implant) brought hypernasal-flat pitch occasional monosyllalbes to the threshold of non-nasal, inflected, first words. Single utterances of up to five entrained syllables were being produced with growth from glottal stops only to 20 total approximants [m, ɰ, j, n, ŋ, ɹ] and obstruents [t, d, v, b, h, p, g, k, χ] and eight different vowels [i, ɪ, ɛ, ʌ, æ, ʊ, oʊ, a] by the last session. This is a rich phonological inventory typical of a normal 3-year-old (Vihman,1996) Equally interesting reduplicated and variegated babble appeared for the first time along with tripling of the number of syllable types. The child clearly took conversational turns with monosyllabic commentary upon auditory stimulation and physical movements. The child's use of visible silent imitations of syllables/words spoken by the therapist was a prelude to verbal imitation in the last three sessions.

For child 'B', 7;6 years old at implantation, after five years of wearing a bilateral hearing aid in a total communication setting, substantial but less rapid growth occurred. Among attainments during the 18-month-long post-implant training were the following: a doubling of the number of different clusters used, a quadrupling of utterances used in a session, a tripling of the number of approximate consonants and near doubling of the number of obstruents — along with a near tripling of the child's MLU. The percentage of simple, open CV forms declined by about 27%. The child's rated intelligibility had more than doubled, and continues to increase. This reflects remarkable progress in the acquisition of phonetic forms.

For child 'C', who was only 2;7 at the time of the implant, the results present a record of more-or-less smoothly incremental acquisition of phonetic forms across the board. The percentage increases ranged from

260% to about 860%. The increases were relatively monotonic, and the formal training sessions underestimated the richness of production manifested by the child in the family home. This child was successfully mainstreamed into a normal hearing classroom.

It should be emphasized that the didactic AV lessons make use of specific visual and sometimes tactile sensations and experiences to accompany the ever-present emphasized auditory stimulation. This bi- and tri-modal stimulation is important in early stages of AV training, as are many exercises in which vocal pitch, intonation, and the rhythm of many vocalizations are heavily stylized and emphasized to facilitate the child's perception and to stimulate the development of an auditory feedback system.

Whereas detailed acoustic, pragmatic, syntactic and lexical analyses are under way on double the number of implanted children, we can say with confidence that children as old as 7 or 8 can profit greatly from one to 1½ years of AV training. Five months of such training brought a 24-month-old from occasional nasal vowels to the edge of the first word stage. Child 'C', an otherwise normal 33-month-old, was successfully mainstreamed six years later. These data, coupled with a clinical record of 16 clients who only wore hearing aids and who were successfully mainstreamed after four to six years of AV therapy, suggest that AV therapy permits the therapist to use cochlear prosthesis' power so that communication based on speaking and listening is attainable. Some implanted children can maintain face-to-face conversations with natural speech; others require their interlocutors to use 'clear speech' input for maximum message comprehension. The financial and social investment of the parents is very great, but so are the rewards and outcomes.

References

Bertram B (1995) Importance of auditory-verbal education and parents participation after cochlear implantation of very young children. In Clark GM, Cowan RSC (Eds) International Cochlear Implant, Speech and Hearing Symposium-Melbourne, 1994. In Supplement 166 Vol. 104(9), part 2 – Annals of Otology, Rhinology and Laryngology. St Louis: Annals Publishing Co, pp 97–100.

Clark GM, Cowan RSC (1995) International Cochlear Implant, Speech and Hearing Symposium, Melbourne, 1994. In: Supplement 166 Vol. 104(9), part 2 – Annals of Otology, Rhinology and Laryngology. St. Louis: Annals Publishing Co.

Daniel L (1990) The Auditory – Verbal philosophy. In The Auditory – Verbal Network, Inc, pp. 2–4.

Daniel L (1996) An auditory processing approach to aural rehabilitation. Seminar presented at American Academy of Audiology workshop, Salt Lake City.

Daniel, L (1997) Personal communication with AV Society members, M Ernst, K Vivian-Rothwell, J Hutchinson.

Grogan ML, Barker EJ, Dettman SJ, Blamey PJ (1995). In Clark GM, Cowan, RSC (Eds) International Cochlear Implant, Speech and Hearing Symposium –

Melbourne, 1994. In Supplement 166 Vol.104(9) Part 2 – Annals of Otology, Rhinology and Laryngology. St.Louis: Annals Publishing Co, pp. 390–3.

Hasenstab MS, Tobey E (1991) Language development in children receiving Nucleus multichannel cochlear implants. Ear and Hearing 12: 555–655.

Norris J, Hoffman P (1993) Whole Language Intervention for School-Age Children. San Diego, CA: Singular Publishing Co.

Okon MR (1995) Early communicative behaviors in a two year old child with a cochlear implant in an Auditory-Verbal program. Thesis: University of North Texas.

Pollack D (1985) Educational Audiology for the Limited-Hearing Infant and Preschooler. Springfield, IL: CC Thomas.

Rice JC, Gibki SJ, Marciano T, Shakes RK, Bissaker KA (1995) Implants in children: the first two years of the South Australian Program. In Clark GM, Cowan RSC (Eds) Cochlear Implant, Speech and Hearing Symposium – Melbourne, 1994. In Supplement 166 Vol. 104(9), Part 2 – Annals of Otology, Rhinology and Laryngology. St. Louis: Annals Publishing Co., pp. 83–5.

Tait DM (1993) Video analysis: a method of assessing changes in pre-verbal and early linguistic communication after cochlear implantation. Ear and Hearing 14: 378–89.

Tait DM, Lutman ME (1994) Comparisons of early communicative behavior in young children with cochlear implants and with hearing aids. Ear and Hearing 15: 352–61.

Tobey E, Angelette S, Marchison C (1991) Speech production performances in children with multichannel cochlear implants. American Journal of Otology 12 (supp.): 165–73.

Tobey E, Pancamo S, Steller S, Brimacombe J, Beiter A (1991) Consonant production in children receiving a multichannel cochlear implant. Ear and Hearing 12: 23–31.

Tye-Murray N, Spencer L, Woodworth G (1995) Acquisition of speech by children who have prolonged cochlear implant experience. Journal of Speech and Hearing Research 38: 327–37.

Tyler R (1991) What can we learn about hearing aids from cochlear implants? Ear and Hearing Vol 6 Suppl. 177–86.

Tyler R (1993) Cochlear Implants: Audiological Foundations. San Diego, CA: Singular Publishing Co.

Vihman M (1996) Phonological Development: The Origins of Language in the Child. Oxford: Blackwell.

Non-linguistic aspects

Chapter 21
The Cognitive Basis of Pragmatic Disability

MICHAEL R. PERKINS

Introduction

The problem

'Pragmatic disability' and other cognate terms are used to describe an excessively wide range of disparate conditions and are often used inconsistently. A typical example is the diagnostic label 'semantic-pragmatic disorder' (Rapin and Allen, 1983) which is sometimes used to describe poor conversational performance resulting from sociocognitive dysfunction (i.e. non-linguistic impairment) and at others to describe similar behaviour caused by problems with lexical access and sentence formulation (i.e. linguistic impairment). Problems have arisen with the clinical use of pragmatic labels because the terminology and conceptual apparatus of pragmatics are derived from linguistics, the philosophy of language and sociology, which are more concerned with abstract models on the one hand and with the description of social behaviour on the other. This apparatus has been imported wholesale and without adaptation into clinical linguistics but it is not generally well suited to the needs of language pathologists. It has led to a great deal of confusion in the clinical diagnosis of pragmatic disability and in regard to the nature of pragmatic disability itself.

A solution

In this paper I will propose a shift of focus and emphasis in the study of pragmatic disability from pragmatic theory to cognitive science. More specifically, I will show how impaired communicative behaviour may be characterized in terms of an imbalance between a range of underlying cognitive systems rather than purely in terms of its pragmatic features. As well as making it possible to distinguish between different types of pragmatic disability in cognitive terms, this approach has the potential to clarify and facilitate the clinician's remedial task by targeting the causes of pragmatic impairment instead of merely focusing on its behavioural symptoms.

Limitations in current approaches to pragmatic disability

Clinicians and language pathologists generally adopt one of two alternative approaches to the description of pragmatic disability. The first is to make use of the conceptual apparatus and terminology of a specific theoretical framework such as speech act theory (e.g. McDonald, 1992), Gricean implicature (e.g. Ahlsén, 1993), conversation analysis (e.g. Willcox and Mogford-Bevan, 1995), relevance theory (e.g. Happé, 1993) or cohesion analysis (e.g. Armstrong, 1991). Such approaches are highly selective in that they limit themselves to the specific types of phenomena identified by the theory in question and are not geared to the requirements of clinicians who need to know what gives rise to such phenomena.

An alternative method that favours comprehensiveness over theoretical coherence is to use a profile or checklist approach. Prutting and Kirchner's (1983) 'pragmatic protocol' includes seven general categories: speech acts, topic, turn taking, lexical selection, stylistic variation, intelligibility and prosodics, kinesics and proxemics, and these in turn are broken down into a further 30 subcategories. A similar degree of comprehensiveness is sought by Penn (1985) in her 'profile of communicative appropriateness' which includes the six general categories of response to interlocutor, control of semantic content, cohesion, fluency, sociolinguistic sensitivity and non-verbal communication, which are subdivided into a further 51 subcategories. Although both checklists have been used successfully to characterize and distinguish different impaired populations, comparing them makes it evident that their criteria for what counts as pragmatic disability are eclectic and somewhat arbitrary. For example, the 30 and 51 subcategories of each respective profile have no more than 12 or so items in common.

A cognitive approach to pragmatic disability

Pragmatic theorists have for the most part considered language use in linguistic, sociological or philosophical terms — for example, what are the characteristics of language in use and what are the sociolinguistic and logical principles that govern it? So far there have been few attempts to look at pragmatic ability — let alone disability — from a cognitive perspective (for a review, see Perkins, in press) and these have tended to use pragmatic theory as their starting point. The cognitive approach proposed here has more in common with cognitive neuropsychology in that it focuses on the various cognitive systems and processes that underlie and contribute to language behaviour. Table 21.1 is a schematic summary of the cognitive and sensorimotor systems

Table 21.1. *The cognitive and sensorimotor bases of pragmatic ability*

PRAGMATIC ABILITY

Linguistic systems	Nonlinguistic systems Cognitive systems	Sensorimotor inpuit and output systems
	inferential reasoning	
phonology	social cognition	
prosody	theory of mind	vocal-auditory
morphology	executive function	visual
syntax	memory	tactile
lexis	affect	
	conceptual knowledge	

that form the basis of pragmatic ability. It should be noted that the category labels are merely illustrative and are not intended to suggest that each cell constitutes a distinct module in a Fodorean sense.

The linguistic cognitive systems shown provide us with the means of encoding and decoding meaning. The non-linguistic cognitive systems interact with the linguistic systems to determine the 'what, why, when, where and how' of the encoding and decoding processes. The sensorimotor input and output systems allow for the transmission and reception of linguistic information through different modalities. Interaction between these various systems determines the behaviour that we describe in pragmatic terms.

In the rest of the paper I will outline a classification system for pragmatic disability based on cognitive and sensorimotor systems, rather than on pragmatic theory. In doing so I will briefly discuss the role played by each of these cognitive systems in pragmatic dysfunction.

A cognitive classification system for pragmatic disability

Table 21.2 provides an outline of a classification system for pragmatic disability in which the diagnostic categories are determined by the type of cognitive or sensorimotor system that is impaired, rather than being based purely on the type of pragmatic behaviour resulting from such an impairment. I will discuss each of the three major categories in turn.

Primary pragmatic disability (PPD)

Primary pragmatic disability (PPD) describes a condition in which the linguistic system is essentially intact but communicative performance is

Table 21.2. A *cognitive classification system for pragmatic ability*

Type of pragmatic ability	Underlying cause
Primary Pragmatic Disability (PPD)	**Dysfunction of:**
	– inferential reasoning – social cognition – theory of mind – executive function – memory – affect – conceptual knowledge
Secondary Pragmatic Disability (SPD)	**a) linguistic dysfunction**
	– phonology – prosody – morphology – syntax – lexis
	b) Sensorimotor dysfunction
	– auditory perception – visual perception – motor/articulatory ability
Complex Pragmatic Disability (CPD)	**Combination of PPD and SPD**

impaired as a result of non-linguistic cognitive dysfunction. It is described as 'primary' because the behaviours associated with such dysfunction constitute the primary focus of pragmatic theory.

Inferential reasoning

Poor inferential reasoning leads to behaviours such as 'missing the point' and 'drawing the wrong conclusions' that are found in conditions such as right brain damage, autism and semantic-pragmatic disorder. Inferential reasoning is also implicated in several of the other non-linguistic cognitive systems discussed below.

Social cognition and theory of mind

Impaired social cognition and theory of mind underlie behaviours such as being unable to explain and predict the actions of others within a social context and difficulties in taking the perspective of other people.

These are also found in people with right brain damage, autism and semantic-pragmatic disorder.

Executive function

Executive function is an umbrella term for mental operations such as intentionality, planning, attention and flexibility. Its dysfunction can give rise to repetitiveness and poor topic control in people with frontal lobe damage, schizophrenia, autism and closed head injury.

Memory

Poor memory can also be implicated in repetitiveness and in problems with conversational coherence found across a range of disorders including schizophrenia, aphasia, specific language impairment in children, autism and closed head injury.

Affect

Pragmatically inappropriate behaviour can arise in conditions such as right brain damage as a result of emotional lability and in autism as a result of being unable to read the emotions of others.

Conceptual knowledge

A circumscribed knowledge base can give rise to conversational repetitiveness and topic bias in people with low intelligence, mental handicap and autism.

Secondary pragmatic disability (SPD)

Secondary pragmatic disability (SPD) is a communicative impairment that is a consequence of either linguistic dysfunction or sensorimotor dysfunction. It is 'secondary' in the sense that such dysfunction has an indirect effect on pragmatic disability — i.e. the pragmatic disability is a concomitantly resultant behaviour. Linguistic and sensorimotor disabilities are very different and distinct but are linked under a common heading because they both restrict the range of choices available for encoding what one wishes to say and for decoding the utterances of others.

Linguistic dysfunction

Any speech or language disorder inevitably reduces communicative effectiveness, and there is therefore a clear sense in which linguistic dysfunction can also be described as incurring a concomitant pragmatic disorder (i.e. SPD). Secondary pragmatic disability can result from impairment in any linguistic system including morphology, syntax, lexis, phonology, prosody. The interpersonal context is also important here in that the more the linguistic system is reduced, the greater the pragmatic burden on the interlocutor (Perkins, 1996).

Sensorimotor dysfunction

Sensorimotor dysfunction also has clear pragmatic consequences. It may initially appear slightly odd to include such phenomena in a discussion of pragmatic disability. If we regard pragmatic functioning as a consequence of interactions between cognitive systems rather than as a primary cognitive system in its own right, however, then sensory and motor systems play a role that is just as crucial as those described above in that they permit a range of choices for the encoding and decoding of communicative behaviour, and their dysfunction can seriously reduce the effectiveness of such behaviour by limiting the available choices. This has been clearly shown in the case of hearing impairment that can lead to shorter conversational turns, fewer initiations and a higher degree of conversational control by interlocutors (Mogford-Bevan, 1993). Likewise, visual impairment can result in atypical turn-taking patterns in adults, echolalia and overly formulaic language in children and more frequent topic initiation by interlocutors (Mills, 1993; Perez-Pereira, 1994). An inability to effect a full range of physical movement, whether for anatomical or neurological reasons, can also severely affect pragmatic ability. In particular, motor/articulatory impairment makes it difficult to make pragmatically appropriate use of intact linguistic and cognitive abilities in conditions such as cerebral palsy, Parkinson's disease, dyspraxia and dysarthria.

Complex pragmatic disability (CPD)

Cases where pragmatic difficulties are not the result of a single underlying cognitive, linguistic or sensorimotor deficit come under the heading of complex pragmatic disability (CPD). Interactions between underlying systems can be extremely complex and many communicative disorders that can be described in pragmatic terms are of this type. For example, the sociocognitive deficits found in autism and which limit understanding of affect and social interaction inevitably mean that the areas of the lexicon where such notions are represented will be underspecified. Although the resulting lexical deficit is at least partly linguistic in nature, the cause of the deficit is non-linguistic.

There are several different ways in which disordered underlying systems may interact to produce CPD. I will give examples of four by way of illustration.

Developmental interactions

There is evidence to suggest that the linguistic deficits found in children with specific language impairment may be a consequence of problems with sequential verbal memory and auditory perception (Bates, Dale and Thal, 1995).

On-line processing interactions

Some have argued that agrammatism in aphasia is not a unitary impairment but may be a consequence of problems with timing and co-ordination during syntactic processing. In other words, grammatical competence may be intact but it may be the case that it cannot be successfully deployed because of disruption in other cognitive systems (Kolk, 1995).

Compensatory interactions

Receptive aphasics will often try to hold on to their conversational turn in order to reduce the number of occasions where they might misunderstand what their interlocutors say to them. Although such behaviour may initially appear to be an instance of PPD (e.g. a sociocognitive deficit) it often makes more sense to describe it as the result of a strategy to compensate for an underlying linguistic deficit.

Unrelated linguistic and non-linguistic deficits

There are also cases where pragmatic disability results both from a linguistic and a non-linguistic deficit that exist simultaneously but unconnectedly. It might be more accurate to describe these in terms of 'compound' rather than 'complex' pragmatic disability.

Conclusion

The classificatory system presented above and summarized in Table 21.2 is a reaction to the fact that the term 'pragmatic disability' is too broad and vague to be of much use in the diagnosis and remediation of communicative impairments. The cognitive approach to pragmatics described here distinguishes between (a) the behavioural symptoms of communicative dysfunction (as described by pragmatic theory), and (b) the cognitive, linguistic and sensorimotor impairments that underlie them. A strong implication of this approach for clinical practice is that instead of focusing exclusively on the linguistic behaviours identified by pragmatic theory, therapy should be directed at the underlying causes. For example, rather than simply noting whether a patient may be described as having problems with Grice's maxim of quantity, indirect speech acts, topic management or turn-taking, we should also be trying to ascertain whether this is a result of, say, a deficit in social cognition or memory (PPD), a problem with sentence formulation or visuo-spatial perception (SPD) or some combination (CPD).

References

Ahlsén E (1993) Conversational principles and aphasic communication. Journal of Pragmatics 19: 57–70.

Armstrong, E. M. (1991) The potential of cohesion analysis in the analysis and treatment of aphasic discourse. Clinical linguistics and phonetics 5: 39–51.

Bates E, Dale PS and Thal D (1995) Individual differences and their implications for theories of language development. In Fletcher P and MacWhinney B (Eds) The Handbook of Child Language. Oxford: Blackwell, pp. 96–151.

Happé FGE (1993) Communicative competence and theory of mind in autism: a test of relevance theory. Cognition 48: 101–19.

Kolk H (1995) A time-based approach to agrammatic production. Brain and Language 50: 282–303.

McDonald S (1992) Differential pragmatic language loss after closed head injury: ability to comprehend conversational implicature. Applied Psycholinguistics 13: 295–312.

Mills AE (1993) Language acquisition and development with sensory impairment: blind children. In Blanken G, Dittmann J, Grimm H, Marshall JC and Wallesch C-W (Eds) Linguistic Disorders and Pathologies: An International Handbook. Berlin: Walter de Gruyter, pp 679–87.

Mogford-Bevan K (1993) Language acquisition and development with sensory impairment: hearing-impaired children. In Blanken C, Dittman J, Grimm H, Marshall JC and Wallesch C-W (eds). Linguistic Disorders and Pathologies: an International Handbook. Berlin: Walter de Gruyter, pp 660–79.

Penn C (1985) The profile of communicative appropriateness. The South African Journal of Communication Disorders 32: 18–23.

Perez-Pereira M (1994) Imitations, repetitions, routines, and the child's analysis of language: insights from the blind. Journal of Child Language 21: 317–38.

Perkins MR (1996) The compensations of an unbalanced mind: a cognitive – interactive account of disorders of language and thought. Paper presented at the Hang Seng Conference on Language and Thought, University of Sheffield, Sheffield, UK.

Perkins MR (in press) The scope of pragmatic disability: a cognitive approach. In Muller (Ed) Pragmatics and Clinical Applications. Amsterdam: John Benjamins.

Prutting CA and Kirchner DM (1983) Applied Pragmatics. In Gallagher TM and Prutting CA (Eds) Pragmatic Assessment and Intervention Issues in Language. San Diego: College Hill Press, pp 29–64.

Rapin I and Allen DA (1983) Developmental language disorders: Nosologic considerations. In U Kirk (Ed) Neuropsychology of Language, Reading, and Spelling. New York: Academic Press, pp 155–84.

Willcox A and Mogford-Bevan K (1995) Conversational disability: assessment and remediation. In Perkins MR and Howard SJ (Eds) Case Studies in Clinical Linguistics. London: Whurr, pp 146–78.

Chapter 22
Is Motor Performance Related to Memory Performance in Children with Specific Language Impairment?

SABINE PREIS AND MARKUS HASSELHORN

Introduction

Children with specific language impairment (SLI) by definition have no underlying neurological disease, normal non-verbal intelligence, and no hearing loss. The term 'specific' implies a selective language deficit. Van der Lely and Howard (1993) have recently presented evidence in a non-word repetition memory test showing that some SLI children have no short-term memory deficits in comparison to a language-matched control group. Nevertheless, the underlying nature of SLI has not yet been identified (Bishop, 1992) and most SLI children have additional non-linguistic deficits, such as motor deficits (Bishop and Edmundson, 1987; Nickisch, 1988; Powell and Bishop, 1992) and memory deficits (Eisenson, 1968; Gathercole and Baddeley, 1990; Gillam, Cowan and Day, 1995; Rice, Oetting, Marquis, Bode and Pae, 1994).

In the framework of Baddeley's (1986) generally accepted working memory model it was shown that 'fast articulators are good rememberers'. Baddeley has suggested the relevance of an articulatory loop in verbal working memory. The current view of the articulatory loop is that it comprises a phonological store and an articulatory rehearsal process. The velocity with which rehearsal processes can be accomplished determines the capacity of the articulatory rehearsal.

In this study we examined whether there is a relationship between memory processing and motor performance in SLI children with mainly grammatical deficits.

Method

Selection of the SLI children

The children were tested with two non-verbal intelligence tests (CFT 1, Raven Matrices Test). The mean IQ of the 16 right-handed SLI (eight girls, eight boys) (mean age 8;8, range 8;1 to 9;0) was 90.5 for the CFT 1 and 99.6 for the Raven Matrices Test.

A definite language deficit in the 16 SLI children was proven by two grammatical subtests (VS and IS) of the Heidelberger Sprachentwicklungstest (Grimm and Schöler, 1978). The mean percentile rank was 15.6% for the VS subtest, which assessed receptive grammatical abilities, and the mean percentile rank was 6.5% for the IS subtest, which assessed expressive grammatical abilities.

Motor performance series

Three different kinds of voluntary movements were used on a standardized computer-based motor performance series (Schoppe, 1974) in a fixed order.

1. In the tapping task children were instructed to tap repetitively and as fast as possible with a stylus on a contact plate. The number of repetitive taps was counted over a period of 10 seconds. The tapping rate was estimated as the average repetition frequency over two runs for both hands.
2. In the aiming movements test the children had to move a stylus over a total distance of 32 cm over 20 consecutive targets from a starting point to a target zone. The computer measured the time from the starting position to the target zone and counted the hits and the errors.
3. For the pegboard movement task the children were asked to move small pegs (length 5 cm, diameter 2 mm) from a home matrix containing 25 pegs into a vertical line of target holes, with the home matrix positioned 30 cm from the target line. The time taken to transfer all pegs was measured.

Test of memory processing

1. For the speech rate test the children were instructed to repeat a triplet of phonetically dissimilar one-syllabic German words 10 times as quickly as possible. The time needed to do this was recorded. The mean of these 10 trials was then transformed to give a measure of speech rate in words per second.
2. To assess memory span, word sets were created from eight phonetically dissimilar one-syllable German words. On each trial, the child

was presented with a sequence of words (one word per second) and was instructed to attempt to repeat the words in the given order immediately. Two lists of words were given at each list length, starting with a list length of two. Testing was discontinued if the child failed to reproduce both sequences of a given length in the correct order. Span was scored as the maximum length at which the child correctly recalled at least one of the two sequences. If the subject recalled both of the successive sequences of this length, a bonus of 0.5 points was credited.

3. For the non-word repetition task a set of 12 non-words, four each containing two, three, and four syllables, was constructed. The phoneme sequences within each non-word were all phonotactically and prosodically legal. The non-words were presented to each child in randomized sequence on a cassette recorder. There was a three-second interval between non-words providing sufficient time for the child to complete a repetition attempt. If an attempt was not made, the experimenter stopped the cassette recorder and allowed the child as much time as was needed to make the response. The test was completed when the child had attempted to repeat the full set of 12 non-words. The number of correct repetitions of the four-syllable non-words provided the total score for repetition of four-syllable non-words.

The data of the grammatical SLI children were compared to an age, gender and RAVEN-IQ matched control group.

Statistical analysis

Independent t-tests for all variables as well as bivariate correlation analysis were performed. Furthermore, with respect to group differences, an analysis of covariance was calculated.

Results

Motor performance

The results of the motor performance series are shown in Table 22.1.

The performance of the SLI children tended to be poorer than that of the control group in some motor tasks. In pegboard movement with the right hand (Figure 22.1) the one-tail t-test reached significance.

Memory processing

The SLI children were significantly impaired in speech rate, memory span and non-word repetition (see Table 22.2 and Figure 22.1).

Table 22.1. Results of the motor performance series

Subtest	16 control children		16 SLI children		2–tail t–test p<0.1
	Mean	SD	Mean	SD	
Tapping					
Hits, right	45.7	±5.4	43.0	±8.6	ns
Hits, left	39.3	±5.3	38.9	±7.1	ns
Aiming					
Hits, right	20.0	±2.2	20.0	±1.5	ns
Hits, left	21.7	±3.4	21.6	±1.4	ns
Errors, right	5.2	±3.2	5.7	±3.0	ns
Errors, left	9.5	±5.2	8.7	±4.0	ns
Total time (s), right	12.0	±2.8	12.2	±1.9	ns
Total time (s), left	13.7	±2.2	14.7	±2.0	ns
Pegboard					
Total time (s), right	58.8	±8.0	64.7	±10.6	<0.09
Total time (s), left	61.2	±7.4	66.1	±10.1	ns

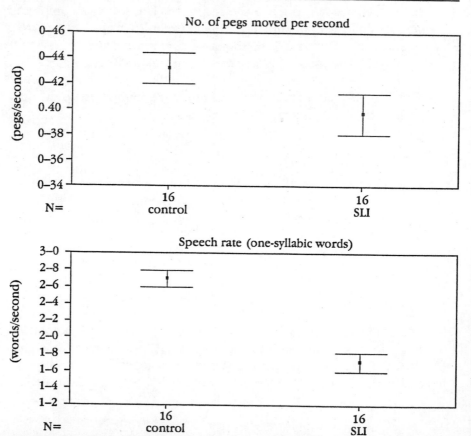

Figure 22.1. Mean plus or minus one standard error of the number of pegs moved per second with the right hand, speech rate, memory span, and non-word repetition in 16 SLI and 16 control children.

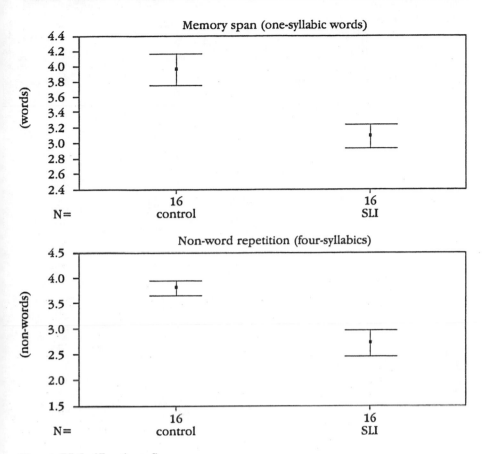

Figure 22.1. (Continued)

Table 22.2. Results of the examination of memory processing

Subtest	16 control children		16 SLI children		2–tail t–test p<
	Mean	SD	Mean	SD	
speech rate (words/second)	2.7	±0.4	1.7	±0.5	0.000
Memory span (words)	3.9	±0.8	3.1	±0.6	0.001
non-word repetition (words)	3.8	±0.5	2.7	±1.0	0.001

Table 22.3. Bivariate correlation analyses revealed significant coefficients among motor, among memory and between motor and memory data

Correlation coefficient significance	hits, tapping right hand	hits, tapping left hand	time, aiming right hand	time, aiming left hand	tim, pegboard right hand	time, pegboard left hand	speech rate	memory span
hits, tapping right hand								
time, tapping left hand	0.66 p=0.00							
time, aiming right hand	-0.41 p=0.02	-0.42 p=0.02						
time, aiming left hand	-0.35 p=0.05	-0.36 p=0.05	0.72 p=0.00					
tim, pegboard right hand	-0.58 p=0.00	0.44 p=0.01	0.48 p=0.00	0.56 p=0.00				
time, pegboard left hand	-0.35 p=0.05	-0.56 p=0.00	0.45 p=0.01	0.41 p=0.02	0.59 p=0.00			
speech rate	0.35 p=0.05	0.11 p=0.54	-0.10 p=0.58	-0.36 p=0.04	-0.38 p=0.03	-0.20 p=0.26		
memory span	0.08 p=0.67	-0.14 p=0.44	0.24 p=0.18	-0.06 p=0.75	-0.09 p=0.63	0.15 p=0.42	0.55 p=0.00	
non-word repetition	-0.11 p=0.56	-0.26 p=0.15	0.28 p=0.13	-0.15 p=0.41	-0.07 p=0.68	0.13 p=0.48	0.51 p=0.00	0.46 p=0.00

Correlations between motor and memory data

Table 22.3 shows the correlation coefficients of the bivariate correlation analyses.

The correlation between speech rate and right hand pegboard movement (Figure 22.2A) and the left hand aiming movement and between speech rate and memory span (Figure 22.2B) is significant. With respect

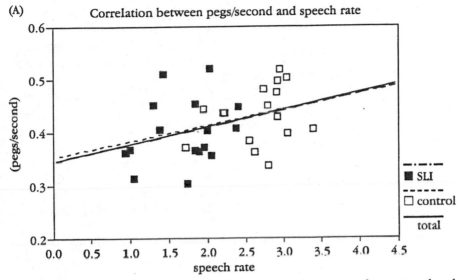

Figure 22.2A The correlation between the number of pegs moved per second and speech rate. The SLI children were slower in right-hand peg movement and in speech rate.

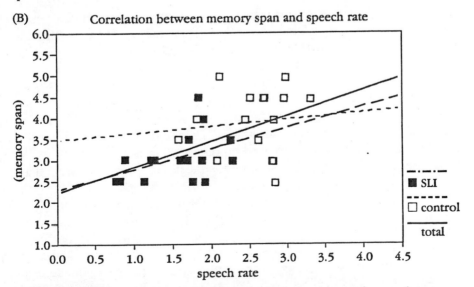

Figure 22.2B The correlation between memory span and speech rate. Performance in speech rate correlated to memory span, which was poorer in the SLI children.

to group differences, right-hand pegboard movement was an important covariate of speech rate for one-syllabic words (p<0.012).

Discussion

In this study we found a significant correlation between motor performances and speech rate. With respect to group differences, right-hand pegboard movement was an important covariate of speech rate. In Baddeley's memory model, speech rate determines the efficiency of the phonological working memory. Our SLI children performed worse than the control group in all three memory-processing tasks, which also showed a significant intercorrelation.

The deficits found in our SLI children support the hypothesis that SLI children have difficulties in the performance and information processing of sequences (Bishop, 1992). These difficulties are shown when successive stimuli are:

1. presented as tones (Tallal and Piercy, 1973);
2. presented as word lists (Gathercole and Baddeley, 1990);
3. presented as digits (Gillam et al., 1995; Shields, Varley, Broks and Simpson, 1996) and
4. in the performance of coordinated sequences of motor movements (Bishop, 1992).

This indicates a supramodal deficit in SLI, probably in timing of information processing as was recently assumed in the case of dyslexia (Frith and Frith, 1996), since functional MRI studies in dyslexics revealed beneath difficulties in phonological processing and also difficulties in the processing of visual motions (Eden, Van Meter, Rumsey, Maisog, Woods, Zeffiro, 1996). Nevertheless in SLI children the learning of sequences does not seem to be impaired in the visual modality – e.g. they perform normally in the Corsi block span (Shields et al., 1996). Furthermore Fazio (1994) compared oral and gestural counting in four-to-five-year-old SLI children and found that oral counting especially and not gestural counting was vulnerable. Therefore beneath the timing problem additional factors have to be regarded in SLI.

There are indications that left hemispheric functions, in particular, are impaired in SLI children with mainly phonological and/or grammatical deficits (Shields et al., 1996). In right-handed and in most left-handed persons the performance of word-list memory and digit span are left hemispheric functions whereas the Corsi block span is a right hemispheric function (Shields et al., 1996). Neuropsychological examinations alone will not clarify the question about changed hemispheric function in SLI. Neuropathological studies (Cohen, Campbell and Yaghmai, 1989) and recent MRI examinations point to a changed hemispheric asymmetry in SLI (e.g. Plante, Swisher and Vance, 1991).

The working memory model provided by Baddeley is a generally accepted one and is supported by many studies (Baddeley, 1986). Our results again indicate a complex connection of apparently independent processes like fine motor performance and cognitive processing. With the memory tests there is the caveat that the interpretation of a verbal test is always confounded by the language impairment of the SLI group but the aim of our study was to describe SLI children's strengths and weaknesses with regard to motor and memory areas and their correlations. Finally our data give support to the hypothesis that the cause of SLI may be a supramodal one and the term 'specific' language impairment may be misleading, as already stated by Stark and Tallal (1981).

References

Baddeley AD (1986) (Ed) Working Memory, Oxford, Oxford University Press.

Bishop DVM, Edmundson A (1987) Specific language impairment as a maturational lag: evidence from longitudinal data on language and motor development. Developmental Medicine and Child Neurology 29: 442–59.

Bishop DVM (1992) The underlying nature of specific language impairment. Journal of Child Psychology and Psychiatry 33: 3–66.

Cohen M, Campbell R, Yaghmai F (1989) Neuropathological abnormalities in developmental dysphasia. Annals of Neurology 25: 567–70.

Eden GF, VanMeter JW, Rumsey JM, Maisog JM, Woods RP, Zeffiro TA (1996) Abnormal processing of visual motion in dyslexia revealed by functional brain imaging. Nature 382: 66–9.

Eisenson J (1968) Developmental aphasia: a speculative view with therapeutic implications. Journal of Speech and Hearing Disorders 33: 3–13.

Fazio BB (1994) The counting abilities of children with specific language impairment: a comparison of oral and gestural tasks. Journal of Speech and Hearing Research 37: 358–68.

Frith C, Firth U (1996) A biological marker for dyslexia. Nature 382: 19–20.

Gathercole SE, Baddeley AD (1990) Phonological memory deficits in language disordered children: is there a causal connection? Journal of Memory and Language 29: 336–60.

Gillam RB, Cowan N, Day l (1995) Sequential memory in children with and without language impairment. Journal of Speech and Hearing Research: 38: 393–402.

Grimm H, Schöler H (1978) (Eds) Heidelberger Sprachentwicklungstest (HSET). Göttingen, Hogrefe.

Nickisch A (1988) Motorische Störungen bei Kindern mit verzögerter Sprachentwicklung. Folia Phoniatrica 40: 147–52.

Plante E, Swisher L, Vance R (1991) MRI findings in boys with specific language impairment. Brain and Language 41: 52–66.

Powell RP, Bishop DVM (1992) Clumsiness and perceptual problems in children with specific language impairment. Developmental Medicine and Child Neurology 34: 755–65.

Rice ML, Oetting JB, Marquis J, Bode J, Pae S (1994) Frequency of input effects on word comprehension of children with specific language impairment. Journal of Speech and Hearing Research 37: 106–22.

Schoppe HJ (1974) Das MLS Gerät: Ein neuer Testapparat zur Messung fein-
   motorischer Leistungen. Diagnostica 20: 43–6.

Shields J, Varley R, Broks P, Simpson A (1996) Hemispheric function in developmental language disorders and high-level autism. Developmental Medicine and
   Child Neurology 38: 473–86.

Stark RE, Tallal P (1981) Selection of children with specific language deficits.
   Journal of Speech and Hearing Disorders 46: 114–22.

Tallal P, Piercy M (1973) Defects of non-verbal auditory perception in children with
   developmental aphasia. Nature 241: 468–9.

Van der Lely HKJ, Howard D (1993) Children with specific language impairment:
   Linguistic impairment or short-term memory deficit? Journal of Speech and
   Hearing Research 36: 1193–207.

Chapter 23
Dyscalculia: Clinical Linguistics?

JOHN VAN BORSEL

Few would deny that speaking, reading and writing are linguistic skills and that disorders in the acquisition of these skills can be appropriately studied within the field of clinical linguistics. A more provocative idea is that mathematics is also a linguistic skill and that linguistics can significantly contribute to the management of mathematical skill disorders. At any rate, it is not common to study mathematics from a linguistic perspective nor is it common to assess and treat problems in mathematics achievement within a linguistic framework. Mathematics and mathematical skill disorders are usually dealt with by teachers, educationists and psychologists, not by linguists. Logically, studies of mathematics and mathematics disorders from a clinical perspective have focused primarily on non-linguistic neuropsychological aspects of mathematical skills such as working memory, visuo-constructive skills and spatial-perceptual skills. The occurrence of mathematical skill disorders in adults consequent upon brain damage, in particular, has received considerable interest (see Levin and Spiers 1985 for a review). More recently, there seems to be a growing interest from cognitive neuropsychology in mathematics and mathematical skill disorders (see for instance Cohen and Dehaene, 1991; Temple, 1991; Macaruso, McCloskey and Aliminosa, 1993; Noel and Seron, 1993). In the latter approach the focus is on the mental processes that are presumed to underlie mathematical activities.

The present paper must be considered as an exercise in clinical linguistics that aims to explore the possibility of a linguistic approach in the management of mathematical skill disorders. We will start this exercise with a descriptive analysis of the language and symbols used in mathematics and some reflections on the nature of mathematics and mathematical tasks. Incorporating the findings and ideas of this first section we will then present a tentative model for the description of mathematics tasks from a linguistic perspective. A linguistic classification of problems in mathematics achievement, referring to this model, is proposed along with some illustrations of how the model could be used in assessment and treatment.

Language, mathematics and mathematics tasks

Numbers play an important role in everyday life. We use numbers when we make purchases, when we tell the time, when we drive a car, when we step on the scales etc. The range of activities involving the use of numbers is very wide. Yet, what we do when we use numbers in all these activities is in essence always the same: we always refer to quantities.

In a shop we ask for a certain quantity of eggs or sandwiches, which cost a certain amount of money. The numbers on the counter in the car refer to a certain quantity of kilometres or miles. The numbers on a scale indicate a certain quantity of pounds or kilograms, those on a watch a certain number of hours etc.

Within the vocabulary of a language, numbers seem to constitute a somewhat particular class of words. More than any other class of words they most naturally appear in a written form. This written form is, moreover, quite different from the one that is normally used. To record spoken words, in the Western world, an alphabetic writing system is normally used in which each written sign represents a spoken sound. Numbers can also be represented in this way (one, two, three, . . .). It is far more usual, however, to represent numbers by means of logographic symbols (signs that each symbolize an entire word) (1, 2, 3. . .).

Using a logographic writing system to record numbers has at least one enormous advantage. As logographic symbols refer to the meaning of words and not to the sounds of words, they can be used by speakers of a great many different languages. Symbols such as '3' or '4' for instance are just as meaningful for a French speaker as they are for a speaker of Italian, Spanish or English and these symbols also mean exactly the same thing for the various speakers.

A well-known weakness of logographic writing systems, however, is that they usually require a very large number of symbols (Crane, Yeager and Whitman, 1981). One needs a different sign for each word of the spoken language with a different meaning. Since the word class of numbers is an open class, being as large as the amount of units contained in the largest quantity thinkable, which is infinite, one would virtually need an infinite number of logographic signs for number writing. Yet, the set of signs we use to represent numbers is extremely limited, actually comprising no more than 10 different items. Quantities of none to nine are each represented by a different symbol (0, 1, 2 . . . 9). For quantities larger than nine the same 10 symbols are combined into sequences of two, three or more signs as required and receive a meaning according to their position (from left to right) in the sequence. When the sign '1' appears in the first position of a two-sign sequence it means a quantity of 10; when it occurs in the first position of a three sign sequence it means 'a quantity of hundred' and so forth. In other words, in the logographic system used to represent numbers, position appears to function as a distinctive feature.

To a large extent the enormous economy of the logographic system for number writing is a reflection of the linguistic make-up of numbers, which in turn resulted from the way man has arranged to deal with quantities. In the development of a system to indicate or determine the magnitude of a quantity, reference to parts of the body, especially the 10 fingers of the hands, seems to have played a significant role (McLeish, 1993). The use of the hands almost certainly lies at the origin of the decimal scale by which we express the magnitude of quantities as multiples of 10. In English the use of parts of the body for determining quantities is shown for instance in the double meaning of a word such as 'digit' ('finger', 'figure'). Expressing magnitude as a function of the number of amounts of 10 prevented the need to invent a new verbal label for every different quantity possible. One word to indicate the number of 10s in a given quantity combined with one word to indicate the number of units not completing a full set of ten is then sufficient. Still further economy was achieved from the use of words to indicate a set of ten tens (hundred), a set of ten times ten tens (thousand) and so forth. In this way the lexicon for quantities became a collection of words shaped according to very logical and predictable patterns, which easily lent itself to recording in a logographic way as outlined above.

Worldwide acceptance of the decimal scale has resulted in a comparable organization of the lexicon for quantities in many different languages. Many languages, however, also show some particularities. At this point it is important to note that the organization of the lexicon for quantities in a given language and the structure of the universally agreed logographic writing system for numbers do not always match completely.

Compare for instance the numbers from twenty to a hundred in English with the same numbers in Dutch or German. These numbers have two constituents in English: a first constituent specifying the tens and a second constituent specifying the units (e.g. *twenty-nine, thirty-one* . . .) This structure (two constituents, the first one specifying the tens, the second one specifying the units) matches exactly the structure of the logographic symbolization (29, 31 . . .). In Dutch and German, however, the structure of numbers between twenty and hundred is different from that in logographic writing. Not only is there an additional constituent (viz. a conjunction) but also the constituent specifying the units precedes the constituent specifying the tens (for instance 42: *tweeënveertig, zweiundvierzig.* . . .).

Another example of such an imperfect match is found in French with numbers between 70 and 100. With these numbers the principle of specifying a quantity by indicating the number of tens and the number of remaining units is abandoned. Instead, quantities between seventy and eighty are treated as compositions of a set of sixty and a number of units, and quantities from eighty to a hundred are treated as compositions of four times twenty and a number of units. The verbal labels for these quantities are formed accordingly (for instance *soixante-douze, soixante-treize* and *quatre-vingt-douze, quatre-vingt-treize* etc.) which is quite unlike the representation in the logographic writing system. As we will illustrate later, incongruities like these between the lexicon and the logographic representation may be an important source of difficulty in mathematics achievement in some languages.

So far we have been discussing numbers as a special subset of the lexicon of languages for referring to quantities. This lexicon for quantities, with its logographic symbolization, is one of the things children learn in mathematics classes as part of the more general skill of handling quantities. Handling quantities, as it is taught in primary school, and also as it takes place in real-life situations, fundamentally seems to imply no more than three different things.

The first thing one can do with a quantity is to specify its magnitude. Actually, this comes down to associating a given quantity with the appropriate verbal label (or logographic symbol). Specifying the magnitude of a quantity could, in other words, be considered a naming task. With small quantities, say smaller than six or seven, this naming task is fairly easy and one can immediately say (or write down) which quantity is shown. With a larger quantity, however, it is no longer possible to determine its magnitude immediately. One then has to resort to the strategy of counting. Counting can be considered a special kind of naming. It is the sequential naming of a systematically increasing quantity. Usually the sequence increases by one unit at a time but it is, of course, also possible to count in twos or in threes for instance (skip counting). The ability to count requires knowledge of the organization of the lexicon for quantities. One has to know the logic and patterns applied in the make-up of numbers. Children's acquisition of this lexicon normally starts before they enter primary school with songs and nursery rhymes containing series of numbers. Although at this age these numbers are for the greater part still void of a precise meaning, they are none the less a first step towards the skill of specifying the magnitude of quantities.

A second thing one can do with a quantity is to determine its magnitude relative to that of another quantity – i.e. compare it with another quantity. The outcome of such a comparison is always limited to one of two possibilities. Either two quantities are equal or they are not. And when two quantities are not equal one is always larger and the other is always smaller. In mathematics these possible relationships between two quantities are, just like numbers, symbolized by means of logographic signs (=, ≠, > and <).

Finally, one can also change the magnitude of a quantity. A quantity can be enlarged by adding items or it can be reduced by taking away items. Either enlarging or reducing a quantity results in a new quantity, the magnitude of which has then to be determined and labelled. These changes of a quantity, known as the operations 'addition' and 'subtraction', are normally symbolized in mathematics by logographic signs: the plus sign (+) and minus sign (–). Exercises in which a quantity is changed and the resulting quantity has to be determined are among the most common problems children learn to solve in basic mathematics. In spoken language the change of the magnitude of a quantity is worded in several ways. A logographic number statement such as 22 – 7 = 15 reads as 'twenty-two minus seven equals fifteen' but also as 'seven from twenty-two leaves fifteen' or as ' twenty-two take away seven is fifteen'.

Sometimes quantities are changed a number of times in succession in a very systematic way. In the logographic writing system these changes are commonly represented in a shortened manner. Successive enlargements of a quantity by adding each time a quantity similar to the original quantity can be represented by using the plus sign (4 + 4 + 4). The more usual way to symbolize such a series of systematic additions in logographic writing, however, is by means of the multiplication sign (3 × 4). Similarly, the division sign '÷' is used instead of the minus sign to represent reduction of a quantity by successive subtraction (12 ÷ 4 rather than 12 – 3 – 3 – 3).

Mathematics and mathematical disorders

It appears that mathematics is concerned with handling quantities (specifying quantities, comparing quantities and changing quantities) and that the preferred symbolization for quantities and specification, comparison or change of quantities is by means of logographic signs. The consistent use of logographic signs and the special organization of the lexicon for quantities make mathematics a highly linguistic skill that can be represented schematically as follows:

reality of quantities	lexicon	logographic signs
specification	number words	
	one, two, three ...	1, 2, 3
	twenty-one, thirty-three	21, 33
	two-hundred and sixty-five	265
comparison	equal	=
	unequal	≠
	more than	>
	less than	<
change	add	+ (×)
	take away	– (÷)

Figure 23.1.

Viewing mathematics as a linguistic skill one can deduce, from the above model, the possible existence of at least two different categories of problem in mathematics achievement. One type of problem results from inadequate knowledge of the logographic system for number writing, and for this we would suggest the name *logographic dyscalculia*. The second type of problem relates to the acquisition of the lexicon for quantities and this could be called *semantic dyscalculia*. Further classification of both disorders into an expressive and a receptive subtype may be warranted as well as more specific indication of the problem areas in accordance with the three possible kinds of activities involving quantities (specification, comparison or change).

Clinical observation of children with problems in mathematics achievement would seem to suggest that the proposed classification scheme might be applicable both in assessment and treatment. By way of illustration let us now look at some examples of errors and how these can be interpreted within the model outlined. All the examples shown are real examples collected from elementary school pupils with problems in mathematics achievement.

Figure 23.2 shows some examples of logographic errors. One type of logographic error consists of those in which a child shows inadequate knowledge of the notational conventions of the logographic number signs, as in the examples under (a). In these two examples the operation itself (reduction of a quantity or a subtraction) was no problem for the pupil. The pupil could correctly identify the amount obtained after reducing the original quantity but he wrote the logographic symbol for 'five' in reverse each time.

(a) $14 - 9 = $ ʑ   (b) $58 + 6 = 52$ (c) $3 \neq 3$
       $12 - 7 = $ ʑ $63 + 8 = 55$ $6 = 7$
                               $44 - 31 = 75$
                               $66 - 15 = 81$

(d) $12 + 3 = 24$ (e)   25   18
       $16 - 5 = 65$ $+ 17$ $\times 3$
                                       $\overline{312}$ $\overline{324}$

       Dictation: 136 (target 163)
                  742 (target 724)

Figure 23.2.

The examples under (b) come from a boy who constantly mistook the minus sign for a plus sign and vice versa. Again, the operations (either enlarging a quantity or reducing a quantity) posed no difficulty. It is faulty comprehension of the meaning of operator signs themselves that generated the error. Orally, problems of this kind were always solved correctly.

A similar error is found in the examples under (c) in which a child had to choose the appropriate sign to indicate whether two quantities were equal or not. Memorizing the meaning of the signs of a logographic writing system is not easy as the signs are normally purely conventional and bear no resemblance to what they are meant to represent. Hence, confusion of signs, especially when they represent polar opposites (such as the signs for 'equal' or 'not equal', or the plus and minus sign), are likely to occur in some children. In the examples under (c) the problem is really one of comprehension of the logographic signs and not of comprehension of the concept 'equal' versus 'not equal' and is in such cases again easily demonstrated by having the child solve the problem orally.

Sometimes problems with the logographic system for number writing may also lead to answers which at first seem bizarre and inexplicable. The solutions to the first two problems under (d) don't seem to make much sense unless one knows that these are examples from a Dutch-speaking pupil. As explained above, in Dutch the lexicon for quantities between 20 and 100 does not match the logographic symbolization. In words to indicate quantities between 20 and 100 the constituent specifying the units precedes the constituent specifying the tens, which is exactly the opposite to the logographic representation of these quantities. Given this, the first two examples under (d) become quite understandable. Apparently the pupil in these examples followed the direction of alphabetic writing, from left to right, and read '12' in the first example as 'twenty-one' ('een/en/twintig' in Dutch) and '16' in the second example as 'sixty-one' ('een/en/zestig' in Dutch). In the latter example he also adopted the alphabetic direction in writing down his answer so that '65' actually represents 'fifty-six' (in Dutch 'zes/en/vijftig'). The next two examples under (d) also illustrate the difficulty some pupils (in Dutch) have with the imperfect match between the organization of the lexicon for quantities and the logographic writing system for numbers. Again the organization of the lexicon (in Dutch 163 = honderd/drie/en/zestig, 724 = zevenhonderd/vier/en/twintig) was followed instead of that the logographic writing system.

The examples under (e) illustrate yet another type of problem that children may have with logographic number writing. What happened in these examples was that the pupil did not respect the principle that in logographic number writing position functions as a distinctive feature. The individual computations as such are correct (five plus seven is indeed 12, and two plus one is three; three times eight is indeed 24 and three times one is indeed three). It is the final notation of the results (the sum total of the individual steps) that is defective.

In our experience many children's problems in mathematical achievement amount to difficulties with the logographic writing system for numbers of the kind illustrated above. The problem for these children is not an inability to handle quantities. They can determine the magnitude of quantities, compare quantities or change the magnitude of quantities as requested. They also have a good command of the lexicon involved in specifying, comparing and changing quantities and are able to put acts relating to quantities into words. What is difficult for them is merely the use of the logographic signs and the notational conventions by which the lexicon and acts relating to quantities are usually symbolized in script. In these cases, the exact determination of which of the notational signs and conventions have not been mastered (those for specification, comparison or change) provides the starting point for remediation.

In other children the problem of mathematics achievement cannot be explained as a difficulty with the logographic signs and notational conventions. Rather, the problem seems to be that of acquiring the lexicon involved in mathematics. Children with this kind of problem do not succeed in determining the magnitude of a quantity, they cannot select a given number of items from a set, they don't seem to grasp the meaning of words such as equal, unequal, more, or less, they cannot correctly reduce or enlarge a given quantity by a number of items. Their problem is that of (correctly) associating the lexicon that is used in mathematics with the factual reality. In these children, approaches that aim to enhance understanding of the basic mathematical terms (terms for specification, comparison and change of quantity) by multiple factual experiences seem to be indicated.

Conclusion

Looking at mathematics with a linguist's eye may prove a valuable approach in both assessment and treatment of mathematics achievement disorders. At any rate, the model outlined above allows one to distinguish between various errors and to classify errors in a logical way. Classification of an error also makes it clear which goals remediation should aim to achieve. Of course, the model presented is but a basic scheme that awaits further exploration and refinement by confrontation with more clinical data and experimentation. We hope this exercise has aroused some interest in an area that, thus far, has been largely neglected in clinical linguistics.

References

Cohen L, Dehaene S (1991) Neglect dyslexia for numbers? A case report. Cognitive Neuropsychology 8: 39–58.

Crane BL, Yeager E, Whitman RL (1981) An introduction to linguistics. Boston, Toronto: Little, Brown & Company.

Levin HS, Spiers PA (1985) Acalculia. In Heilman KM, Valenstein E (Eds) Clinical Neuropsychology. New York, Oxford: Oxford University Press, pp.97–114.

Macaruso P, McCloskey M, Aliminosa D (1993) The functional architecture of the cognitive numerical-processing system: evidence from a patient with multiple impairments. Cognitive Neuropsychology 10: 341–76.

McLeish J (1993) Het getal. Van kleitablet tot computer. Amsterdam: Amber.

Noel M-P, Seron X (1993) Arabic number reading deficit: a single case study or when 236 is read (2306) and judged superior to 1258. Cognitive Neuropsychology 10: 317–39.

Temple CM (1991) Procedural dyscalculia and number fact dyscalculia: double dissociation in developmental dyscalculia. Cognitive Neuropsychology 8: 155–76.

PART II
SPEECH AND LANGUAGE
DISORDERS IN ADULTS

SPEECH AND LANGUAGE PROCESSING IN NORMALS

Chapter 24
The Relevance of Temporal Resolution for Functional Neuroimaging Studies of Speech and Language Processing

DAVID POEPPEL

Introduction

Our knowledge of the neural basis of speech and language processing derives primarily from more than a century of deficit-lesion correlation analysis. In the past few years, the development of functional neuro-imaging methods has provided the field with a new tool to examine where and how cognitive processes are represented *in vivo*. Functional brain imaging approaches can be categorized into the hemodynamically based methods, positron emission tomography (PET) and functional magnetic resonance imaging (fMRI), as well as the electromagnetically based methods, electroencephalography (EEG) and magneto-encephalography (MEG). PET and fMRI both have excellent spatial resolving power (2–5 mm), whereas their temporal resolution lies in the range of 1 (fMRI) to 30 (PET) seconds, depending, for example, on the hemodynamic lag (fMRI) or parameters constraining image acquisition time (PET). EEG and MEG, in contrast, both have millisecond temporal resolution — appropriate to the measurement of neural activity — but are limited in the extent to which they can spatially resolve sources (typ-ically >5 mm). Extensive discussions of the functional neuroimaging methods and their respective strengths and limitations are provided by George, Aine, Mosher, Schmidt, Ranken, Schlitt, Wood, Lewine, Sanders and Belliveau (1995), Gevins, Le, Martin, Brickett, Desmond and Reutter (1994), Hämäläinen, Hari, Ilmoniemi, Knuutila and Lounasmaa (1993), Kwong (1995), Näätänen, Ilmoniemi and Alho (1994); Nadeau and Crosson (1995), Orrison, Lewine, Sanders and Hartshorne (1995), Posner and Raichle (1994), Raichle (1994) Roland (1993).

PET and fMRI have clearly extended our understanding of the functional neuroanatomy of speech and language processing (Binder, Frost, Hammeke, Cox, Rao and Prieto, 1997; Binder, Frost, Hammeke, Rao and Cox, 1996; Démonet, Price, Wise and Frackowiak, 1994; Démonet, Chollet, Ramsay, Cardebat, Nespoulous, Wise, Rascol and Frackowiak, 1992; Fiez, 1996; Fiez, Raichle, Miezin, Petersen, Tallal and Katz, 1995; Mazoyer, Dehaene, Tzourio, Frak, Murayama, Cohen, Levrier, Salamon, Syrota, and Mehler, 1993; Petersen, Fox, Posner, Mintun and Raichle, 1989; Stromswold, Caplan, Alpert and Rauch, 1996; Zatorre, Evans, Meyer and Gjedde, 1992). There is no question that PET and fMRI at the current level of technical and analytic sophistication constitute the cornerstone of functional brain imaging. The relative success of this new enterprise notwithstanding, a number of critical evaluations have also been put forth. The critiques have focused on issues of experimental design, on the one hand, and technical shortcomings of the methods for studying cognitive brain function on the other (Friston, Price, Fletcher, Moore, Frackowiak and Dolan, 1996; Nadeau and Crosson, 1995; Poeppel, 1996; Sarter, Berntson and Cacioppo, 1996; Sergent, 1994; Whitaker, Poeppel and Hochman, 1997). Nevertheless, with regard to questions of functional localization, fMRI and PET will continue to dominate the field.

There are a number of phenomena in the domain of speech and language processing that crucially require the temporal resolution of electromagnetic recording techniques. In this chapter I review briefly the basis of magnetoencephalography (MEG) and magnetic source imaging (MSI) and then highlight the importance of temporal resolution by illustrating some MEG findings on speech and language processing that are not — at least in any obvious way — visible to hemodynamically based methods.

The basics of MEG

Magnetoencephalography detects the minute magnetic fields associated with neuronal current flow (Hämäläinen *et al.*, 1993). Biophysical considerations suggest that the extracranially measured signals are not the reflection of action potentials but are rather generated by post-synaptic current flow in the apical dendrites of pyramidal cells (Lewine and Orrison, 1995). The magnetic field associated with such current flow is, of course, extraordinarily small (~10 orders of magnitude smaller than the Earth's steady field) and thus requires extremely sensitive detectors. Superconducting Quantum Interference Devices (SQUIDs) form the basis of MEG signal detection by acting as low-noise, high-gain amplifiers for the signals picked up in special detection coils. Data acquisition is typically performed in magnetically shielded rooms to further attenuate the effects of surrounding magnetic fields. Current MEG recording set-ups range from single channel to large-array (e.g. 37 channel) to 300 channel whole-head devices.

The output of a given detector is a time-varying evoked neuro-magnetic field, which resembles an electrically recorded field potential (Figure 24.1a). Because (a) the head can be modelled as a roughly spherically symmetric conductor, and (b) magnetic fields are not significantly attenuated by nervous tissue, cerebrospinal fluid and bone, it is possible to estimate the origin of sources with remarkable accuracy. (It is important to note, however, that source modelling of electromagnetic data is an ill-posed computational problem — i.e. for a given field distribution there are no unique solutions in the absence of explicit constraints.) The standard source estimation method is equivalent-current dipole modelling (Hämäläinen *et al.*, 1993; Scherg, Vajsar and Picton, 1989), although other methods are being applied with increasing success as well (Ioannides, 1993; Ioannides, Singh, Hasson, Baumann, Rogers, Guinto Jr. and Papanicolaou, 1993; Mosher, Lewis and Leahy, 1992). The dipole modelling strategy is predicated on the fact that one can, at each recorded time sample, reconstruct the distribution of the magnetic field (Figure 24.1b). For a given distribution, one can subsequently compute the well-described magnetic 'forward' equations and then, for example, using an iterative least squares minimization procedure, find the best fit for the (a) location, (b) direction, and (c)

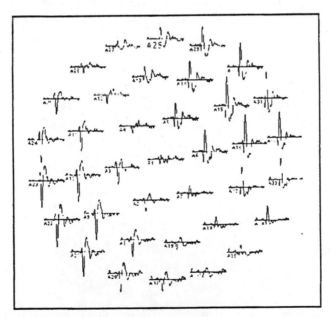

Figure 24.1(a) Sensor layout display. The hexagonal array of 37 SQUID-based detectors can be positioned to record over the desired part of cortex. An auditory stimulus such as a tone or speech sound elicits a series of time-varying evoked responses in sensors. The largest response, peaking at a latency of 100 ms post stimulus onset, is the M100 — related to the electrically observed N1 response. The polarity reversal across channels indicates that the underlying current source is approximately in the middle of the sensor array at a depth that needs to be reconstructed (cf. Figure 24.1b).

amplitude of an underlying dipole. Given an estimated source (in each time sample), one can now co-register the MEG data for each time point with independently obtained magnetic resonance images (MRIs). The combination of MRI and MEG data sets is known as magnetic source imaging (MSI; Figure 24.1c).

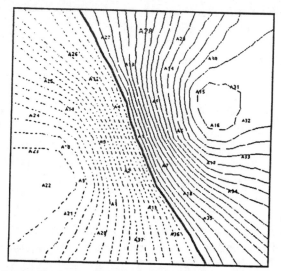

Figure 24.1.(b) Contour map at M100 peak. The current source underlying the extracranially evoked activity can be reconstructed by computing the magnetic field distribution at a given sample point. These data can be used to estimate the location of the source (e.g. a dipole).

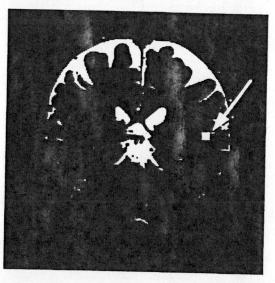

Figure 24.1(c) Magnetic source image. The M100 dipole as recorded (1a) and reconstructed (1b) is overlaid onto a coronal MR image (FSE sequence). The stimulus was presented to the right ear and the recording was performed over the left temporal lobe. The dipole localizes to the upper bank of the superior temporal gyrus in the left hemisphere.

Some experiments illustrating time-based phenomena

In what follows I provide, in a very brief fashion, four examples of speech and language data obtained with MEG that underscore the importance of temporal resolution.

1. Perhaps the most compelling example of how both the spatial and temporal aspects of MEG can be harnessed is provided by the work of Salmelin and her colleagues (Salmelin, Hari, Lounasmaa and Sams, 1994; Salmelin, Service, Kiesilä, Uutela and Salonen, 1996). Using a biomagnetometer that covers most of the head (Neuromag™, 122 channels), these investigators examine what they have been calling the 'brain dynamics' associated with processing a variety of stimuli: their data provide the spatio-temporal sequence of activation in the whole brain. In a recent experiment (Salmelin et al., 1996) they reported the activation generated by the processing of visual words (in a comparison between normal controls and adult dyslexics). Using a sophisticated multiple dipole modelling scheme, a precise cortical activation sequence was determined (0–200 ms: striate and extrastriate visual cortices, >200 ms: spread to temporal and frontal cortices, 200–400 ms strong left temporal activations) and the behaviour of the sources in time was carefully reconstructed and coregistered to individual subjects' MRIs. Two aspects of this study are particularly noteworthy in the context of the present discussion: first, the signal attributable to word processing can be 'followed', allowing one to study the sequence of processing in real time; secondly, it was shown that activity spread to virtually the entire cortex within 400 ms. The reason to be cognisant of this is that even the fastest hemodynamic methods (fMRI) are subject to a hemodynamic lag that prevents the effective registration of such signals, particularly if they are transient (cf. section 3). Whole-head MEG promises not just to supplement insights obtained by fMRI and PET but to be a true competitor to these methods, especially insofar as source localization schemes are improved.

2. A second example of time-based data is provided by effects that are limited to particular frequency bands. Eulitz, Pulvermüller and their colleagues (Eulitz, Maess, Pantev, Friederici, Feige, Elbert (1996); Pulvermüller, Eulitz, Pantev, Mohr, Feige, Lutzenberger, Elbert and Birbaumer, 1996) have looked at stimulus-related changes in regional (e.g. temporal lobe) spectral power in MEG recordings. For example, they have studied how the distinction between words or non-words in a lexical decision task modulates the spectral power in the 30 Hz, or gamma band (Pulvermüller et al., 1996) or how language versus non-language stimuli affect the spectral activity in cer-

tain time and frequency bins (Eulitz et al., 1996). Eulitz et al. presented subjects with visual or auditory words or non-words, or matched control items. Subjects had to attend and respond to the presence or absence of a specific distractor item in each stimulus. Using a 37-channel biomagnetometer (Magnes™), they measured responses from the temporal lobe and analysed, for various time- and frequency bins, the (normalized) spectral power and its regional variation across the conditions. One of the core results of the study was that, for auditory words, there were significant spectral power changes over the left hemisphere: for example, at ~130 ms post-stimulus onset there was a significant increase in the 9–18 Hz band, and at ~900 ms after stimulus onset there was a significant increase in the 14–32Hz band. Stimulus-specific decreases were observed as well. Coupled with the localization of the sources that underlie these spectral changes, such studies afford the opportunity to observe the responses of neuronal populations to language-specific stimulus attributes. Such observations must certainly be tied closely to models of word processing, but the fact that there were differential spectral changes highlights that a full description of language-related phenomena requires these types of electromagnetic data.

3. There are speech-specific effects that occur early and are transient and thus probably not detectable in hemodynamic responses. One such example is provided by the experiment presented in Poeppel, Yellin, Phillips, Roberts, Rowley, Wexler, and Marantz (1996). Subjects were presented with synthesized speech syllables (/ba/, /pa/, /da/, /ta/) and asked to listen passively in one run and categorize them by voicing in a second run (e.g. categorize /ba/ and /da/ versus /pa/ and /ta/). The analysis of the dominant auditory evoked neuromagnetic response, the M100, revealed that the execution of the task increased the response amplitude in left auditory cortex. In the right auditory cortex, however, the execution of the very simple speech discrimination and categorization task was associated with an amplitude decrease. Such a task-induced asymmetry was not observed in a similar experiment using tones (Arthur, Lewis, Medvick and Flynn, 1991) suggesting that there exist speech-specific lateralized responses in cortex as early as 100 ms after stimulus onset that might be no longer as clearly visible at later measurement points (e.g. 200 ms). Importantly, the responses in both the passive-listening and task-dependent conditions completely co-localized in the superior temporal cortex, ruling out the interpretation that the execution of an experimental task demands selectively engaged different cortical areas, thus making amplitude comparisons invalid. That such fast and transient speech-specific phenomena necessitate an electrophysiological recording method is obvious.

4. A different set of considerations is introduced by some recent work that suggests that latency may play a role in coding auditory information. The dominant way in which one thinks about stimulus representation in the central nervous system is spatial: the visual system has retinotopic areas, the somatosensory system has somatotopic areas and the auditory system has tonotopic areas. Are such spatial representations sufficient? We have been investigating whether one can observe a time-based encoding of stimuli – in other words 'time-o-topic' representational mechanisms in hearing and speech perception. There are two ways in which a temporal framework might encode stimulus information: as stimulus-related oscillations (Eulitz et al., 1996; Pulvermüller et al., 1996; Salmelin and Hari, 1994; Salmelin and Mäkelä, 1995) or as latencies of peak responses associated with specific stimulus attributes (Roberts and Poeppel, 1996). A clear example of latency-based coding is provided by the repres-

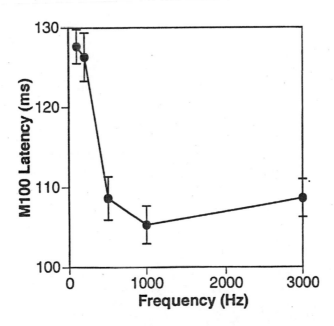

Figure 24.2. The most prominent auditory evoked neuromagnetic field, the M100 (cf. Figure 24.1), is reliably elicited by a variety of auditory stimuli. The figure shows the peak latency of the M100 response for pure tones (400 ms duration) of varying frequencies (100—3000 Hz), presented to the right ear (128 repetitions/stimulus). All tones were presented at 40 dB SL. There is a dramatic latency difference as a function of frequency, with low frequencies being associated with significantly longer latencies (>20 ms).]

entation of tone frequency. We have observed a systematic relationship between tone frequency and the latency of the major cortical
auditory evoked (M100) response (Roberts and Poeppel, 1996). As
shown in Figure 24.2, low frequency sounds (100–200 Hz, characteristic of the pitch of speech sounds) are associated with up to 30
ms longer latencies than the middle frequencies (1000–3000 Hz,
associated with the formants of speech sounds). It thus appears that
the auditory system can code frequency in the spatial and time
domains. We have been able to extend these findings to speech
sound processing (latency is associated with formant frequency, not
fundamental frequency, Poeppel, Phillips, Yellin, Rowley, Roberts
and Marantz, 1997), which suggests that a latency-based coding
mechanism is perhaps a general feature of auditory processing.
Indeed, it has been argued that using latency to encode sensory
objects is an effective way to help the nervous system disentangle
the multitude of simultanously processed information (Eysel, 1996).
Should information be coded as latency variation in the range of
tens of milliseconds, only electrophysiologic methods will be appropriate.

Conclusion

Cortical dynamics, spectral changes and oscillations, speech-specific
transient effects and latency-based codes are electrophysiological phenomena that are quite clearly tied to electrophysiological methods.
These briefly-presented examples thus merely serve to illustrate that
there are speech- and language-related phenomena that crucially
require the time resolution of electromagnetic methods. Insofar as
one will want to localize the activity, thus connecting with spatially
based imaging such as fMRI or PET, data obtained in MEG recordings
appear especially useful. Insofar as it is desirable to connect non-
invasive functional imaging data with systems-level electrophysiology,
the data obtained by MEG and EEG also seem particularly well suited
to de-velop an integrated perspective that combines the localization
of cerebral processes underlying cognition (provided primarily by
PET and fMRI) with the temporal structure of cerebral events (typically provided by electrophysiology). Of course, it is important to bear
in mind that even an exhaustive spatio-temporal description will in
the end not be satisfactory without a comprehensive explanatory theoretical account of how speech and language are represented and
processed.

References

Arthur D, Lewis P, Medvick P, Flynn E (1991) A neuromagnetic study of selective auditory attention. Electroenceph Clin Neurophysiol 78: 348–60.

Binder JR, Frost JA, Hammeke TA, Cox RW, Rao SM, Prieto T (1997) Human brain language areas identified by functional magnetic resonance imaging. Journal of Neuroscience 17(1): 353–62.

Binder JR, Frost JA, Hammeke TA, Rao SM, Cox RW (1996) Function of the left planum temporale in auditory and linguistic processing. Brain 119: 1239–47.

Démonet J, Price C, Wise R, Frackowiak R (1994) A PET study of cognitive strategies in normal subjects during language tasks: influence of phonetic ambiguity and sequence processing of phoneme monitoring. Brain 117: 671–82.

Démonet J, Chollet F, Ramsay S, Cardebat D, Nespoulous J-L, Wise R, Rascol A, Frackowiak R (1992) The anatomy of phonological and semantic processing in normal subjects. Brain 115: 1753–68.

Eulitz C, Maess B, Pantev C, Friederici A, Feige B, Elbert T (1996) Oscillatory neuro-magnetic activity induced by language and non-language stimuli. Cognitive Brain Research 4: 121–32.

Eysel U (1996) Latency as additional dimension for object encoding in sensory systems. Neuroreport 7: 1113.

Fiez J (1996) Cerebellar contributions to cognition. Neuron 16: 13–15.

Fiez J, Raichle ME, Miezin FM, Petersen SE, Tallal P, Katz WF (1995) Studies of auditory and phonological processing: effects of stimulus characteristics and task demands. Journal of Cognitive Neuroscience 7(3): 357–75.

Friston KJ, Price CJ, Fletcher P, Moore C, Frackowiak RSJ, Dolan RJ (1996) The trouble with cognitive subtraction. NeuroImage 4(2): 97–104.

George JS, Aine CJ, Mosher JC, Schmidt DM, Ranken DM, Schlitt HA, Wood CC, Lewine JD, Sanders JA, Belliveau JW (1995) Mapping function in the human brain with magnetoencephalography, anatomical magnetic resonance imaging, and functional magnetic resonance imaging. J Clin Neurophysiol 12(5): 406–31.

Gevins A, Le J, Martin NK, Brickett P, Desmond J, Reutter B (1994) High resolution EEG: 124-channel recording, spatial deblurring and MRI integration methods. Electroencephalogr Clin Neurophysiol 90(5): 337–58.

Hämäläinen M, Hari R, Ilmoniemi R, Knuutila J, Lounasmaa OV (1993) Magnetoencephalography–theory, instrumentation, and applications to non-invasive studies of the working human brain. Rev Mod Phys 65(2): 413–97.

Ioannides AA (1993) Brain function as revealed by current density analysis of magnetoencephalography signals. Physiol Meas 14 Suppl 4A: A75–80.

Ioannides AA, Singh KD, Hasson R, Baumann SB, Rogers RL, Guinto FC, Jr., Papanicolaou AC (1993) Comparison of single current dipole and magnetic field tomography analyses of the cortical response to auditory stimuli. Brain Topogr 6(1): 27–34.

Kwong KK (1995) Functional magnetic resonance imaging with echo planar imaging. Magnetic Resonance Quarterly 11(1): 1–20.

Lewine J, Orrison W. (1995). Magnetoencephalography and magnetic source imaging. In Orrison W, Lewine J, Sanders J, Hartshorne M (Eds) Functional Brain Imaging. St. Louis: Mosby.

Mazoyer BM, Dehaene S, Tzourio N, Frak J, Murayama N, Cohen L, Levrier O, Salamon G, Syrota A, Mehler J (1993) The cortical representation of speech. Journal of Cognitive Neuroscience 5(4): 467–79.

Mosher JC, Lewis PS, Leahy RM (1992) Multiple dipole modeling and localization from spatio-temporal MEG data. IEEE Trans Biomed Eng 39(6) 541–57.

Näätänen R, Ilmoniemi R, Alho K (1994) Magnetoencephalography in studies of human cognitive brain function. Trends in Neurosciences 17(9): 389–95.

Nadeau S, Crosson B (1995) A guide to the functional imaging of cognitive processes. Neuropsychiatry, Neuropsychology, and Behavioral Neurology 8(3): 143–62.

Orrison W, Lewine J, Sanders J, Hartshorne M (Eds) (1995). Functional Brain Imaging. St Louis: Mosby.

Petersen S, Fox P, Posner M, Mintun M, Raichle M (1989) Positron emission tomographic studies of the processing of single words. Journal of Cognitive Neuroscience 1(2): 153–70.

Poeppel D (1996) A critical review of PET studies of phonological processing. Brain and Language 55: 317–51.

Poeppel D, Phillips C, Yellin E, Rowley HA, Roberts TPL, Marantz A (1997) Processing of vowels in supratemporal auditory cortex. Neuroscience Letters 221: 145–8.

Poeppel D, Yellin E, Phillips C, Roberts TPL, Rowley HA, Wexler K, Marantz A (1996) Task-induced asymmetry of the auditory evoked M100 neuromagnetic field elicited by speech sounds. Cognitive Brain Research 4: 231–42.

Posner M, Raichle M (1994) Images of Mind. New York: Freeman.

Pulvermüller F, Eulitz C, Pantev C, Mohr B, Feige B, Lutzenberger W, Elbert T, Birbaumer N (1996) High-frequency cortical responses reflect lexical processing: an MEG study. EEG and Clin Neurophysiol 98: 76–85.

Raichle ME (1994) Visualizing the mind. Sci Am 270(4): 58–64.

Roberts TPL, Poeppel D (1996) Latency of auditory evoked M100 as a function of tone frequency. NeuroReport 7: 1138–40.

Roland P (1993) Brain Activation. New York: Wiley-Liss.

Salmelin R, Hari R (1994) Characterization of spontaneous MEG rhythms in healthy adults. Electroencephalogr Clin Neurophysiol 91(4): 237–48.

Salmelin R, Hari R, Lounasmaa OV, Sams M (1994) Dynamics of brain activation during picture naming. Nature 368(6470): 463–5.

Salmelin R, Mäkelä J (1995) Magnetic signals in the study of human brain dynamics. Rivista di Neuroradiologia 8: 329–44.

Salmelin R, Service E, Kiesilä P, Uutela K, Salonen O (1996) Impaired visual word processing in dyslexia revealed with magnetoencephalography. Ann. Neurol. 40: 157–62.

Sarter M, Berntson GG, Cacioppo JT (1996) Brain imaging and cognitive neuroscience: toward strong inference in attributing function to structure. American Psychologist 51(1): 13–21.

Scherg M, Vajsar J, Pickton T (1989) A source analysis of the late human auditory evoked potentials. Journal of Cognitive Neuroscience 1(4): 336–55.

Sergent J (1994) Brain-imaging studies of cognitive functions. TINS 17(6): 221–7.

Stromswold K, Caplan D, Alpert N, Rauch S (1996) Localization of syntactic comprehension by positron emission tomography. Brain and Language 52(3): 1974–91.

Whitaker HA, Poeppel D, Hochman D (1997) A logical problem in the interpretation of functional brain images: the need for independent evidence. Journal of the International Neuropsychological Society 3(1): 1.

Zatorre R, Evans A, Meyer E, Gjedde A (1992) Lateralization of phonetic and pitch discrimination in speech processing. Science 256: 846–9.

Chapter 25
Hemispheric Lateralization of Speech Production and Singing at the Level of the Motor Cortex in fMRI

DIRK WILDGRUBER, HERMANN ACKERMANN, UWE KLOSE, BERND KARDATZKI AND WOLFGANG GRODD

Introduction

A variety of studies has demonstrated lateralization of language functions to the left hemisphere of the human brain. For example Penfield and Rasmussen (1949) observed that, as a rule, speech was arrested following electrical stimulation of the inferior frontal and parietal cortex of the left hemisphere. Right-sided exploration of these areas left speech unimpaired. At the level of the Rolandic cortex, however, vocalizations and speech arrest were produced by electrical stimulation with similar frequency and at approximately symmetrical locations within both hemispheres. On the basis of these findings it was concluded that there is no lateralization of speech production at the level of the primary sensorimotor cortex.

In contrast to this hypothesis, Geschwind (1969) observed that lesions restricted to the left internal capsule may give rise to transient dysarthria whereas damage to the right internal capsule is not followed by articulatory impairments. He explained the complete recovery of articulatory functions after left-sided damage in terms of compensatory activation of an alternative pathway projecting from Broca's area to the cranial nerve nuclei via the corpus callosum, Broca-analogon of the non-dominant hemisphere and right Rolandic cortex. Permanent articulatory disorders following lesions restricted to the left motor cortex or pathways have been reported (Schiff, Alexander, Naeser and Galaburda, 1983; Alexander, Benson and Stuss, 1989). Schiff et al., for example presented a sample of cases suffering from dysarthria without aphasia following focal lesions of the frontal lobe. In four out of 12 cases the lesion was restricted to the primary motor area. The lesion was localized within the left hemisphere in all but one case.

In contrast, impaired singing and monotonous speech, lacking emotional expression, concomitant with mainly preserved articulatory performance at the phonemic level, have been observed in patients with damage to the right motor cortex or the respective cortico-bulbar projections (Ross, 1981; Ross et al., 1981; Alexander et al., 1989). Assuming that prosodic aspects of spoken language depend upon the non-dominant hemisphere, verbal utterances lacking any relevant melodic modulation must be considered in order to evaluate functional lateralization of speech motor control at the level of the primary motor cortex.

Methods

Continuous recitation of highly automated word strings such as the names of the months of the year seem to represent a feasible task in this regard. This condition was labeled 'automatic speech'. As control conditions non-speech tongue movements (vertical excursions inside the closed mouth - the 'tongue movement' condition) and singing of a well-known melody ('Oh Tannenbaum') with the syllable 'la' as its carrier were considered (the 'syllable singing' condition). All tasks were carried out by 10 healthy right-handed subjects (five males and five females aged 20—36 years). Handedness was assessed by means of the Edinburgh Inventory (Oldfield, 1971). Since it has been demonstrated (Yetkin et al., 1995) that speaking aloud produces considerable artifacts in the fMRI activation maps due to head motion during the activation period, while the same pattern of activation within the speech areas was found during silent speech, the administered tasks were carried out silently and the backs of the subjects' heads were snuggly surrounded with foam rubber within the head coil and a strap was placed over the forehead. Since the tasks were carried out silently, it seemed to be impossible to control quality and quantity of 'internal' speech production during rest and activation periods. To reduce speech production during rest, we asked the participants to refrain from 'internal speech' as far as possible during the rest periods and told them to visualize a black wall instead to make it more comfortable.

Using the blood oxygen level dependent (bold) contrast effect as an indirect marker of local neuronal activity (Ogawa, Lee, Kay and Tank, 1990), functional magnetic resonance imaging (fMRI) was carried out to evaluate hemispheric lateralization under the three tasks considered. The measurements were performed with a 1.5 Tesla whole-body scanner (Siemens Vision) by means of a multislice echo-planar imaging (EPI) sequence (TE = 72 ms, alpha = 90 deg, FOV = 260 × 163 mm, 128 × 80 matrix). Twenty-seven parallel axial slices of 4 mm thickness and 1 mm gap were acquired covering the whole brain volume. Each measurement across the 27 slices required 7 s; the interval in between amounted to 3 s giving an effective TR of 10 s. Absence of observable head motion during task administration was ensured for all participants by their viewing the series of images in cine mode. As an anatomical reference, T_1-weighted images of the same axial slice positions were obtained using a spin echo sequence (TR 600 ms, TE 15 ms).

Each task comprised eight successive groups of five measurements, alternately performed during 'rest' and 'activation'. To assess individual task-specific activation in terms of signal-to-noise units, z-values were calculated separately for each pixel (mean difference of signal intensities during rest and activation divided by the root mean square deviation of the signal intensities; Le Bihan, Jezzard, Turner, Cuenod, Pannier and Prinster, 1993). A pixel was considered 'activated' if it belonged to a circular area of 2.5 pixels radius characterized by a mean z-value above 0.3. This spatial filter was introduced to minimize false negative and false positive entries into the activation-map due to random signal variations caused by the measurement procedure.

For the purpose of this study, the lower half of the precentral gyrus was considered the relevant part of the motor strip. To identify this region of interest (ROI) within individual subjects unbiased by knowledge of the activation maps, the area between the precentral and the central sulcus was surrounded on each set of T1 weighted anatomical images (Rademacher, Galaburda, Kennedy, Filipek and Caviness, 1992). These regions were assigned to the corresponding EPI-activation maps, and the numbers of activated pixels within these ROIs covering multiple slices were calculated for both hemispheres of each participant and statistically evaluated with a t-test for paired samples.

Results

A highly significant lateralization of the hemodynamic response towards the left hemisphere emerged at the lower half of the motor strip under the automatic speech condition. The mean number of activated pixels within the left lower motor cortex amounted to 48.4 (SD = 26.0) as opposed to 19.1 (SD = 13.9) on the right side (t = 3.6, p = 0.006). Syllable singing led to a significant lateralization effect towards the right motor cortex (t = −2.9, p = 0.02) with a mean value of 32.7 (SD = 30.9) activated pixels in the left and 52.9 (SD = 29.9) in the right oro-facial area of the motor cortex.

Symmetrical bilateral activation within the same areas during tongue movement confirms the correct identification of the oro-facial sensory-motor area during the parcellation procedure (see figures of the fMRI activation maps during the different tasks in Wildgruber, Ackermann, Klose, Kardatzki and Grodd, 1996). The mean number of activated pixels during tongue movement amounted to 149.7 (SD = 79.4) at the left and 135.8 (SD = 74.5) at the right side. Statistical analysis (two-tailed t-test for paired samples) did not reveal significant lateralization differences (t = 1.0, p = 0.36).

The number of activated pixels obtained from each subject under the various task conditions is given in Table 25.1. Since the absolute number of activated pixels showed considerable variance, the percentage of lateralized activation to either motor strip was calculated for each participant (number of activated pixels on either side divided by their total number) in order to normalize the observed lateralization effects. Considering the individual data, in nine out of ten cases (all but subject no. 3) a lateralization to the left was obtained during automatic speech, whereas syllable singing yielded a lateralization towards the right hemisphere in eight out of 10 cases (all but subjects no. 4 and no. 7).

Table 25.1. Number of activated pixels within the lower half of the pre-central gyrus of the left and right hemisphere, obtained during the various tasks. Percentage of activated pixels within the left and right motor cortices are printed in brackets. The respective mean values and standard deviations are shown at the bottom of the table

Subject No.	Gender m/f	AUTOMATIC SPEECH left no. (%)	right no. (%)	TONGUE MOVEMENT left no. (%)	right no. (%)	SYLLABLE SINGING left no. (%)	right no. (%)
1	f	56 (84%)	11 (16%)	157 (59%)	107 (41%)	30 (33%)	61 (67%)
2	f	16 (100%)	0 (0%)	81 (47%)	93 (53%)	16 (36%)	28 (64%)
3	f	27 (39%)	42 (61%)	55 (52%)	50 (48 %)	9 (24%)	29 (76%)
4	f	87 (86%)	14 (14%)	156 (61%)	98 (39%)	79 (54%)	68 (46%)
5	f	56 (69%)	25 (31%)	124 (45%)	149 (55%)	4 (15%)	22 (85%)
6	m	21 (60%)	14 (40%)	107 (44%)	134 (56%)	8 (25%)	24 (75%)
7	m	29 (100%)	0 (0%)	165 (51%)	157 (49%)	56 (57%)	43 (43%)
8	m	91 (75%)	30 (25%)	85 (50%)	86 (50%)	34 (27%)	92 (73%)
9	m	46 (68%)	22 (32%)	237 (63%)	162 (37%)	86 (44%)	109 (56%)
10	m	56 (63%)	33 (37%)	294 (48%)	322 (52%)	5 (14%)	31 (86%)
mean		74.3%	25.7%	52.1%	47.9%	32.3%	67.7%
std. dev.		± 18.9	± 18.9	± 6.8	± 6.8	± 15.7	± 15.7

Discussion

Non-speech tongue movements yielded a rather symmetrical activation of the lower Rolandic cortex whereas, in contrast, a significantly stronger hemodynamic response of the left-sided motor strip emerged during the production of word strings. These findings corroborate the suggestion, derived from clinical data, of a functional lateralization of speech production at the level of the primary motor cortex.

It might be argued that this observed lateralization effect simply reflects activation of Broca's area during speech production. Admittedly, there is no clear-cut anatomical landmark that unambiguously demarcates the transition between lower motor cortex and the posterior part of the inferior frontal gyrus at MR scans. The hemodynamic response during automatic speech was, however, located within the region activated by non-speech tongue movements. It can be assumed, therefore, that the documented lateralization effect during speech refers to the motor cortex.

In contrast to production of verbal utterances, syllable singing resulted in a functional lateralization towards the right motor strip. There is considerable clinical and experimental evidence that the processing of pitch predominantly involves the non-dominant hemisphere. Gordon and Bogen (1974), for instance, observed a monotonous quality of singing after injection of amytal into the right carotid artery, whereas articulation remained relatively intact. The left-sided Wada-test, by contrast, did not significantly interfere with the production of melodies. Since right-sided damage to the precentral cortex or the respective cortico-bulbar projections may give rise to monotonous speech lacking emotional modulation ('affective aprosodia'), the non-dominant hemisphere seems to be more efficient in the processing of speech melody as well (Alexander et al., 1989; Ross, 1981; Ross and Harney, 1981). With respect to hemispheric lateralization, thus, a dissociation between articulatory and affective prosodic aspects of verbal utterances can be assumed.

Singing yielded a less pronounced lateralization effect than aprosodic speech. It is conceivably easier voluntarily to refrain from prosodic modulation of highly automated word strings than to avoid verbal representations during syllable singing. This suggestion is corroborated by the report of some participants that they had to refer to the text of the song in order to remember the melody.

To avoid movement artifacts, the subjects of the present study were asked to perform the tasks silently. Since action potentials can be recorded from the speech musculature during silent speaking, motor cortex activation must be assumed under these conditions (Sokolov, 1972). Yetkin, Hammeke, Swanson, Morris, Mueller, McAuliffe and Haughton (1995) found similar fMRI activation patterns during covert and audible word generation. In comparison to spoken language, a smaller number of motor units are recruited during inner speech. These observations may explain the smaller areas of activation and the less pronounced signal increase during silent speaking as opposed to non-speech tongue movements.

Conceivably, the asymmetric organization of speech production at the level of the primary motor cortex prevents mistiming of motor impulses to the speech muscles. Compared to the left motor strip, transfer of information originating in Broca's region to the right pre-central gyrus via callosal pathways should require more time. This extra delay must be expected to result in asynchronous input to the bulbar nuclei, a mechanism that has been assumed to produce stuttering (Van Riper, 1971). Functional lateralization to the left pre-central cortex might represent a compensatory mechanism in this regard.

References

Alexander MP, Benson DF, Stuss DT (1989) Frontal lobes and language. Brain & Language, 37: 656–91.

Geschwind N (1969) Problems in the anatomical understanding of the aphasias. In Benton AL (Ed) Contributions to Clinical Neuropsychology. Chicago: Aldine, 107–28.

Gordon HW, Bogen JE (1974) Hemispheric lateralization of singing after intra-carotid sodium amylobarbitone. J Neurol Neurosurg Psychiatry, 37: 727–38.

Le Bihan D, Jezzard P, Turner R, Cuenod CA, Pannier L, Prinster A (1993) Practical Problems and Limitations in Using Z-Maps for Processing of Brain Function MR Images. SMRM 12th meeting, Abstracts: 11.

Ogawa S, Lee TM, Kay AR, Tank DW (1990) Brain magnetic resonance imaging with contrast dependent on blood oxygenation. Proc Natl Acad Sci USA. 87: 9868–72.

Oldfield RC (1971) The Assessment and Analysis of Handedness: The Edinburgh Inventory. Neuropsychologia 9: 97–113.

Penfield W, Rasmussen T (1949) Vocalization and arrest of speech. Arch Neurol Psychiat. 61: 21–7.

Rademacher J, Galaburda AM, Kennedy DN, Filipek PA, Caviness VS (1992) Human cerebral cortex: localization, parcellation, and morphometry with magnetic resonance imaging. J Cogn Neurosci 4: 352–74.

Ross ED (1981) The aprosodias: functional-anatomic organization of the affective components of language in the right hemisphere. Arch Neurol 38: 561–9.

Ross ED, Harney JH (1981) How the brain integrates affective and propositional language into a unified behavioral function. Arch Neurol 38: 745–8.

Schiff HB, Alexander MP, Naeser MA, Galaburda AM (1983) Aphemia: clinical-anatomic correlations. Arch Neurol, 40: 720–7.

Sokolov AN (1972) Inner Speech and Thought. New York: Plenium Press.

Van Riper C (1971) The Nature of Stuttering. London: Prentice-Hall.

Wildgruber D, Ackermann H, Klose U, Kardatzki B, Grodd W (1996) Functional lateralization of speech production at primary motor cortex: a fMRI study. Neuroreport 7: 2791–5.

Yetkin FZ, Hammeke TA, Swanson SJ, Morris GL, Mueller WM, McAuliffe TL, Haughton VM (1995) A comparision of functional MR activation patterns during silent and audible language tasks. AJNR 16: 1087–92

Chapter 26
Articulation of Spoken and Sung Sentences

CREIGHTON J. MILLER, LEE HARRIS, RAY DANILOFF AND KYM SCHULZE

Introduction

Vocal research has characterized systematic differences in the carriage of vocal organs — lips, mandible, tongue, pharynx, larynx, etc. – adopted for singing in the 'classical' mode (Appelman, 1967). The pedagogue, Vennard (1967, p. 163) characterized the vocal differences between singers of classical music and entertainers who 'violate the canons both of good singing and of good music'. The latter appear to rely upon 'diction' and 'dramatic projection'. He claimed that, 'in singing, when we want the voice to be a musical instrument (classical) we shape the resonators to be in tune with the fundamental and so our vowel formants are harmonics, whereas in speech (and popular singing) this need not be the case'. Indeed, Apelman's (1967) study of systematic articulatory-laryngeal shifts across the range of vocal frequencies and intensities for English vowels characterizes such classically trained articulatory-vocal adjustments for song. In a review decades later, (Sundberg, 1987) a wealth of new literature explored singers' source characteristics and intonation patterns, whose highly stylized forms can be differentiated on the basis of conveyed emotional status and force. Two poles of intonational-rhythmic extremes are, Schonstimme-Sprechstimme (sparing voice) and Kraftstimme (Trojan, 1952 as quoted in Sundberg, 1987). Inspection of Titze's (1994) text reveals an absence of studies designed to contrast articulatory patterns between spoken and classically sung text.

The purpose of the current study was to examine the distribution of intrinsic and extrinsic allophone productions in spoken and sung English sentences. Ladefoged's (1993) list of 23 pronunciation rules that characterize the candid articulatory behaviour of typical speakers of American English was used to probe possible shifts in allophone production characteristic of sung versus spoken articulation of sentences.

Method

Four students (ages 24–34; two males, two females), enrolled in the Doctorate of Musical Arts programme at the University of North Texas, were recruited as speaker-singers. Each had normal articulation and passed a hearing screening at 20 dB HL. Each had sung academically/professionally for a minimum of seven years.

Thirty-six sentences containing multiple examples of 23 allophonic processes said to characterize typical American English pronunciation were devised (Daniloff and Wolfe, 1995, see Table 26.1). The second author composed different, simple melodic patterns to accompany each sentence. The second author sang the melodic phrases; his modelling of the 'songs' was not intended to be a stylistic norm. One might say that he sang 'vanilla' versions of the songs.

Table 26.1. Examples of sentences spoken and sung

1.	He wants to lay around very lazily.
2.	Betty is praising her lacy skirt.
3.	Can you praise God as you pray?
4	Put a piece of lace on the windows.
5.	Be nice to the bees my lad.
6.	Play with my cousin Buzz.
7.	I'm going with Tad soon.
8.	The lazy man lays in a bed.
9.	Swirls of frost lacily cover the leaves.
10.	Cotton shirts wear pretty well.

In composing the short melodies for each sentence, LH followed a rhythmic sense that flowed out of syntax, prosody, and the usual emphasis given to English sentences, similar to that in operatic recitative, which is typically more speech-like than an aria. The range and key used in each melody was limited so that there would be few technical demands placed on the singers that might interfere with their execution of the phrases.

Singers are taught that the beauty of the vocal sound is of paramount importance. Although the meaning in the text must be conveyed to the listener, vocal diction is a balancing act between aesthetic and communicative criteria. An emphasis on tone quality is usually expressed in *legato* (smooth, flowing) singing, a greater emphasis on vowels than consonants, and the elision of consonants and vowels in some cases. Whereas speakers, such as radio announcers, might have a pleasing vocal quality, their primary emphasis is on communicating a text as clearly as possible. Trained singers, on the other hand, seek first to optimize vocal quality; conveying the meaning of the text is subordinate to the aesthetic standards that they and the listener share. Participants were recorded as they read each sentence aloud at moderate tempo. Then each singer imitated a tape recording of the second author's sung versions of the sentences, reproducing his sung sentences at the indicated moderate tempo. The recordings were phonetically transcribed and selected sentences, contexts, and subjects were analysed using the signal analysis programs WavEdit (Miller, 1991), and Soundscope 16 (GW Instruments, 1991).

Results

Table 26.2 compares sung versus spoken percentages of occurrence for the allophones tracked in the study. Although individual data are included in this figure for reference, our considerations below address only the mean data for all participants.

Phonetic analysis of the allophones not routinely produced during song, revealed significant reductions in spoken vs. sung frequency of occurrence only for syllabic /n/ (41.7% decrease) and glottal stops (62% decrease). Substantial, though nonsignificant differences also occured for unreleased stop in stop + stop sequence (62% decrease), word final unexploded stop (30% decrease) and flap of alveolar stop (25% reduction). Of the singers examined, LH and RW produced a statistically significant spoken vs. sung difference in the percentage of allophones produced.

The following allophonic variations, with few exceptions, were honoured almost without exception in spoken/sung sentences, by all subjects: (a) devoicing of approximant in voiceless, obstruent, and approximate clusters, (b) partial devoicing of utterance final obstruents (except in a few cases where /ə/ was appended), (c) vowel duration open syllables (range 51– 8.1%) exceeded durations in closed syllables, etc. Overall, subjects singing produced 34% fewer allophones than when speaking (range 62–25%). Overall, the subjects produced fewer allophones during singing than during speaking.

Table 26.3 displays other allophonic variations observed in sung sentences for all four subjects. Syllabification (schwa epenthesis) of final stops and other consonants, strengthening and substitution of vowels, loss of ambisyllabicity of a consonant, etc. occurred. The number of instances was very small, but perceptually highly noticeable. Two of four subjects were responsible for the unsought allophonic variations.

Temporal measures

All sentence durations were normalized as follows: subjects' mean spoken and mean sung sentence durations were computed. Subject LH's two means, spoken and sung, were chosen as the standard sentence durations. The ratios of LH's mean values to those of the other

Table 26.2. Percentage of allophones uttered

Allophones	LH(M) read	LH(M) sung	RW(M) read	RW(M) sung	KB(F) read	KB(F) sung	SP(F) read	SP(F) sung	X read	X sung	mean difference r vs. s
syllabic /n̩/ (3)	100	66.6	66.6	33.3	100	66.6	100	33.3	91.7	50.0	*41.7
stop + stop /c c/ (16)	93.7	62.5	91.3	12.5	87.5	68.7	62.5	43.7	81.2	46.9	34.3
utterance final unreleased stop /-c #/ (10)	70.0	20.0	50.0	0.00	20.0	0.00	0.00	0.00	35.0	5.00	30.0
flap of alveolar stop /ɾ/ (6)	100	100	100	0.00	100	100	100	83.3	100	75.0	25.0
glottal stop /ʔ/ (2) /stop + homorg nasal/	100	50.0	100	0.00	100	50.0	50.0	0.00	87.5	25.0	*62.0
X	94.6	57.8	75.7	8.10	72.9	54.0	54.0	35.0	73.0	39.0	
difference	*36.8%		*67.6%		18.9%		19.0%		34.0%		

* Differences marked with asterisks are significant (p<0.05)

singers (x_{LH}sung/x_{KB}sung) = 0.90, etc. were computed, and used as multipliers of individual sentence duration to bring subjects KB, SP, and RW's sentences into alignment with LH's. These normalized values were used in the computations below.

Table 26.3. Minor allophonic variations of sung sentences.

In the transcriptions, the following unexpected allophonic variations occurred for one or two of the four subjects.

					Subjects
1.	/əɹ aund/	→	[ə.ɹaun]	d-deletion	RW
2.	/vɛɹi/	→	[vɛ.ɹi]	ambisyllabicity deleted	RW
3.	/leɪ.zɪ.li/	→	[leɪ.zʌ.li]	stress-induced vowel	
	/koɹ.səz/	→	[koɹ.sʌz]	change	RW
4.	/bæd, pæd, kæd/	→	[bæ.də, pæ.də, kæ.də]		RW
	/mæn, bɛd, ðiz/	→	[mæ.nə bɛ.də, ði.zə]		SP
				six cases of syllabification of word final consonants	
5.	/əv/	→	[ɔv]	substitution	RW, SP
	/ðə/	→	[ðʌ]	substitution	RW, SP
	/ðʌ/	→	[ði]	substitution	RW, SP
	/'ɛm.fə.sɪs/	→	['ɛm.fɪ.sɪs]	substitution	RW
	/spoɹts/	→	[spaɹts]	substitution	SP
6.	/skɜ˞t/	→	[skɑɪt]	loss of rhotacized vowel	SP

1. Subject KB produced larger sung/spoken sentence ratios than subject SP on 21/29 sentence comparisons; similarly subject RW's ratios exceed LH's on 27/29 comparisons. Clearly, the extent of sung sentence lengthening is substantial and subject dependent. Figure 26.1 shows a pair of regression lines fitted to KB's and SP's spoken and sung sentence durations. The slopes are nearly identical at 1.7, $p < 0.003$, that is, singing produces an elongation of sung sentences as contrasted with spoken sentences of roughly 1.7/1.

2. In the 21 sentences where sung sentences were longer, sung syllables and words were also longer in every case, suggesting that articulated-sung syllables and words, not filled or silent pauses, were part of the lengthening. The word and syllable lengthening was also subject dependent.

3. For both sung and spoken sentences, Spearman correlations between sentence duration (msec) and the number of words in the sentence ranged from 0.350 to 0.490 ($p < 0.01$). For spoken sentences, correlations between sentence duration and number of syllables in the sentence ranged from 0.705 to 0.765 ($p < 0.001$).

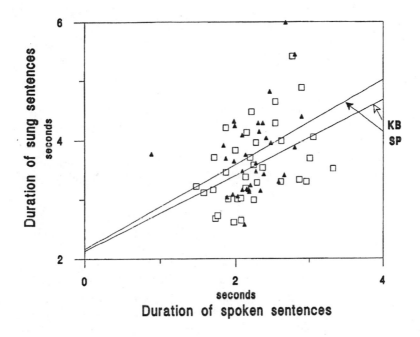

Figure 26.1 Duration of sung versus spoken sentences

Considered together, these results suggest that phonetic/phonological factors and the singing act may have an interactive influence upon sentence durations. Spoken sentence durations were also significant, and generally, much higher (e.g. 0.765 for subject KB, 0.705 for subject SP). These results suggest that with sentence duration, syllable count is more strongly correlated with spoken sentence duration than with sung sentence duration. The phonetic structure of the word and the act of singing appear capable of weakening the temporal relationship.

Discussion

Frequency of production of intrinsic allophones, relatively involuntary variants dictated by articulatory constraints, etc., did not change in any notable fashion for singing versus speaking contexts in this study. This result stands in direct contrast to our findings for the extrinsic allophones, those that are acquired by speakers for volitional phonetic/phonological reasons. Our analyses revealed a consistent and noteable tendency towards reduction in frequency of occurrence in sung, versus spoken spech (statistically significant in three cases). Although this effect was smallest for subject RW (male) his singing voice is also that

judged to have been most 'operatic-florid', including the fewest occurrences of extrinsic allophones among all participants. Perhaps the most
formal, operatic, singing style also demands the most formal, standard
(e.g. non-allophonic) phoneme production. Subject LH (male) produced more allophones during singing than any other participant in
the study and, interestingly, his singing was judged to be the most
'speech-like', possessing most of the qualities of 'pop' vocalization.

Temporal analyses of our data further indicate that singing elicits a
durational increase in sentences of about 1.7 for the two female subjects analysed and roughly 1.8 for the two males.

Our results indicate that the articulatory perturbations introduced
by singing alter characteristic relationship between syllable count and
total sentence duration (msec).

We interpret this as an indication that the expressive temporal
demands of vocal artistry can override the simple duration patterns of
speech.

In conclusion, this study indicates that simple articulatory probes of
singing will reveal widespread intrasubject and intersubject differences
in phonetic behaviour between speech and song and, perhaps, types of
singing style. These differences can be used to probe the temporal-
intonation-stylistic sources of such behaviour, and suggest that a
modest part of what is identified by listeners as characteristic of song is
phonetic-phonological in nature. We are currently exploring popular/
classical singer differences with regard to such allophonic behaviour.

References

Appelman DR (1967) The Science of Vocal Pedagogy. Bloomington, IN: Indiana
    University Press.
Daniloff R, Wolfe K (1995) Contribution of allophonic processes to the accent of
    English spoken by Chinese speakers. In Powell MT (Ed.) Pathologies of Speech
    and Language: Contribution of Clinical Linguistics and Phonetics. New Orleans
    ICPLA, pp 187–192.
GW Instruments (1991) Soundscope user's manual vol. 1.2. Sommerville, MA: GW
    Instruments, Inc.
Ladefoged P (1993) A Course in Phonetics, 3rd edn. New York: Harcourt Brace
    Jovanovich.
Miller CJ (1991) WavEdit: General purpose program for waveform capture/manip-
    ulation/analysis. Users' Manual. Baton Rouge: Creighton J. Miller.
Sundberg J (1987) The Science of the Singing Voice. DeKalb, IL: Northern Illinois
    University Press.
Titze I (1994) Principles of Voice Production. Englewood Cliffs, NJ: Prentice-Hall.
Trojan E (1952) Experimentalle Untersuchungen über den Zusammenhang zwis-
    chen dem Ausdruck der Sprechstimme und dem vegetativen Nervensystem.
    Folia Phoniatrica 4, 65–92.
Vennard W (1967) Singing: The Mechanism and the Technique. New York: Carl
    Fisher.

LANGUAGE PROCESSING IN APHASIA AND DEMENTIA

Chapter 27
The English Language Version of the Aachen Aphasia Test[1]

NICK MILLER, RIA DE BLESER, KLAUS WILLMES

Introduction

The Aachen Aphasia Test (AAT) is a test of language functioning after brain damage. Its aim is to identify reliably the presence of aphasia in people with any kind of brain damage, to provide a detailed profile of speakers' language functioning according to the different language modalities (speaking, listening, reading, writing) and different levels of linguistic description (phonology, morphology, semantics and syntax) and from this offer indications for more detailed testing and/or therapeutic intervention. It also provides a means of assembling speakers into naturally occurring diagnostic groups for performance in the different modalities on the range of linguistic units (sounds, words, phrases . . .) that exist in language. For each unit the AAT samples a number of the regularities or 'rules' used in English for the combination of sounds and words and signalling of meaning distinctions.

Format and content of the EAAT

The English AAT (EAAT) comprises five subtests (Table 27.2 column 1) preceded by a semi-standardized interview to establish rapport with the speaker and to elicit a spontaneous language sample.

The token test (TT), an adaptation by Orgass (1976) of De Renzi and Vignolo (1962), consists of five subparts, each 10 items long. The TT was designed to detect mild language comprehension disturbances. The (age-adjusted) error score provides an indication of the presence or absence of aphasia and a measure of overall severity of aphasic symptoms.

The repetition subtest has five parts, all 10 items long, as in the rest of the test. Each requires the subject to repeat a different unit of language after the examiner: isolated sounds (e.g. /f/, /a:/); monosyllabic, monomorphemic words with consonant clusters (e.g. *axe, splodge*);

monomorphemic words of increasing length but simple (CV) syllable structure (*lee* to *hippopotamus*), with the criteria for selection being that words are loanwords into English (e.g. *salami*) or do not have English roots (e.g. *telephone*); words of increasing bound morphemes (*teacher* to *unconventionality*); and sentences with an increasing number of constituents.

The three subsections of the written language subtest investigate respectively reading of words and phrases, making up a given word or phrase using letter and word tiles, and writing to dictation. Items in the three parts parallel each other in syllable/phrase structure and as closely as possible in word frequency to enable a precise comparison across tasks.

Naming is examined using four tasks: naming pictures of common simple nouns (e.g. *table; belt*); colours; compound nouns (e.g. *hairdryer; typewriter*); and producing a sentence to describe 10 pictured situations. The latter are designed to elicit phrases with an increasing number of obligatory constituents, as is the case with the repetition subtest. Words are chosen to cover a range of semantic categories and to fulfil criteria of unambiguousness of lexical label and visual-perceptual distinctness. The compound nouns are made up from noun-noun and noun-verb combinations where correct naming cannot be achieved by naming only a subfeature of the picture or only one part of the compound.

The final subtest covers comprehension of spoken and written words and sentences in four separate parts. Speakers must point to the target from a selection of four pictures, one or other of which is a close semantic, phonemic, or syntactic distracter; one a picture thematically related to the target, but not close semantically or syntactically; and the fourth unrelated in any way. The sentence stimuli items are constructed so that the target cannot be deduced by attention to a keyword in the sentence. Again, in order to maximize comparability across subparts, the corresponding auditory and reading tasks are structured to parallel each other in the linguistic feature being probed. Amongst categories covered is discrimination between semantically similar words (e.g. according to function or the semantic ambiguity of homonymous words) and inference of sentence meaning from highly pronominalized phrases.

Subtests and subsections are administered in the order shown in Table 27.2 column 2, with the exception of writing to dictation which comes between the naming and comprehension subtests. The sequence of parts within subtests follows a gradient of rising difficulty (cf. Table 27.2 column 4). Subtests are ordered so that those that are generally difficult for speakers with aphasia are followed by subtests that are generally found to be easy. Further, the modality of presentation and response is alternated.

Scoring

Each TT section is marked on a right-wrong basis and the score is interpreted from the total number of errors. The repetition, written language, naming and comprehension subtests are all scored on a four-point scale, where '3' represents correct performance and '0' no response, perseveration, automatism, or a response that is totally unrelated to the target. The scale is intended to add scoring sensitivity that would not be available with a simple pass-fail convention. Thus, in general, '2' represents a correct response, but after a long reaction time, hesitancy, self-correction, or with minor deviation from the target; '1' represents in general a response with weak similarity to the target. Examples and criteria for these distinctions are provided and are defined in the manual.

The spontaneous language sample is evaluated according to six criteria. The communicative behaviour scale (adopted from the Boston Diagnostic Aphasia Examination, Goodglass and Kaplan, 1972) gives an indication of overall communicative success. The other scales pertain to: (a) segmental and suprasegmental aspects of articulation — in general these scales are designed to highlight the presence and degree of dysarthria or speech dyspraxia; (b) the extent to which the speaker relies on formulaic language, or is restricted to recurrent utterances or echolalia; (c) semantic production (frequency of semantic paraphasias; information conveyed); (d) phonological production (frequency and extent of phonemic paraphasias); and (e) syntactic production (range and integrity of syntactic structures). Each level is rated on a six-point scale, where '0' represents non-scorable and '5' represents normal performance. Intermediate scores are clearly defined in the manual on the basis of qualitative symptoms and their severity.

Construction of the EAAT

The rationale underlying the AAT is that aphasia represents a dysfunction of language and that breakdown may affect components of language differentially independent of modality whereas, on occasions, impairment may vary according to modality. In turn, determination of subgroups of speakers with dysphasia and distinguishing between individual speakers must be on the basis of linguistic performance.

Correspondingly, the basis for the construction of items and grouping into subparts and subtests in the AAT is that of linguistic structure and processing. The AAT is built on the principle of investigating the levels (phonology, semantics, syntax) and units of language (phonemes, morphemes, syntactic structures), the regularities that apply for a given language for the combination and differentiation of these units and the different modalities in which they are used. Hence the different subtests vary according to modality (e.g. written, spoken) used and transcoding between modalities (e.g. grapheme-phoneme conversion and vice versa, auditory to spoken conversion) and subtests progress through the various units of analysis (sound, syllables, morphemes, words, phrases).

The emphasis on purely linguistic criteria means that the AAT does not contain sections demanding recall of stories, copying of letters, performance of so-called automatic sequences (counting, months of the year, etc.) or direct investigation of praxis. These are rejected on the basis of performance being highly dependent on educational level, susceptible to disruption by neuropsychological dysfunction other than linguistic (e.g. attention, memory, visual-spatial functioning) and being uninformative as regards language performance or specific variables within language.

Adaptation into English

All languages employ sounds that are combined into words and these, in turn, are combined into phrases. However the precise range of sounds and words and the rules that dictate their contrasts, combination and use clearly differ across languages. For this reason it is not possible simply to translate a test from one language into another and still expect to test the same variables. An item investigating word-final morpheme contrasts in the differentiation of number or tense in one language may end up a test of function word usage, and/or involve complex adjective-noun-verb agreement across a whole phrase in another language. A lexical item with a high frequency and simple syllable structure in German may have a complex multisyllable structure in English and demand the choice of a low frequency word. So, in deriving the EAAT from the German original, the tactic was not simply to translate items. Rather, the aim was to preserve the underlying rationale for the division of subtests and the characteristics of subtasks within a subtest, while at the same time adapting these to the structure and regularities of English.

Thus, for example, where the German test was tapping speakers' ability to comprehend, read or repeat an interrogative or relative clause structure, the English item followed this, even though the precise morpho-syntactic expression may be different in English. In the written language and comprehension subtests where corresponding items across all subtasks parallel each other exactly, this element of design was preserved using English words and structures that did not always translate the German meaning but did retain as nearly as possible the properties of length, complexity and frequency. Where German items could be taken over (e.g. *Schüssel/bowl*, *Star/star* in the auditory comprehension subtest) necessary alterations of distracters were made to reflect English phonemic and semantic structure.

Further examples illustrate other adaptations. *Viereck* is the high-frequency word used in the German AAT for the rectangular shapes in the TT. It translates into English strictly speaking as *quadrilateral*. Such a low-frequency word would be unacceptable. *Rectangle* was chosen as an appropriate translation but piloting showed that not all English speakers knew this low-frequency word. The shapes were therefore changed to squares. The word *square* was recognized by everyone. *Stern* and *Schokolade* appear in the German word repetition sections. *Stern* could have been rendered as *stern* (albeit with a different meaning) in the EAAT, except that it would then alter the criterion of having words all of the same class. *Chocolate* would have preserved meaning and class, but transformed the syllable structure and stress pattern of the item.

Psychometric properties of the EAAT

The EAAT has been standardized to date on 135 speakers with aphasia and 93 without the condition. The aetiology of all the cases of aphasia was a single vascular episode. Descriptive statistics for the groups involved appear in Table 27.1. The key psychometric data are summarized in the following paragraphs. Full details are given in Miller, De Bleser and Willmes (in preparation).

Table 27.1. Descriptive statistics for the groups of speakers with aphasia and the control groups.

	N	F	M	Mean age (yrs)	Age range	Mean education (yrs)	Education range
Aphasia	135	41	94	60.03	29–74	9.21	4–14
Controls	93	51	42	54.20	21–72	9.82	8–22

The constructional validity of the EAAT and its subtests and subparts, reflecting the different linguistic units and modalities, is demonstrated from the results of a complete linkage hierarchical cluster analysis conducted on an intercorrelation matrix of the 120 speakers with a clearly classifiable aphasia syndrome. This is illustrated in Figure 27.2. It can be seen that links between subtests and parts deemed linguistically similar are stronger than between unrelated elements. The only subtest with all its parts not appearing on the same main branch is the written language subtest. The element of comprehension required to compose or write words and phrases to dictation places these tasks under the

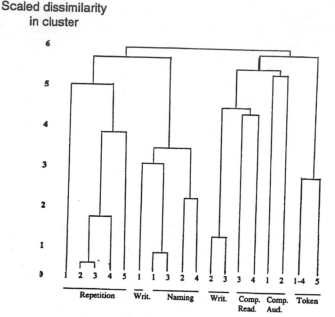

Figure 27.1. Grouping of EAAT subtests (hierarchical cluster analysis complete linkage method).

comprehension branch. Reading words and phrases comes out as closer to the naming and repetition tasks.

The consistency coefficients (Cronbach's α coefficient; see Table 27.2 column 3) obtained for each subtest and each part indicate a similar gradation of subjects across items and show these are measuring the same linguistic variable from speaker to speaker.

The results in Table 27.2 column 4 illustrate that the rising difficulty across the subtasks of subtests in the German AAT is preserved in the EAAT.

As regards the ability of the EAAT to distinguish speakers with and without aphasia and to identify subgroups of speakers with aphasia, the following results are noted. Using results just from the TT linear discriminant analysis demonstrates 92% accuracy in separating participants with and without aphasia. Entering all subtests into the discriminatory equation gives an overall classificatory level of 93%.

It is possible to establish subgroups of speakers using the (E)AAT. Although the AAT, across the different language versions, retains the traditional terms Broca's, Wernicke's, Amnestic and Global aphasia for the main subgroups of speakers identifiable with the test, the definitions for these syndromes are based on linguistic criteria (Poeck, Kerschensteiner, Stachowiak and Huber, 1975; Poeck, 1983) and are not synonymous with 'classical' definitions of these labels. Syndrome assignment takes place on the basis of evaluation of performance in the semi-structured interview at the start of the test.

Table 27.2 Consistency coefficients for subpart and subtests of the EAAT, and mean correct items per subpart for the combined (n=135) groups with aphasia.

		Cronbach's α	Mean Correct Items for Speakers with Aphasia
Token Test	Part 1	.90	6.52
	Part 2	.90	5.24
	Part 3	.91	3.36
	Part 4	.92	2.64
	Part 5	.91	2.49
	Parts 1–4	.97	–
	Token Test Overall:	.98	–
Repetition:	Sounds	.96	21.62
	Single syllable words	.96	20.07
	Multisyllable words	.96	19.06
	Morphologically complex words	.96	15.71
	Sentences	.97	13.26
	Repetition Subtest Overall	.99	–
Witten Language:	Reading aloud (words, phrases)	.97	16.27
	Composing words/phrases	.97	13.13
	Writing words/phrases to dictation	.97	10.77
	Written Language Overall	.98	–
Naming:	Pictured objects	.95	16.37
	Colours	.96	16.45
	Pictured compound nouns	.95	13.34
	Pictured sentences	.96	11.39
	Naming Subtest Overall	.97	–
Comprehension:	Auditory, words	.72	24.30
	Auditory, sentences	.79	21.28
	Reading, words	.86	18.86
	Reading, sentences	.87	16.79
	Comprehension Subtest Overall	.94	–

Table 27.3 shows that, by and large, speaker-groups identified as clinically separate score significantly differently on the spontaneous speech-language rating scales and the formal subtests. The results are based on a one-factorial ANOVA with subsequent multiple pairwise comparisons according to Tukey's 'honestly significant differences' method. Groups linked with an underline do not score significantly differently to each others, while unlinked groups do ($p = <0.05$). Results relate to quantitative scores. Groups not separable on this basis can nevertheless remain distinguishable on qualitative grounds.

Future work with the raw data will enable clinicians to relate speakers' performances to standard scores, percentile ranks and sta-nine severity scales for the various subtests. The EAAT will thus be able

Table 27.3 Differencess in EAAT performance of the different syndrome groups according to the spontaneous language rating scales and the separate subtests. G=Global; W=Wernicke's B=Broca's; A=Amnestic; C=CNS lesion without aphasia; H=Hospitalized, no CNS involvement, no aphasia; N=healthy non-hospitalized controls.

Spontaneous language rating scales:

Communication	G	W	B	A	C	H	N
Articulation	G	B	W	A	C	H	N
Formulaic lang.	G	W	B	A	C	H	N
Semantics	G	W	B	A	C	H	N
Phonology	G	B	W	A	C	H	N
Syntax	G	W	B	A	C	H	N

Subtests of EAAT:

Token Test	G	W	B	A	C	H	N
Repetition	G	W	B	A	C	H	N
Written lang.	G	W	B	A	C	H	N
Naming	G	W	B	A	C	H	N
Comprehension	G	W	B	A	C	H	N

to serve as a sensitive measure for changes in individual speakers and for comparison across and between groups of people with aphasia.

Conclusions

The psychometric studies demonstrate that the properties of validity and reliability of the original version are maintained in the EAAT. In this sense the adaptation into English can therefore be considered successful. Apart from offering clinicians a detailed screening test based on linguistic principles and with demonstrated validity and reliability, the fact that there is tight correspondence between versions in different languages opens new doors. The different versions of the AAT may serve as the basis for cross-language studies of aphasia and for multicentre trials of therapy which cross language boundaries.

References

De Renzi E, Vignolo L (1962) The token test. Brain 85: 665–78.
Goodglass H, Kaplan E (1972) Boston Diagnostic Aphasia Examination. Philadelphia PA: Lea Febiger.
Miller N, De Bleser R, Willmes K (in preparation) Psychometric Properties of the English Language Aachen Aphasia Test.

Orgass B. (1976) Eine Revision des Token Tests, Teil I und II. Diagnostika 22: 70–87, 141–56.

Poeck K, Kerschensteiner M, Stachowiak F, Huber W (1975) Die Aphasien. Aktuelle Neurologie 2: 159–69.

Poeck K (1983) What do we mean by 'aphasic syndromes'? Brain and Language 20: 79–89.

Note

1   The research for this project was supported in part by UCB Pharma, Belgium. Thanks also to F. Stewart who assisted with the initial pilot versions of the EAAT and later data collection. The following speech language therapists also kindly supplied tests: A Cameron; T Catcherside; C Davison; J Douglas; C Finlayson; M Goodger; J Goodson; C Heffer; F Kevan; E Khairuddin; R March; M Metcalf; C O'Neill; J Roberts; M. Robinson; L Rodriguez; F Wendon; N Woodyatt.

Chapter 28
Word Formation versus Inflection: Processing of 'Binding Morpheme' in German Aphasics

SYLVIA ELSNER AND WALTER HUBER

Introduction

Word formation and inflection in grammar

Spencer (1991) describes compounding as 'the interface between morphology and syntax par excellence'. Both phrases and compounds are concatenations of words. There are properties like constituent structure, binary branching, recursiveness, head, argument structure and feature percolation that link compounding with syntax. Phrases and compounds are very productive – they are permanently used to create new phrases or words (cf. *Ozon-loch* 'ozone-hole' 'hole in the ozone layer'). There are no restrictions on the semantic interpretation of compounds: the relations between both constituents are variable and often vague. In German, type N+N is one of the most productive compounding processes. The formation rule for N-N-root compounds is given in (1):

(1)　　[N] → [[N] [N]]

There are two kinds of N-N compounds: those that merely consist of two nouns (2a) and those that contain a 'binding morpheme' (*Fugenmorphem, linking element*) between the constituents (2b):

(2)　a.　Ohr-ring　　　　　　b.　Arbeit-s-platz
　　　　　'ear-ring'　　　　　　　　'work- . . . -place'
　　　　　'earring'　　　　　　　　　'place of work, job'

Incidentally, we even find this phenomenon in English compounds such as *teethmarks* and *systems analyst* (Spencer, 1991).

In the theoretical literature there is disagreement on the status of binding morphemes. Two approaches are discussed: the theory that binding morphemes are plural affixes and are therefore predicted by inflectional operations, and the theory that they are not, and therefore are determined by word formation rules. Depending on whether the binding morpheme marks the plural or not we find different views on the morphological structure of compounds like *Nervenfaser* 'nerve fibre'. In the first case, we have two morphemes, namely the stem *Nerv-* and the plural affix *-en*. In this case, the binding morpheme may be determined by morpho-syntactic factors (Wiese, 1993). In the second case, the structure *Nerven-* is regarded as variant of *Nerv* 'nerve', and is therefore a stem allomorph of *Nerv* (Anderson, 1992). The occurrence of the stem allomorphs may be determined by morphological or phonological factors, or may not be predictable at all. Hence we have structure (3a) in contrast with structure (3b):

(3) a. [[Nerv]$_{stem}$·[en]]$_{word}$]]·[faser]·[∅].]$_{word}$ 'nerv-Nom.Pl.-fibre-Nom.Sg.'

(3) b. [[[Nerven]$_{stem}$·[faser]]$_{stem}$]·[∅].]$_{word}$ 'nerv-fibre-Nom.Sg.'

Binding morphemes in compounds: word formation or inflection?

Traditionally, morphology is divided into inflection and word formation. Inflection is assumed to work differently from the other subdomains of morphology since it creates forms of words that are syntactically relevant (cf. agreement, government). It is a subject of intense debate whether morphology belongs to the lexicon, syntax, or phonology, or whether it is split across different grammatical components. According to the 'strong lexicalist hypothesis' (Selkirk, 1982, Di Sciullo and Williams, 1987), word formation and inflection are properties of the lexicon. One of the consequences of this view is that word formation and inflection can interact: inflection may occur inside compounds or derived words. On the other hand, this leads to a set of morphological and syntactic redundancies, which one does not want on general theoretical grounds. According to the weak lexicalist hypothesis (Anderson, 1982; Roeper, 1988), only word formation takes part in the lexicon, while inflection is part of the syntax (split-morphology hypothesis). The point is that syntax has no access to the internal structure of words. Inflection therefore always takes place after word formation, and inflectional affixes can never occur inside morphologically complex words (4):

(4) a. [Licht-bild]-∅]   'light-picture'-Nom.Sg.   1. 'photo', 2. 'slide'
    b. [[Licht-bild]-er]   'light-picture'-Nom.Pl   1. 'photos', 2. 'slides'

This will cause problems when binding morphemes have to be regarded as inflectional affixes. The phenomenon of 'binding morphemes' is of great theoretical interest for exactly this reason. In current morphological theory, the plural view is widely accepted (cf. Wiese, 1993; Clahsen, Eisenbeiss, Sonnenstuhl-Henning, 1996 for German; Selkirk, 1982 for English) but also rejected (cf. Anderson, 1992, Becker, 1992, Plank, 1974).

In German, about 30% of N-N-compounds occur with binding morphemes (Ortner, Müller-Bollhagen, Ortner, Wellmann, Pümpel-Mader and Gärtner, 1991). The number of binding morphemes is limited (5):

(5) -e-	1. Tag-e-buch	'day-. . . -book'	'diary'
-er-	1. Männ-er-stimme	'man-. . . -voice'	'man's voice'
-(e)n-	1. Nerv-en-bahn	'nerve-. . . -tract'	'nerve tract'
-s-	Arbeit-s-platz	'work-. . . -place'	'place of work, job'

The choice of binding morphemes cannot be predicted. In most cases, binding morphemes are formally identical with the inflectional ending of the nominative or genitive (singular or plural) of the first constituent. One and the same first constituent can occur with or without a binding morpheme (6a). Furthermore, some nouns may take the same binding morpheme in all compounds (6b), or there may be alternations depending on the compound in which it is used (6c). Plank (1974) found that speakers vary in the use of binding morphemes inter- and intra-individually. Depending on the local dialect, the use of binding-morphemes may differ as in Bavarian *Schwein-s-braten* 'roast pork', as opposed to high German *Schwein-e-braten*.

(6) a. Ohr-Ø-ring 'ear-ring'; Ohr-en-schmerzen 'earpain'
    b. Pferd-e-decke 'horse-blanket', Pferd-e-rennen 'horse-race'
    c. Kind-s-kopf 'child-head'; Kind-es-kind 'child-child' (i.e. grand child), Kind-er-geburtstag 'child -birthday'

In most cases, the forms of binding morphemes are identical to plural affixes. Furthermore, binding morphemes correspond with the semantics of the inflectional affix in some cases (7a, b) but not in others. For example, *Kindergeburtstag* has the meaning of a child's birthday party, not of 'children's birthday party' (cf. 7c) despite the superficial plural form of the first constituent *(die) Kinder*.

(7) (a) Kind-es-kind	'child-Gen.Sg.-child'	'child of one´s child'
(b) Kind-er-buch	'child-Akk.Pl.-book'	'book for children'
(c) Kind-er-geburtstag	'child-Gen.Pl-birthday'	'birthday party of a child'

In still other cases, binding morphemes are not identical with any inflectional ending of the first constituent. This is demonstrated in (8); note that there does not exist a word *Liebes or *Schwanen in German. In addition, as Wiese (1993) pointed out, the binding morpheme -s- may occur with feminine nouns like (die) Arbeit, which in general do not have an inflectional affix -s in their paradigm, e.g. Arbeit-s-raum, 'workroom'. On the other hand, nouns that form their plural with -s never occur with binding morpheme -s in compounds (9).

(8) Liebe-s-brief   'love- . . . letter'   'love letter'
     Schwan-en-gesang   'swan- . . . -song'   'swan song'

(9) Auto-s, Auto-∅-schlange
     Champignon-s; Champignon-∅-pizza

Moreover, not all potential affixes are used as binding morphemes, and we find alternations for the genitive suffixes -s and -es (10a), but not for the corresponding binding morphemes (10b) (Becker, 1992; Plank, 1974; Augst, 1975; Becker, 1992):

(10) (a) Tag-s, Tag-es
     (b) Tag-es-plan; *Tag-s-plan

There are numerous reports in the literature on word processing in conditions of aphasia, which give important insights into the functional architecture of the mental lexicon. Most research, however, has focused either on morphologically simple words or on derived words (Badecker and Caramazza, 1993). Research on compounds is restricted to a few case studies (De Bleser and Bayer, 1990; Blanken, 1990); to date no study has examined binding morphemes. There are three different possibilites for binding morphemes to be formally embedded in N-N-compounds (11) (cf.3):

(11) a. [Nervenfaser]
     b. [[[Nerve] [n]] [faser]]
     c. [[Nerven] [faser]]

Empirical evidence for choosing among these alternatives may come from studies of aphasic patients. We assume the following pathological conditions to be found among the aphasic population:

(a) preference for lexical processing due to an impairment of segmental phonology;
(b) preserved lexical decomposition;
(c) omission of bound morphemes.

These three conditions are likely to co-occur in patients with chronic Broca's aphasia, which evolved from initial global aphasia. These patients usually show deep dyslexia and deep dysphasia with agrammatism, i.e. they read and repeat words in a holistic fashion and they omit function words and inflectional endings (Katz and Goodglass, 1990). The binding morpheme is expected to be ignored by these patients if its morphological status is indeed a plural ending.

Methods

Subjects

Subjects consisted of 11 aphasic patients who were chosen from the aphasia ward at the University Hospital of the RWTH Aachen (Table 28.1). The group was composed of five Broca's aphasics, four Wernicke's aphasics and two patients with conduction aphasia. The diagnosis was based on the Aachen Aphasia Test (Huber, Weniger, Poeck and Willmes, 1983; Huber, Poeck and Willmes, 1984). A total number of 20 controls participated in the study, consisting of 10 subjects who were matched with the aphasic patients in age, education and gender (median in years = 52; range 27–73), and 10 young male students (median in years = 26; range 22–30). The controls were free of any neurological, visual, or motor impairment.

Table 28.1 Clinical data of patients

	Aphasia	Age (years)	Sex[1]	Aet.[2]	Paresis	Cerebral CT-/MRI- scan[3]	Duration (month)
B1	Broca	24	f	i	brach.fac., mild	A.c.media, complete	10
B2	Broca	35	m	i	brach.fac., mod.	A.c.media, complete	58
B3	Broca	46	f	i	brach.fac., mod.	A.c.media, complete	7
B4	Broca	54	f	h	complete, mod.	basalganglia, complete	11
B5	Broca	59	m	i	brach.fac., mild.	A.c.media, ant., part.	32
W1	Wernikle	34	f	i/h	-	A.c.media, post., part.	9
W2	Wernikle	52	m	h	complete, mod	basalganglia, large	3
W3	Wernikle	59	m	h	-	A.c.media, post., part.	2
W4	Wernikle	74	m	i	-	A.c.media, post., part.	7
L1	Conduct.	35	m	i	-	A.c.media, post., part.	19
L2	Conduct.	53	m	j	-	A.c.media, post., part.	49
Total: median		52	7m,4f				10
	range	(24-74)					(2-58)

1 Sex: m=male, f=female 2 Aetiology: i=infarct, h=haemorrhage 3: Exclusively left hemisphere.

Stimuli

A total of 160 N-N-compounds were used as stimuli in each of three tasks: repetition, reading aloud and lexical judgement. 50 stimuli showed correct forms of the German language, 10 having binding morphemes, 40 having no binding morphemes. The other 110 stimuli deviated in one of the following aspects:

– LINKING POSITION
– binding morpheme
20 compounds with a binding morpheme incorrectly added (n=10) or missing (n=10) in the linking position, e.g.
* Ei-becher (instead of 'Ei-er-becher' 'egg- . . . cup' 'egg cup'),
* Ohr-en-ring (instead of 'Ohr-ring' 'ear-ring' 'earring')
– phoneme / grapheme
20 compounds with a phoneme / grapheme added or missing in the linking position, e.g.
* Somme-regen (instead of 'Sommer-regen' 'summer shower' 'summer shower')
* Wagent-rad (instead of 'Wagen-rad' 'car-wheel' 'wheel of a car')

– CONSTITUENT STRUCTURE
– order
30 compounds with first and second constituent reversed
    e.g., *Nagel-finger (instead of 'Finger-nagel' ´finger-nail´ 'fingernail'
- - phoneme / grapheme
2 x 20 compounds with a phoneme / grapheme added or missing in the first constituent (n=20) or in the second constituent (n = 20), e.g.
    * Figer-nagel (instead of 'Finger-nagel' ´finger-nail´ 'fingernail')
    * Apftel-saft (instead of 'Apfel-saft' 'apple-juice' 'apple juice')
    *Land-staße (instead of 'Land-straße' 'country-road' 'country road')
    *Käse-eckte (instead of 'Käse-ecke' 'cheese-piece' 'cheese triangle')

The compounds were matched in length and frequency across stimulus type. The total set of stimuli was presented in a different randomized order for each task.

Procedure

The aphasic performance was assessed in three tasks, which were each given in a full hour session on three consecutive days in the following order:

(a) Repetition
(b) Reading aloud
(c) Lexical judgement

In the repetition and reading task, subjects were instructed to reproduce the stimuli verbatim; for example if the stimulus *Eibecher* was presented, they had to reproduce it as *Eibecher* without correcting it to *Eierbecher*. In the lexical judgement task, compounds were presented both auditorily and visually. Subjects were asked to decide whether the stimulus word existed in the vocabulary of German. Furthermore, any deviation had to be marked on the written stimulus. With the help of practice trials, the instructions to each task were repeated until it was clear that the subject fully understood them. All spoken responses were tape-recorded.

Response analysis

The responses obtained in the repetition and reading task were subclassified into three different types:

1. 'Reproduction': the subject was able to reproduce *Eibecher* as *Eibecher*, as required;
2. 'Correction': a word like *Eibecher* was substituted by the existing word Eierbecher; i.e. the subject was not able to reproduce the stimulus;
3. 'Others': no reaction, perseveration, circumlocution etc.

In the lexical judgement task, responses were classified as:

1. 'Rejection': a compound like *Eibecher* was not accepted and the deviation was identified;
2. 'Acceptance': a compound like *Eibecher* was accepted and not rejected.

Results and discussion

Reproduction tasks: repetition and reading aloud

Controls always performed according to the instruction – they never corrected any of the deviant stimuli. The performance obtained in the two patient groups is given in Table 28.2. We first consider the processing of the control stimuli, which either contained wrong order of constituents (*Nagelfinger*) or wrong phonemic structure of the first or second constituent (*Apftelsaft*, *Käseeckte*). Both patient groups reproduced the wrong constituent order when required, which shows that lexical decomposition was possible for the majority of patients. If compounds were only available as whole words (full listing hypothesis, Manelis and Tharp, 1977, Butterworth, 1983, Henderson, 1985), one would have mainly obtained corrections, no responses or visual/lexical expansions on the first constituent – e.g. *Nagellack* 'nail-varnish'.

Table 28.2. Corrections (*Ohrenring → Ohrring) in reproduction tasks

Stimulus deviation	Corrections			Repetition task	Reading task	
	Broca	Wernicke, conduction.	DIFF. (p-values)[2]	Broca	Wernickle conduction.	DIFF (p-values)[2]
	n=5	n=6		n=5	n=6	
Linking position						
-binding morpheme (20 items)	2.0 (1-7)	2.0 (0-5)	0.5121	9.0 (3-11)	2.0 (1-4)	0.0131*
-phoneme (20 items)	13.0 (6-15)	5.5 (2-9)	0.0277*	14.0 (11-17)	10.0 (2-11)	0.0074*
DIFF. (exact p-values)[1]	0.0431*	0.1250		0.0422*	0.03125*	
-Constituent structure						
-order (30 items)	0.0 (0-1)	0.0 (0-9)	0.4860	1.0 (1-6)	0.0 (0-1)	0.0080*
-phoneme (20 items)	16.0 (11-18)	6.5 (3-18)	0.0427*	28.0 (23-36)	9.5 (3-21)	0.0062*
DIFF. (exact p-values)[1]	0.0422*	0.0277*		0.0431*	0.0277*	

median range
1 Wilcoxon Matched Pairs Signed-Ranks Test, 2-tailed; 2 Mann Whitney U-Test, 2-tailed

Stimuli with deviating phonemic structure of first or second constituent were processed differently. The four Wernicke's aphasics and the two conduction aphasics performed significantly better than the Broca's aphasics – they reproduced the given phonemic non-word rather than substituting in the corresponding real word. In contrast, the Broca's aphasics made lexical corrections in about 40% of the items. As expected, Broca's aphasics relied on lexical rather than sublexical processing.

A parallel group effect was found for processing compounds with a wrong phoneme in the linking position. Broca's aphasics corrected them in 60–70% of the items. In other words, Broca's aphasics again relied on lexical routes of processing.

What happened when the deviation was due to the binding morpheme being either incorrectly added or dropped? Corrections occurred in very few instances, even in the group of Broca's aphasics. Both patient groups made substantially fewer corrections of the binding morpheme than of a deviant phoneme/grapheme in the linking position. As illustrated in Figures 28.1 and 28.2, this difference was observed for each individual patient in both groups in both tasks (with the exception of one conduction aphasic in the repetition task). This difference was unexpected for Broca's aphasics given their pathological reliance on lexical routes of processing.

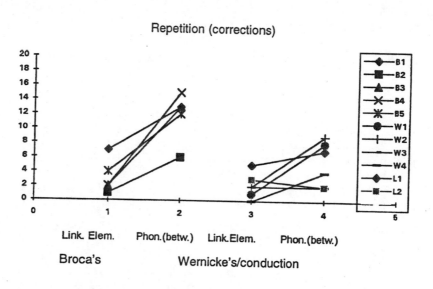

Figure 28.1. Corrections (*Ohrenring → Ohrring) in Repetition task (n = 20 Items)

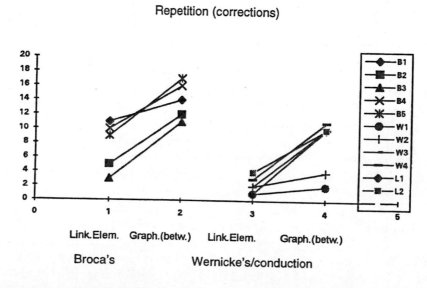

Figure 28.2. Corrections (*Ohrenring → Ohrring) in Reading Task (n = 20)

Lexical judgement task

In the judgement task we found outstandingly poor performance on compounds with deviation in binding morpheme as opposed to almost perfect performance on compounds with linkage that was otherwise incorrect (Figure 28.3). Apparently all aphasic patients relied on a decomposition strategy. They were able to identify the two basic lexemes and to reject any misspellings between the two lexemes as long as they were not possible candidates of a binding morpheme.

Table 28.3. Rejections (*Ohrenring → Ohrring) in lexical judgement task

Stimulus deviation	Broca	Wernicke, conduction.	DIFF. (p-values)[2]	Controls	
				old	young
	n=5	n=6		n=10	n=10
Linking position					
-binding morpheme					
(20 items)	12.0 (6-15)	6.5 (3-9)	0.0432*	19.0 (14-20)	2.0 (18-20)
-phoneme/grapheme					
(20 items)	20.0 (20-20)	19.5 (17-20)	0.2419	20.0 (20-20)	19.0 (19-20)
DIFF. (exact p-values)[1]	0.0431*	0.03/25			
-Constituent structure					
-order (30 items)	28.0 (16-29)	13.0 (6-21)	0.0171*	2.90 (21-30)	30.0 (28-30)
-phoneme/grapheme					
(40 items)	40.0 (36-40)	39.0 (32-40)	0.5006	40.0 (38-40)	40.0 (39-40)
DIFF. (exact p-values)[1]	0.1756	0.0277*			

median range
1 Wilcoxon Matched Pairs Signed-Ranks Test, 2-tailed; 2 Mann-Whitney U-Test, 2-tailed

Similarly, all patients, even the Broca's aphasics, were able to identify phonemic and/or graphemic deviations within the individual lexemes in both the first and second components (Table 28.3). Apparently, Broca's aphasics had access to sublexical segmentation under the controlled processing conditions of the judgement task, but not when more automatic processing was required as in repetition and reading aloud.

Patients with Wernicke's aphasia found remarkable difficulties with reversed constituent order (Table 28.3). Obviously, these patients had only limited access to the full listing of the N-N-compounds but were able to identify and judge its individual lexemes. This is shown by their significantly better performance when the wrong phonemic structure of the individual constituents had to be identified. In contrast, most Broca's aphasics rejected reversed constituent order successfully – i.e. they had good access to N-N-compounds as a whole.

So far we have argued that both patient groups were able to decompose N-N-compounds and that only Broca's aphasics rejected reversed constituent order successfully – i.e. they had also access to the whole word entry. Nevertheless, their judgement on compounds with erroneous binding morphemes was poor (Figure 28.3). How can this be explained? The full listing approach in these patients seems to be semantically based, but not formally, so the deviant morphological linkage is not detected. Semantically based processing of N-N-compounds was previously found for naming (Stachowiak, 1979).

Lexical judgement (rejections)

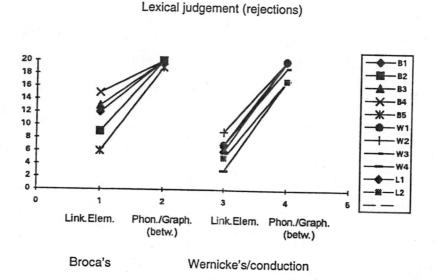

Figure 28.3. Rejections (*Ohrenring → Ohrring) in Lexical Decision Task (n = 20)

Are the difficulties of the Broca's aphasics derived from their agrammatism – from their tendency to omit or to confuse inflectional endings? As a consequence, they would give a random response when a morphological linkage was present. If this is the case, we should obtain differences between incorrectly added and omitted binding morphemes. Non-existing compounds due to an added binding morpheme like *Ohrenring* would lead to rejections, whereas stimuli with omitted binding morpheme like *Ohrsausen* should be as likely accepted as existing N-N-compounds without linking elements (e.g. *Ohrring*). This interpretation was not substantiated by the data for Broca's aphasics nor for Wernicke's aphasics (Table 28.4). Taking all three tasks together, we found median values of seven and eight corrections/rejections of omitted and added binding morphemes respectively per patient. Furthermore, correct compounds were always accepted, whether they had a binding morpheme or not. Thus, the binding elements hardly have the status of inflectional endings, otherwise they would be specifically affected by the agrammatisms of Broca's aphasics.

Table 28.4. Comparisons between deviantly omitted and added binding morphemes

Absolute number of response and median, range per patient		Deviation in binding morpheme					
		Omission			Addition		
		Broca $n=5$	Wern/con. $n=6$	Both $n=11$	Broca $n=5$	Wern/con. $n=6$	Both $n=11$
Repetition	Correction	8	7	15	8	7	15
20 items	Reproduction	38	33	71	41	37	78
	Other	4	20	24	1	16	17
Reading Aloud	Correction	13	7	20	20	6	26
20 items	Reproduction	34	51	85	23	53	76
	Other	3	2	5	7	1	8
Lex. judgement	Rejection	29	15	44	26	22	48
20 items	Acceptance	21	45	66	24	38	62
All 3 tasks	Corr./Reject.	Md = 12	Md=4	Md=7	Md=10	Md=5,5	Md=8
60 items		7–14	3–8	3–13	6–17	3–9	3–17

The data can readily be explained within a stem-based model of word processing. According to this model, binding morphemes are integrated into the first noun, thereby making up the stem. These stems, e.g. *Ohr-, Ohren-, Arbeit-, Arbeits-, Tag-, Tage-, Kind-, Kinds-, Kinder-* are entries of the lexicon and consequently undergo lexical decomposition. In aphasia, formally deviant compounds may not be noticed because the full listing control is generally weak, as in Wernicke's aphasia, and/or semantically biased as in chronic Broca's aphasia. First constituents therefore tend to be accepted irrespectively of the stem form present in a given N-N-compound because they are always processed as an existing stem of the German vocabulary.

In conclusion, the results of this study fit into a growing number of morphological theories that base their models on stems (Anderson, 1992) and not morphemes. Further research has to clarify to what extent this holds true only for those language capacities that are still available or have recovered in aphasia. In the normal brain, additional decomposition of stems might take place in the processing of N-N-compounds.

References

Anderson S (1982) Where's morphology? Linguistic Inquiry 13: 571–612.
Anderson S (1992) A-Morphous Morphology. Cambridge: Cambridge University Press.

Augst G (1975) Untersuchungen zum Morpheminventar der deutschen Gegenwartssprache. Forschungsberichte des Instituts für deutsche Sprache, Tuebingen: Narr.

Badecker W, Caramazza A (1993) Disorders of Lexical Morphology in Aphasia. In Blanken G, Dittmann J, Grimm H, Marshall J, Wallesch CW (Eds) Linguistic Disorders and Pathologies. An International Handbook. Berlin: de Gruyter. (=Handbücher zur Sprach- und Kommunikationswissenschaft, Band 8) 181–6.

Becker T (1992) Compounding in German. Rivista di Linguistica 4: 5–36.

Blanken G (1990) Sprachzerfall. Empirische Studien zur kognitiven Neurolinguistik. Freiburg, unveröff. Habilitationsschrift.

Butterworth BL (1983) Lexical representation. In: Butterworth BL (Ed) Language Production, Volume 2. London: Academic Press, pp. 257–94.

De Bleser R, Bayer J (1990) Morphological reading errors in a German case of deep dyslexia. In Nespoulous JL, Villiard P (Eds) Morphology, Phonology and Aphasia. New York: Springer.

Di Sciullo AM, Williams E (1987) On the Definition of Word. Cambridge: MIT.

Clahsen H, Eisenbeiss S, Sonnenstuhl-Henning (1996) Morphological Structure and the Processing of Inflected Words (Essex Research Reports in Linguistics 13). Essex: Essex University, pp. 1–53.

Henderson L (1985) Towards a psychology of morphemes. In Ellis, AW (Ed) Progress in the Psychology of Language (Vol 1). London: Erlbaum.

Huber W, Weniger D, Poeck K, Willmes K (1983) Der Aachener Aphasie Test. Göttingen: Hogrefe.

Huber W, Poeck K, Willmes K (1984) The Aachen Aphasia Test. In: Rose FC (Ed) Progress in aphasiology. New York: Raven Press.

Katz, R, Goodglass, H (1990) Deep dysphasia: an analysis of a rare form of repetition disorder. Brain and Language 39: 153–85.

Manelis L, Tharp DA (1977) The processing of affixed words. Memory and Cognition 5: 690–5.

Ortner L, Müller-Bollhagen E, Ortner H, Wellmann H, Pümpel-Mader M., Gärtner H (1991) Substantivkomposita. Komposita und kompositionsähnliche Strukturen. Berlin: De Gruyter.

Plank Frans (1974) Die Kompositionsfuge in der neuhochdeutschen Nominalkomposition. Köln: Unveröff. Magisterarbeit.

Roeper T (1988) Compound syntax and head movement. Yearbook of Morphology 1: 187–228.

Selkirk E (1982) The Syntax of Words. Cambridge, Mass: MIT.

Spencer A (1991) Morphological Theory. Oxford: Blackwell.

Stachowiak FJ (1979) Zur semantischen Struktur des subjektiven Lexikons. München: Fink.

Wiese R (1993) The Phonology of German. [MS]. Düsseldorf Universität.

Chapter 29
Modelling Within-Category Function Word Errors in Language Impairment[1]

LOUISE KELLY, RICHARD SHILLCOCK AND
PADRAIC MONAGHAN

Introduction

The function words of a language are those words that have a predominantly syntactic role – 'if', 'of', 'was', 'on', for instance. It is well documented that at a linguistic level they differ from content words along many dimensions: they are non-productive; they rarely undergo semantic change; they typically lack semantic content and have been seen as having a logical rather than denotative interpretation; they are typically the highest frequency words. In spoken English they attract substantial phonological reduction (Cutler, 1993) and can exhibit phonological patterns unique to their class – in English, only function words have word initial /ð/ for instance. In reading text they are often not directly fixated (Carpenter and Just, 1983). In sum, content and function words tend to have different linguistic traits (see Cann (1996) for an extended review of the content/functor distinction).

One additional dimension along which the content and function lexica diverge is in their morphosyntactic properties – functional categories often take the form of bound morphs or clitics: they fail to undergo derivational processes and appear in more restricted syntactic contexts. This greater contextual constraint on function words appears to have an impact on processing. Shillcock and Bard (1993) demonstrate that the access of function words that are homophonous with content words (e.g. 'would/wood', 'will/will') is influenced 'top down' by principally syntactic context. In contrast, Tanenhaus and Donnenwerth-Nolan (1984) have shown content word homophones, like 'rose' (= 'flower' or 'stood up'), are not susceptible to the effects of syntactic context. In sum, (principally syntactic) context typically plays a major part in the access of function words, compared with content words.

This conclusion is supported by an analysis of lexical competitors, involving those words that contain, word-initially, the target word, as /tɪndə/ contains /tɪn/. The target's segmental representation is not unique at offset. Shillcock, Hicks, Cairns, Levy and Chater (in press) studied the incidence of neighbours in the London-Lund corpus of transcribed speech, (Svartvik and Quirk, 1980). Analysis of an idealized transcription of this corpus showed, overall, a difference between function and content words (Shillcock et al. in press). Function words were more likely to have post-offset competitors of any sort, content or function, as is shown in Table 29.1.

Table 29.1. Percentage of words having a post-offset competitor

	function words, e.g., 'not' (contained in 'notting')	content word e.g. 'crow' (contained in 'chromium')
types	38.5%	8.5%
tokens	57.3%	9.3%

The prevalence of post-offset competitors for function words reflects their shortness. The 100 most frequent content words show an equal level of these competitors; however, overall, it is more typical of function words. The fact that function words very often have a post-offset competitor emphasizes the fact that their recognition typically relies on context.

Function word errors in deep dyslexia and deep dysphasia

Within-category function word errors are errors in spoken and written word production in which a function word is erroneously replaced by another function word. In spoken word repetition, 'above' might be repeated as 'enough'. In word naming, 'us' might be read as 'is'. These errors are characteristic of deep dysphasia (Howard and Franklin, 1989) and deep dyslexia (Morton and Patterson, 1980; Patterson and Marcel, 1977). A frequent conclusion is that function and content words are stored in separate lexicons. We present an alternative model, in which we assume common storage and common initial processing for both types of word.

Statistical studies on language corpora

(a) Orthographic representations

Using large corpora we examined the ways in which the sets of competitors of the two word types differ. A variable that shows a consistent effect on recognition time in visual word recognition is that of word neighbourhood (see Andrews, 1992; Grainger and Segui, 1990). Neighbourhood, here, is defined as those words that differ from each other by only one letter, but maintain word length (Coltheart, Davelaar, Jonasson and Besner, 1977). For instance, the neighbourhood for 'hand' includes 'sand', 'wand', 'hind', 'hard', 'hang'.

In our current study the two word types differ in their lexical neighbourhoods (see Table 29.2). A search in the CELEX database (Bayeen, Piepenbrock and Gulikers, 1995) of all word lemmas in the English lexicon of lengths 2 - 12 letters (a corpus of 32 086 words), showed that the ratio of function word neighbours to the total number of neighbours, was greater for function words than for content words ($t = 2.55$, $df = 8$, $p < 0.025$). That is, whereas content words typically have more neighbours than do function words, function words have more (other) function words as neighbours than do content words.

Table 29.2. Neighbours of the two word types in English words of length 2–12 letters

	content words	function words
content word neighbours	36074	732
function word neighbours	732	132

This effect also holds when only a subset of the most frequent content and function words in the lexicon are studied. A set of 44 frequency-matched pairs of three- and four-letter function words from Besner (1989) showed the same distributional difference between content and function words (see Table 29.3). Function words have more function word competitors than do content words ($t = 3.63$, $df = 38$, $p < 0.005$).

Table 29.3. Neighbours of the two word types in words (of length three and four letters) matched for frequency (materials from Besner, 1989)

	content words	function words
content word neighbours	413	198
function word neighbours	14	23

Even when we control for frequency and word length, function words are more likely than content words to have other function words as orthographic neighbours.

(b) Phonological representations

The phonological neighbourhoods for the same set of words taken from Besner (1989) also displays the same clustering of function words, for instance:

'has' /haz/   function word cohort members: /had/ /hav/ /haθ /hɪz/
               content word cohort members: /hak/ /hag/ /ham/
                                                 /haŋ/ /haʃ/ /hat/ /hatʃ/

Table 29.4. Phonological neighbours of the two frequency matched word types (materials from Besner,1989)

	content words	function words
content word neighbours	183	153
function word neighbours	8	17

The distributional difference between the two word classes holds for phonological neighbourhood, shown in Table 29.4 (χ^2= 3.85, df = 1, p < 0.05). The phonological neighbours of function words are more likely to contain other function words than those of content words.

Cross-linguistic data

The pattern we report is not restricted to English: the Dutch lexicon appears to be partitioned in a similar way (see Table 29.5). Examination of the Dutch corpus in the CELEX database (87 064 words) shows that the orthographic competitor sets for function words consists of a greater proportion of function words than would occur by chance. For Dutch words that are two to 12 letters long, t = 2.5, df = 8, p < 0.05.

Table 29.5. Neighbours of the two word types in Dutch words of length 2–12 letters

	content words	function words
content word neighbours	68376	1142
function word neighbours	1142	276

Psychological models

The differing neighbourhood patterns, together with the differential effects of context for function and content words, conspire to create within-category function word errors.

We assume an architecture that takes letter- (or phoneme-) level input and that contains a lexical level and above that, a syntactic level. The following occurs in reading a function word:

(a) The input of the letters 'h-i-s' will activate the function word 'his' and its neighbours 'him', 'hit' . . . etc.
(b) The function words will activate the relevant syntactic information at the syntactic level.
(c) Groups of high-frequency function words will interact with the activated syntactic representations to give 'gang effects' (see Rumelhart and McClelland, 1981) that augment groups of function words.
(d) Top-down activation from the syntactic level will also activate non-sensory-matching members of the relevant category of function word, 'their' in our example.
(e) Noisy representations accompanying impaired processing allow for the target word to be displaced as the most highly activated word by a competing function word. Because of their high frequency, function words make effective competitors.
(f) Comparable content-word gang effects do not occur because content word neighbours are typically low frequency and because these words do not interact with the syntactic level.

Conclusions

The preponderance of intra-category function word errors in linguistic impairments such as deep dyslexia and deep dysphasia can be accounted for in terms of the distributional differences between the function and content words and the evidence for their differing reliance on syntactic context. Content and function words are stored and processed in similar ways; frequency and letter-shape are both important for orthographic representations, for instance. Common processing of the two word-types is advantageous, given that in conversational English, some 55% of word boundaries are between the two different word types (Shillcock et al., in press). However, the two word types differ in that function words typically have access to more constraining syntactic (and semantic) information. (Also, in degraded visual word recognition, lexical neighbourhoods are important for function words but not content words (Shillcock, Kelly, Buntin and Patterson (in preparation).)

This difference in the availability of syntactic context underlies the two word types' different appearance in the language, and their differential breakdown. Specifically, it predicts that function words will be confused with other function words in the dyslexias and dysphasias. Storage in (physically) separate lexica is not required.

References

Andrews S (1992) Frequency and neighbourhood effects on lexical access: lexical similarity or orthographic redundancy? Journal of Experimental Psychology: Learning, Memory and Cognition 18(2): 214–54.

Bayeen RH, Piepenbrock R, Gulikers L. (1995) The CELEX Lexical Database (CD-ROM). Linguistic Data Consortium, University of Pennsylvania, Philadelphia, PA.

Besner D (1989) On the role of outline shape and word-specific visual pattern in the identification of function words: NONE. Quarterly Journal of Experimental Psychology 41A: 91–105.

Cann R (1996) Categories, labels and types: functional versus lexical. Edinburgh Occasional Papers in Linguistics 96-3.

Carpenter PA, Just MA (1983) What our eyes do while our mind is reading? In Rayner K (Ed) Eye movements in reading: Perceptual and Language Processes. New York: Academic Press, pp. 275–307.

Coltheart M, Davelaar E, Jonasson JT, Besner D (1977) Access to the internal lexicon. In S Dornic (Ed) Attention and Performance VI: 535–55. Hillsdale, NJ: Erlbaum.

Cutler A (1993) Phonological cues to open- and closed-class words in the processing of spoken sentences. Journal of Psycholinguistic Research, 22: 109–31.

Grainger J, Segui J (1990) Neighbourhood frequency effects in visual word recognition: a comparison of lexical decision and masked identification latencies. Perception and Psychophysics 47: 191–8.

Howard D, Franklin S (1989) Missing the Meaning? Cambridge, MA: MIT Press.

Morton J, Patterson K (1980) 'Little words – No!' In Coltheart M, Patterson K, Marshall JC (Eds) Deep Dyslexia. London: Routledge & Kegan Paul.

Patterson KE, Marcel AJ (1977) Aphasia, dyslexia and phonological coding of written words. Quarterly Journal of Experimental Psychology 20: 587–608.

Rumelhart DE, McClelland JL (1981) An interactive activation model of context effects in letter perception: Part 2. The contextual enhancement effect and some tests and extensions of the model. Psychological Review 89: 60–94.

Shillcock RC, Bard EG (1993) Modularity and the processing of closed class words. In Altmann GTM, Shillcock, RC (Eds) Cognitive Models of Speech Processing. The Second Sperlonga Meeting. Hillsdale NJ: Erlbaum.

Shillcock RC, Hicks J, Cairns P, Levy J, Chater N. (in press). A statistical analysis of an idealized phonological transcription of the London-Lund corpus. Computer Speech and Language.

Shillcock RC, Kelly ML, Buntin L, Patterson D (in preparation). Neighbourhood effects for function words, but not content words in the Clarity Gating Task.

Svartvik J, Quirk R (Eds) (1980) A Corpus of English Conversation. Lund Studies in English 56. Lund: Lund University Press.

Tanenhaus MK, Donnenwerth-Nolan S (1984). Syntactic context and lexical access. The Quarterly Journal of Experimental Psychology 36a: 649–61.

Note

1 This work was partly supported by MRC grant G9421014 (UK).

Chapter 30
The Processing of Linguistic Emotional Information in Patients with Acquired Brain Lesions

MANUELA SCHWARZ AND WOLFRAM ZIEGLER

Introduction

Right-brain-damaged patients are frequently described as being impaired in processing both linguistic and non-linguistic emotional information (Borod et al. 1992; Bloom, Borod, Obler and Gerstman 1992; Blonder, Bowers and Heilman 1991). As far as left brain damaged aphasic patients are concerned, it has often been observed, since the findings of Hughlings-Jackson (1880), that emotional words and phrases can be spared selectively.

The present study was designed to examine the processing of emotional words, sentences, non-literal and inferential linguistic meaning, as well as the processing of emotional prosody and facial expression in patients with acquired unilateral cerebrovascular lesions. Comparing verbal and non-verbal, emotional and non-emotional paradigms, we tested the hypothesis that there is dissociation between the processing of verbal and non-verbal emotional information.

Methods

Subjects

We examined 11 right-brain-damaged patients (RBD) aged 21–68 (mean 55), three women and eight men. A second patient group consisted of nine left-brain-damaged patients (LBD) aged 30–54 (mean 38), four women and five men. Twenty-five neurologically healthy subjects

(NOR) served as controls. They were matched for age (25–78 years, mean 57), education and gender (nine women, 16 men).

All patients were right-handed, native speakers of German suffering from acquired unilateral cerebrovascular accidents. As to the aphasic patients contained in the LBD group, we took care not to include patients with moderate or severe speech comprehension deficits.

Materials

The materials consisted of verbal and non-verbal (vocal and visual) items. Verbal and vocal items were presented binaurally, visual items in photographs. All verbal items were spoken by a professional radio speaker who tried to realize an emotionally neutral prosody. In a listening task subjects were requested to match each of these utterances to one of five target categories presented on a computer screen. Following each multiple-choice selection, subjects were asked to indicate their degree of certainty on a confidence rating scale.

The target categories for the emotional tasks consisted of five primary emotions. For the non-emotional control tasks, the categories consisted of five human characteristics (Table 30.1).

Table 30.1: Target categories

Emotional		
positive	*negative*	*neutral*
happiness	fear	surprise
	anger	
	sadness	
Non-emotional		
positive	*negative*	*neutral*
friendliness	ugliness	paleness
	stupidity	
	weakness	

We used identification tasks to investigate the processing of word meaning, non-literal meaning, associative meaning, and inferential meaning. To test the processing of word meaning, we selected adjectives denoting one of the target categories (e.g. *scared* for 'fear'). Care was taken to ensure that these adjectives were morphologically unrelated to the category names. To test non-literal meaning, we used metaphors and idioms (e.g. *she was on cloud nine* for the 'happiness' category). The processing of associative meaning was tested by sentences containing associative primes (e.g. the word *loss* priming 'sadness'). As far as inferential meaning was concerned, we constructed short texts consisting of three phrases each. The first phrase contained a lexical distractor referring to a different category (e.g. *tears* in the 'happiness' text). Only by drawing inferences was it possible to choose the appropriate target. Table 30.2 gives an overview over the numeric distribution of items.

Table 30.2: Stimuli

	Verbal				Non-verbal		
	Adjectives	Metaphors	Sentences	Texts	Prosody	Facial Exp	Σ
emotional	N=15	N=15	N=5	N=5	N=20	N=20	N=80
non-emotional	N=15	N=10	N=9	N=5	–	– ·	N=39
Σ	N=30	N=25	N=14	N=10	N=20	N=20	N=119

By testing the processing of emotional prosody and facial expression we aimed to identify patients who were unimpaired in the processing of lexical emotional information but who showed problems identifying emotions communicated prosodically or mimically. A genuine affect-processing deficit was expected to manifest itself here as well as in the verbal tasks. Patients with specifically verbal impairments were expected to solve the task correctly. The material we used for the prosody task was constructed by Tischer (1993). It consists of a sequence of three phrases (*Say it again! I can't believe it! What a day!*), which was spoken with different emotional intonations by four actors (cf. Geigenberger and Ziegler, this volume). The facial expression materials we used were the 'Pictures of facial affect' by Ekman and Friesen (1979). Table 30.2 also includes an overview of the numeric distribution of non-verbal items.

Preliminary results

Verbal emotional tasks

Error matrices for all types of verbal emotional stimuli demonstrate that interchanges with the category 'surprise' were relatively frequent, even for normal subjects. Table 30.3 presents the error matrix for the normals' responses to the text stimuli. It illustrates what was said about the misidentifications of the 'surprise' category (see asterisks). The ratings appearing in the cells marked by asterisks are not counted as errors in the following.

Table 30.3: Error matrix for emotional tests (normal subjects)

Stimulus → Response ↓	sadness	fear	anger	surprise	happiness
sadness	96.0			4.0	8.0
fear		56.0	4.0		
anger		4.0	84.0		
surprise		32.0*	12.0	80.0	40.0*
happiness	4.0	8.0		16.0	52.0

The emotional categories used as distractors in these texts (see the methods section) are marked by shadowed cells. As Table 30.3 shows, the normal listeners were not influenced to any relevant extent by the distractors. In contrast, as shown in Table 30.4, the RBD-group made a greater amount of errors on the distractors, indicating that these patients were unable to draw the required inferences.

Pairwise comparisons over all verbal emotional tasks (Figure 30.1) revealed a significant group effect (Kruskal-Wallis $\chi^2 = 7.63$, $p = 0.02$) between the RBD and the NOR group, but no difference between the two patient groups ($p = 0.38$).

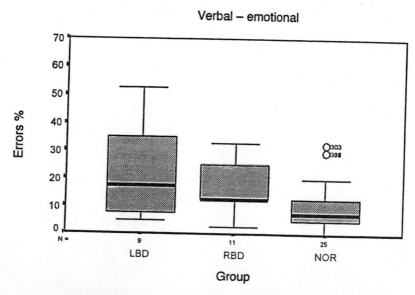

Figure 30.1. Verbal emotional tasks: group comparison of error scores.

Table 30.4: Error matrix for emotional tests (RBD-patients)

Stimulus → Response ↓	sadness	fear	anger	surprise	happiness
sadness	54.5	9.1	9.1	9.1	36.4
fear	9.1	27.3			
anger	9.1		63.6	9.1	
surprise	9.1	45.5*	27.3	63.6	0*
happiness	18.2	18.2		18.2	63.6

Verbal non-emotional tasks

Comparing the three groups on the verbal non-emotional tasks (see Figure 30.2) reveals a very similar pattern, indicating that the poorer performance of RBD patients cannot be attributed to a specific deficit in the processing of verbally communicated emotions.

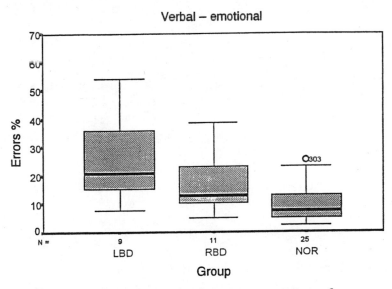

Figure 30.2. Verbal non-emotional tasks: group comparison of error scores.

Non-verbal emotional tasks

As Figure 30.3 shows, the RBD group was clearly impaired. There was a marked difference between the RBD patients and both the NOR group and the LBD group in the processing of facial expression and prosody.

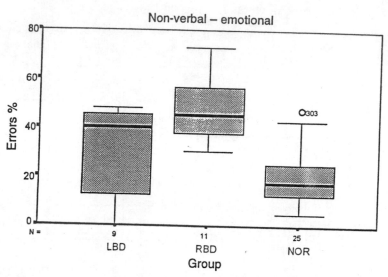

Figure 30.3. Non-verbal emotional tasks: group comparison of error scores.

Deficits were also seen in the LBD group. These might be due to the fact that the task imposed some verbal demands: the categories were verbal and the solution of the categorization-tasks required verbal abilities.

Conclusion

The data suggest that, compared to left-brain-damaged patients and normal controls, right-brain-damaged patients demonstrate deficits in processing emotion on non-verbal tasks. On verbal emotional tasks there was a difference between the performance of the right-brain-damaged patients and the normal control group. However, this difference could also be made out in the non-emotional verbal tasks and thus cannot be interpreted as an emotion-processing deficit. The right-brain-damaged patients' errors in verbal tasks could, to some extent, be attributed to a textual information-processing deficit, insofar as the right-brain-damaged patients had problems drawing the required inferences.

Left-brain-damaged patients showed significant impairments in all verbal tasks, and even in non-verbal tasks they performed worse than the normal control group – a fact that could be seen as a consequence of the linguistic demands contained in all tasks.

References

Blonder LX, Bowers D, Heilman K (1991) The role of the right hemisphere in emotional communication. Brain 114: 1115–27.

Bloom RL, Borod JC, Obler LK, Gerstman LJ (1992) Impact of emotional content on discourse production in patients with unilateral brain damage. Brain and Language 42: 153–64.

Borod JC, Andelman F, Obler LK, Tweedy JR, Welkowitz J (1992) Right hemisphere specialization for the identification of emotional words and sentences. Evidence from stroke patients. Neuropsychologia 30/9: 827–44.

Ekman P, Friesen W (1979) Pictures of facial affect. University of California Medical Center, San Francisco.

Hughlings-Jackson J (1880) On affections of speech from disease of the brain. Brain 2: 323–56.

Tischer B (1993) Die vokale Kommunikation von Gefühlen. Weinheim Beltz: Psychologie Verlags Union.

Chapter 31
Differences between the Left and the Right Hand in Agraphics

RENATA WHURR, MARJORIE LORCH AND
ILIAS PAPATHANASIOU

Introduction

The production of written language requires the formulation of linguistic content, spelling, visual-spatial organization, sequencing, and motoric control of graphemic output. Among the various communication disorders that result from a CNS lesion, acquired disorders of writing have received the least attention from researchers. In clinical practice, speech and language therapists typically train hemiplegic agraphic aphasic patients to write with their non-dominant, non-hemiplegic left hand. In recent years, several centres in the USA and Europe have developed a variety of writing prostheses to aid written language production with the dominant paretic limb (e.g. Leischner, 1983; Brown and Chobor, 1989; Whurr and Lorch, 1991; Lorch, Papathanasiou and Whurr, 1996). These studies have demonstrated that the written language produced by the paretic dominant right hand facilitated with a writing prosthesis is superior to the language produced by the non-dominant intact left hand (see Lorch, 1995 for review).

This paper aims to describe the linguistic and motoric aspects of writing in four moderate aphasic agraphic hemiplegic right-handed patients. Two of the patients received writing therapy with the left non-dominant hand and two of the patients received writing therapy with the prosthesis in the right hand. Written language performance, as evidenced in the pre-treatment baseline assessment (with the left hand), will be compared with left-hand productions and right-hand productions aided by the prosthesis in the post-treatment assessment.

Method

Subjects

Four right-handed agraphic aphasic hemiplegic patients were treated. In two cases, ES and MC, writing therapy was performed with the right hemiplegic limb, facilitated by the use of a writing prosthesis. In the other cases, BE and MR, writing therapy was performed with the left non-dominant, non-paralysed hand – i.e. the common rehabilitation strategy used by speech and language therapists.

Subjects treated with the right hand plus prosthesis.

Subject ES: a 75-year-old, right-handed, wheelchair-bound, retired male electrician. In December 1991 he suffered a left CVA resulting in right hemiplegia, moderate aphasia and agraphia. He received rehabilitation therapy for two years post-onset. Prior to this study, ES had been trained to use the left hand for writing.

Subject MC: a 69-year-old, right-handed wheelchair-bound retired male opera producer. In February 1990, he suffered a left CVA resulting in right hemiplegia, severe aphasia and agraphia. Prior to his entry in this study he had been trained to use his left hand for writing by a speech and language therapist.

Subjects treated with the left hand.

Subject BE: a 58-year-old, right-handed male chartered surveyor from Nigeria (English/Urdu bilingual). In May 1987 he suffered a left CVA resulting in right hemiplegia, severe aphasia and agraphia. Prior to this study he had been trained to use his left hand for writing. In this study, he was initially trained to use the prosthesis with his right dominant paralysed hand, but chose to use his non-dominant, non-paralysed left hand during the therapy period.

Subject MR: a 77-year-old, right-handed, retired, female, wheelchair-bound teacher. In August 1991, she suffered a left CVA resulting in right hemiplegia, severe aphasia and agraphia, and left-limb apraxia.

The prosthesis

The 'Agrafa' writing prosthesis, developed at the National Hospital for Neurology and Neurosurgery, London, facilitates writing through the involvement of the proximal muscles and leads to reduction of spasticity in the hand. Training with this prosthesis has enabled functional distal control of writing in hemiplegic agraphic patients.

Protocol

An initial baseline assessment was carried out. Patients subsequently received training in the use of the prosthesis for writing for two hours each week for four weeks. Writing therapy was then given for two hours a week over the course of 12 weeks. Each patient was reassessed at the end of this period of therapy.

Assessment

The initial pre-training assessment and the post-treatment assessment consisted of both motoric and linguistic tasks. The Jebsen hand function test (Jebsen, Taylor, Treischmann, Trotter and Howard, 1969) which involves skilled motor and motor graphic tasks, and the aphasia screening test (Whurr, 1996) which includes tasks for all four linguistic modalities, were also used to elicit linguistic performance. For the pre-training assessment, writing was examined with the left hand only, due to the lack of motor skills of the right hand. In post-treatment reassessment, writing was examined with both hands on separate occasions to avoid any priming effect.

Training programme

During the prosthesis training sessions, the table and chair height were adjusted to the subject's height in order to reduce trunk flexion and other associated movements and to promote shoulder movements without elbow flexion. The movement patterns used during the training sessions aim to promote and facilitate proximal arm movement. The prosthesis-training tasks included free movement, drawing and copying shapes, letters and words. These tasks were used in the given sequence at the beginning of each training session. During the first 10 minutes of each therapy session, these tasks were used to 'loosen up' the arm and prepare for therapy. The patient initially used the prosthesis supported with the left hand producing bilateral movements. This progressed to unilateral unaided use of the paralysed limb. The therapy materials were designed to take into account the spared and impaired areas of written language functions of each individual patient.

Results

Linguistic function

In all cases, total language performance as measured by the AST

(Whurr, 1996) improved after treatment (see Table 31.1). Written language performance, which was the focus of the present treatment, improved after treatment in all four patients. The superiority of written language production of the right hand was observed in both patients who received treatment with the prosthesis, ES and MC. In the case of BE, initial training was given in using the prosthesis with the right hand, but the patient chose to receive writing therapy with his left hand. It is notable that post-treatment testing indicates superior performance in the right hand productions in this instance as well. Patient MR's writing function with the left hand improved with treatment but could not be compared to the right hand. Qualitative and quantitative differences in error types in the written productions of the two hands were observed (see Table 31.2).

Table 31.1. Aphasia Screening Test

	% VIS PER	% REA COM	% AUD COM	% SP PRD	% LG PRD	% WRT PRD	% CAL	% COM	% PRD	% TOTAL
				Patient ES						
PRE	100	87.5	85	76.4	63.3	41.8	0	89	56	69.2
POST Lt*	100	92.5	97.5	89.1	90	50.9	90	96	69.3	80
POST Rt**	100	92.5	97.5	89.1	90	56.4	90	96	71.3	81.2
				Patient MC						
PRE	100	97.5	85	70.9	66.6	47.2	0	93	56.6	71.2
POST Lt*	100	90	95	63.4	80	41.8	80	94	60	73.6
POST Rt**	100	90	95	63.4	80	52.8	80	94	64	76
				Patient BE						
PRE	100	90	95	76.4	60	60	90	94	68	78.4
POST Lt*	100	87.5	90	78	56.6	69.1	90	79	72	79.6
POST Rt**	100	87.5	90	78	56.6	74.5	90	79	74	80.8
				Patient MR						
PRE	100	85	92.5	90.9	76.6	0	0	91	48.6	65.6
POST Lt*	100	90	87.5	98.1	90.6	58.2	60	91	80.6	86.8
POST Rt**				Not tested						

* Writing was performed with the left hand
** Writing was performed with the right hand plus prosthesis

Table 31.2. Written Object Naming

Target	Pre-Treatment	Post-Treatment Left*	Post-Treatment Right**
Patient ES			
Toothbrush	TPOOB	–	TOOHBRUS
Comb	COB	COMB	COMB
Spoon	Spoon	S	Spoon
Envelopes	EVO	–	E
Pen	–	PEN	PEN
Patient MC			
Toothbrush	Theechsooth	Teethagne	Teenbrush
Comb	Comb	Heir	Comb
Spoon	Speech	Teaproon	Copteen
	Spood		
	Spoob		
	Spoon		
Envelopes	Evolles	Evloppesne	Evnolepes
Pen	pen	Pan	Pen
Patient BE			
Toothbrush	TOOTH	TOOTHBROCH	TOOTHBRUSH
Comb	COMP	COMB	COMB
Spoon	SPOON	SPOON	SPOON
Envelopes	ENVEPENE	ENVELOPE	ENVELOPE
Pen	PEN	PEN	PEN
Patient MR			
Toothbrush	–	toothtbbt	NT
Comb	–	comb	NT
Spoon	–	spoon	NT
Envelopes	–	ee	NT
Pen	–	pen	NT

* Writing was performed with the left hand
** Writing was performed with the right hand and prosthesis
NT Not tested
– No response

Motor function

In the prosthesis users, general reduction of the spasticity of the paralysed hand was observed, which enabled passive movements of the fingers. Improvement in the speed of skilled motor task was also demonstrated (see Table 31.3). At the end of training, sufficient release of spasticity occurred to enable both prosthesis users to hold a pen and write with the hemiplegic hand.

Table 31.3. Jebsen test of hand function

	WR	MAZ TRA	ER	CAR TRN	SMA OBJ	SIM FEE	DRT	ASM	LLO	LHO
				Patient ES						
PRE TREAT	6	13	0	4	2	1	2	11	4	4
POST TREAT	9	7	1	5	2	1	2	9	5	1
				Patient MC						
PRE TREAT	5	4	0	3	2	2	3	21	6	6
POST TREAT	3	4	1	1	1	2	1	22	1	2
				Patient BE						
PRE TREAT	6	14	6	2	13	5	6	NT	5	5
POST TREAT	4	5	2	2	5	2	5	NT	6	6
				Patient MR						
PRE TREAT	7	1	7	3	5	3	10	NT	11	25
POST TREAT	24	1	8	2	4	16	6	15	9	16

The scores represent times of standard deviation away from the mean.
The normal limits are within –2 and 2, shown in bold type.
NT=not tested.

Conclusions

There was an overall improvement for these four patients on treated as well as untreated areas of language performance after receiving writing therapy. The treatment effect demonstrated in these hemiplegic agraphic aphasics replicates findings of superior written language production with the right hand, as compared to the left, after using a prosthesis reported previously (Lorch, 1995). The use of the prosthesis also gave rise to a reduction of spasticity in the paretic hand. Skilled motor tasks demonstrated an improvement in the speed of motor tasks. Our results suggest that training aphasic hemiplegics to write with their dominant hand achieves two rehabilitation effects:

- Linguistic – achieves superior written language production in aphasic agraphia with the right hand.
- Motor – with training the prosthesis can achieve motor gains in the hemiplegic limb.

References

Brown J, Chobor K (1989) Therapy with a prosthesis for writing. Aphasiology 3: 709–15.

Jebsen R, Taylor N, Treischmann T, Trotter M, Howard L (1969) Objective and standardized test of hand function. Archives of Physical Medicine and Rehabilitation 50: 311–19.

Leischner A (1983) Side differences in writing to dictation of aphasics with agraphia: a graphic disconnection syndrome. Brain and Language 18: 1–19.

Lorch M (1995) Laterality and rehabilitation: differences in left and right hand productions in aphasic agraphic hemiplegics. Aphasiology 5: 257–82.

Lorch M, Papathanasiou I and Whurr R (1996) Laterality and written language production: writing with the right hand in an aphasic agraphic hemiplegic patient. In Powell T (Ed) Pathologies of Speech and Language: Contributions of Clinical Phonetics and Linguistics. New Orleans: ICPLA, pp 297–304.

Whurr R (1996) Aphasia Screening Test 2nd Ed. London: Whurr.

Whurr R, Lorch M (1991) The use of a prosthesis to facilitate writing in aphasia and right hemiplegia. Aphasiology 5: 411–18.

Chapter 32
Increased Writing Activity: a Neurolinguistic Perspective[1]

PETER VAN VUGT, PHILIPPE PAQUIER AND PATRICK CRAS

Defining the problem

Increased writing activity (IWA) is a well-studied phenomenon in the psychiatric literature (Trimble, 1986; Ludwig, 1994). In neurological conditions, writing anomalies mostly consist of agraphia – most frequently a substantial reduction of the written output – in combination with important dysfunctions mainly of the lexicographemic processes. However, a considerable increase of writing activity can be observed in a limited number of neurological patients (see Table 32.1). For reasons of clarity, we will confine ourselves to the neurological literature.

In this literature, IWA is discussed under a number of headings: phonographie (Bernard, 1889), echographia (Pick, 1924), graphorrhée (Manuila, Manuila, Nicole and Lambert, 1970), hypergraphia (Trimble, 1986), graphomania (Cambier, Masson, Benammou and Robine, 1988), anosognosic graphomimia (Gil, Neau, Aubert, Fabre, Agbo and Tantot, 1995) compulsive writing behaviour (Van Vugt, Paquier, Kees and Cras, 1996a). The terminology used is far from unequivocal. Firstly, group studies provide very little information on inter-patient differences in the clinical manifestation of IWA. Secondly, comparing a limited number of detailed case reports reveals that one particular term may denote different types of behaviour and that similar IWAs have been labelled differently.

The same equivocal situation holds with regard to the use of the term hypergraphia. The use of hypergraphia to indicate a remarkable or intact orthographic skill in patients with general learning disabilities is perhaps unexpected (Burd and Kerbeshian, 1985). The term here is used as a parallel for the better-known phenomenon of hyperlexia (see

Aram and Healy, 1988). Waxman and Geschwind (1974) described a set of behavioural symptoms that have been observed in patients with temporal lobe epilepsy (TLE): (a) circumstanciality (including a particular form of IWA); (b) altered sexuality (most frequently hyposexuality); (c) increased concern with philosophical or religious issues; and (d) intensification of emotional responses (e.g. irritability) (see Waxman and Geschwind, 1974, 1975; Benson, 1991). Within the conceptual framework of this so-called Geschwind syndrome, hypergraphia refers to an increased written output with generally normal writing skills, syntax and semantics. The IWA is observed in the period separating the clinical seizures. An over-inclusive style is thought to be pathognomonic. However, it remains questionable whether the Geschwind syndrome constitutes a specific entity (Hermann, Whitman, Wyler, Richey and Dells, 1988; Benson, 1991). On the other hand, in descriptions of IWA in epileptic and non-epileptic patients, the term hypergraphia also refers to excessive writing production ranging from (copied) comprehensible text over legible but incomprehensible text to the repetitive use of a symbol or even page-covering scribbling.

Several efforts have been made to distinguish the supposedly TLE-related, 'overinclusive' hypergraphia from other types of IWA (Cambier et al. 1988; Okamura, Fukai, Yamadori, Hidari, Asaba and Sakai, 1993; Kanemoto, Akamatsu, Itagaki and Nishitani, 1990; Gil, Neau, Aubert, Fabre, Agbo and Tantot, 1995). The common feature shared by instances of the 'non-Geschwindian' IWA consists in the involuntary, almost mechanical nature of the writing process. However, varying degrees of 'automaticity' have been described ranging from writing movements, even without pencil, and without looking at the hand (Gil et al. 1995), to attempts to correct the spelling errors made (Pick, 1924). Moreover, varying degrees of preserved communicative abilities in writing have been reported ranging from none (Gil et al. 1995) over servile copy and more-or-less adequately written fairy-tale generation (Cambier et al. 1988), to answering questions (Yamadori, Mori, Tabuchi, Kudo and Mitani, 1986). Differences in input channels (written reproduction of what has been heard or seen) have also led to a multiplicity of terms.

Review

Different lines of approach present themselves when reviewing the literature. First, one needs to check whether differences in aetiology help in distinguishing between the diverse IWA pictures. One has to conclude that IWA is reported in patients suffering from afflictions with different causes, namely in (epileptic and non-epileptic) patients with general learning disabilities (Jancar and Kettle, 1984) in patients known with brain tumours (Cambier et al. 1988; Imamura et al. 1992), cerebral strokes (Yamadori et al. 1986), multiple sclerosis (Kanemoto et al. 1990), or frontal lobe atrophy (Frisoni, Scuratti, Bianchetti and Trabucchi, 1993; Van Vugt, Paquier, Kees and Cras, 1996b). Moreover, we cannot but notice that, even when making abstraction of the problems of reliability and comparability of the different imaging techniques, different cortical and subcortical structures may have an influence on the development of IWA.

Okamura, Motomura, Asaba, Sakai, Fukai, Mori and Yamadori (1989) have suggested that meaningful writing, produced in a conscious, purposeful way, can be related to epilepsy (more precisely to the Geschwind syndrome), while compulsive and absent-minded, almost automatic writing activity can be observed in patients with stroke, and degenerative or space-occupying disease. However, this view of the mechanisms leading to IWA does not clearly distinguish aetiology and symptoms. Moreover, it is contradicted by Joseph's (1986) report of a TLE patient who presented with frequent, ictal and thus sudden-onset, non-volitional writing automatisms, as well as by some of Yamadori et al.'s (1986) right-brain damaged patients who display the overinclusive style in their notes said to be characteristic of Geschwindian hypergraphia. With respect to the lateralization of the causal lesions, hypergraphia (IWA) has been considered a right hemisphere syndrome (Yamadori et al. 1986). However, this finding is not corroborated by our review. The only conclusion we can draw from the table, in relation to hemispheric specialization, is that left-handed subjects, up until now, did not present with IWA. This is indeed a very narrow basis for neuro-anatomical conclusions.

When confronted with samples of written output of neurological patients, it is definitely not easy to determine their informative quality (Pick, 1924; Perkins, 1994). In a number of instances, the patient obviously wants to transmit a message (Roberts, Robertson and Trimble, 1982; Hermann et al. 1988). In other cases, this is much less the case or not the case at all – for instance when a particular phrase is endlessly repeated or linguistic elements are wrongfully omitted (Van Vugt, Paquier, Kees and Cras, 1996a, b). Repetition may be expected to some extent when dealing with increased linguistic production (Perkins, 1994). In most cases, repetitions of verbal material are, indeed, observed. In some samples a rather thematic repetition is seen (Waxman and Geschwind, 1974, 1975; Hermann et al. 1988), whereas in others one observes a formal repetition of syntactic, lexical, and even graphemic elements (Cambier et al. 1988, Van Vugt et al. 1996a, b). Sporadic and even isolated episodes of IWA are described, for example, by Yamadori et al. (1986) and Hermann et al. (1988). Pick (1924), Waxman and Geschwind (1974), Cambier et al. (1988), Gil et al. (1995) and Van Vugt et al. (1996ab) have reported IWA of a more permanent nature.

Discussion and conclusion

In order to avoid confusion when discussing causal mechanisms, we would like to redefine some terms in a behavioural perspective. Firstly, we tend to believe the patient's communicative intention can help to distinguish between the different types of IWA. Secondly, we think that the linguistic level at which the repetitiveness occurs is of great diagnostic importance. In our view, a third question imposes itself: is the IWA permanently present or can it be elicited?

In view of these observations, we would like

> to call hypergraphia all transient IWA with a non-iterative appearance on syntactic or lexico-graphemic level. We suggest to reserve the term automatic writing behaviour (AWB) to indicate a permanently present or elicitable, compulsive, iterative and not necessarily complete written reproduction of visually or orally perceived messages [Van Vugt, 1996a,b, pp. 514].

When patients with general learning disabilities exhibit an unusual orthographic talent, as described by Burd and Kerbeshian (1985), we think a term like hyperorthographia might be more suitable.

We would like to maintain the distinction between AWB and the writing behaviour of aphasic patients who, when confronted with a written question, are unable to answer it either verbally or by writing, although they can indicate that they understood the question by gesturing (Pick, 1924). These patients only succeed in repeatedly transcribing the written question, which attempts reflect their repeated trials to answer, and show that they are aware of their failure. This written reproduction can thus hardly be interpreted as a compulsive or automatic behaviour. This phenomenon is quite similar to what is known in aphasiology as *echolalia*. For this reason we would like to call this particular type of writing behaviour *echographia*.

As can be seen in Table 32.1, the IWA may sometimes combine features of both hypergraphia and AWB. For instance, the symptomatology of Joseph's (1986) patient B who produced religiomystical material in a semi-automatic way during an ictus is strongly reminiscent of the so-called Geschwind syndrome. In spite of the semi-automatic generation of text, this (ictal) instance of IWA might be called *hypergraphia*. Concerning Joseph's (1986) patient A, we have unfortunately not enough information about the thematic content of her writing to characterize the IWA. The report by Yamadori et al. (1986) of a unique IWA episode that was not thematically centred (patient TN) is entirely different. In patient KH (Yamadori et al. 1986) the IWA had obviously no communicative intention, but the phenomenon was observed only occasionally. In other cases there may be insufficient information on the form and content of the writing. For all these cases, it seems appropriate to use a generic term like 'IWA not otherwise specified'.

Table 32.1 Review of detailed reports of increased writing activity in neurological conditions

Report	Case	Sex	Age	Handedness	Aetiology	Localization	TLE	UB	IWA frequency
Cambier et al., 1988	E	f	67	r	tum	bi F			+ not transient
Frisoni et al., 1993	EP*	m	60	r	deg	gen atrophy			not transient
Gil et al., 1995	955	f	93	r	vi	r			not transient
Inamura et al., 1992	X	m	80	r	tum	r P			not transient
Yamadori et al., 1986	CA	f	54	r	vh	r CI			− during 4 days
Waxman and Gerchwind, 1974, 1975	1	f	25	r	?	r T	+		several hours a day
Waxman and Gerchwind 1974	4	m	35	r	?	r T	+		daily
Kanemoto et al., 1990	X	f	22	r	ms	bi T & pv			not transient
Van Vugt et al., 1996	X	m	70	r	deg	gen atrophy			not transient
Herman et al., 1988	TF**	f	28	r	lobectomy	l T	+		transient episodes
Herman et al., 1988	LN**	f	40	r	?	r	+		transient episodes
Herman et al., 1988	NS**	f	51	r	?	r	+		transient episodes
Joseph, 1986	B	f	45	r	deg	bi F and r T	+°		transient episodes
Roberts et al., 1982	JK	m	30	r	infectious	r T	+		transient episodes
Roberts et al., 1982	VG	m	36	r	deg	r F T	+		transient episodes
Roberts et al., 1982	MW	m	33	r	atroph. les. §	r P O		normal EEG	transient episodes
Roberts et al., 1982	PM	f	25	r	?	r	gen E		transient episodes
Roberts et al., 1982	GT	m	48	r	vm	r T th	+		transient episodes
Waxman and Geschwind, 1974	2	m	28	r	lobectomy	l T	+		daily entry in diary
Waxman and Geschwind, 1974	3	m	>40	r	lobectomy	l T	+		daily entry in diary
Waxman and Geschwind, 1974	5	m	37	a	infectious	l T P			daily
Waxman and Geschwind, 1975	2	m	20	r	infectious	r T (P)	+		transient episodes
Waxman and Geschwind, 1975	3	m	28	?	?			normal EEG	transient episodes
Yamadori et al., 1986	TK	m	64	r	vi	r ps	+°°		− during at least 8 days
Joseph, 1986	A	f	17	r	trauma	l	+°°		+ transient episodes
Roberts et al., 1982	WM	f	61	r	?	r F T			transient episodes
Yamadori et al., 1986	TN	f	50	r	vi	r F P			− once
Yamadori et al., 1986	AK	m	70	r	vi	r			− during at least 11 days
Yamadori et al., 1986	KH	m	65	r	vh	r ci			− occasionally in 8 day period
Waxman and Geschwind, 1974	6	m	27	r	atroph. les. §	r and l T			transient episodes
Waxman and Geschwind, 1974	7	m	42	r	lobectomy	r T			?
Pick, 1924	F	f	64	?	vi	l			not transient
Pick, 1924	2	m	58	?	vi	l			not transient

Table 32.1 (cont.) Review of detailed reports of increased writing activity in neurological conditions

IWA communicative value	RWM	ROM	Repetition thematic	Syntact.	Lexical	Graphemic	Original denomination	New IWA typology
poor: page filling	+	+	−	+			graphomanie	AWB
poor: page filling	?	?	−		+	+	H	AWB
poor	?	?				+	graphomimie	AWB
poor: inattentive writing	?	?	−				H	AWB
?	−	−	−				H	AWB
rather poor	+	?	+ lists, songs, mystical issues	+	+		H	AWB
rather poor: automatisms	?	?	+ diary, songs, aphorisms	+	+		H	AWB
meaningless automatisms***	?	?	−		+	+	H	AWB
poor: page filling	+	+	−	+	+		CWB	AWB
Informative	−	−	+ quarrels	−	−	−	H	H
Informative	−	−	+ job, car driving	−	−	−	H	H
Informative	−	−	+ family				H	H
poor: nonvolitional automatisms	−	−	+ religiomystical material	−	−	−	H	H
Informative	?	?	+ minute diaries				H	H
Informative	?	?	+ religious experiences				H	H
Informative	?	?	+ memory aid, spiritual powers				H	H
Informative	?	?	+ diaries				H	H
Informative	?	?	+ diaries, prayers				H.	H
Informative	?	?	+ illness, God				H	H
Informative	?	?	+ meticulous notes on health				H	H
Informative	?	?	+ circumstantial sermons				H	H
Informative	?	?	+ love, life, God				H	H

Informative	?	?		+ poems, essays, prayers	H	H
Informative, overinclusive	–	–		+ illness	H	H
poor: nonvolitional automatisms	–	–			H	IWA
poor: unconnected jottings	?	?		–	H	IWA
?	–	–		–	H	IWA
poor	?	?			H	IWA
poor	?	?			H	IWA
informative	?	?		+ CV, lists (of telephone calls)	H	IWA
hidden outline for a novel	?	?	+		H	IWA
informative	+	?	+		EG	EG
?	+	?		+	phonographia	EG

*: personal communication dd 14-02-1994; **: personal communication and samples provided dd 27-01-1994; ***: personal communication dd 07-06-1996. m: male; f: female; l: left; r: right; a: ambidexter; bi: bilateral; ?: information not provided; §: not otherwise specified; tum: tumour; vi: vascular ischaemic; vh: vascular haemorrhagic; vm: vascular malformation; deg: degenerative disease; ms: multiple sclerosis; F: frontal; P: parietal; T: temporal; O: occipital; ci: capsular; ps: perisylvian; pv: periventricular; th: thalamic; TLE: temporal lobe epilepsy; gen E: generalized epilepsy; +: present; –: absent; °: and bipolar; °°: and depression; RWM: reproduction of written material; ROM: reproduction of oral material; UB: utilization behaviour; AWB: automatic writing behaviour; H: hypergraphia; CWB: compulsive writing behaviour; IWA: increased writing behaviour; EG: echographia.

In Table 32.1, we have regrouped the cases of IWA that have been described in detail up until now. Imaging techniques and neurobehavioural descriptions (cf. inattentive writing, meaningless automatisms) document or suggest an involvement of left or right frontal lobe areas in several case reports of AWB. It seems reasonable to consider AWB a particular, sometimes isolated, form of utilization behaviour (Van Vugt, 1996b) in the sense that the inhibitory function of the frontal lobes is suppressed, thus leaving the subject dependent on the slightest stimulus (Lhermitte, 1983). One has to be less conclusive with respect to the mechanisms leading to the other forms of IWA. When epilepsy-related memory problems are taken into account (Okamura et al. 1993) it seems only natural that patients tend to compensate by writing things down as detailed as possible, in a 'hypergraphic' way (Cambier et al. 1988). In the case of echographia, it is important that the repetitive writing activity can be explained as a pragmatically adequate reaction to a linguistic deficit. Hyperorthographia and hyperlexia can both find a place within the framework of the isolated skills that make the so-called mono-savants so unique.

References

Aram D, Healy J (1988) Hyperlexia: a review of extraordinary word recognition. In Obler L, Fein D (Eds) The Exceptional Brain, Neuropsychology of Talent and Special Abilities. New York: Guilford Press, pp 70–102.

Benson F (1991) The Geschwind syndrome. Advances in Neurology 55: 411–21.

Bernard (1889) De l'Aphasie. Paris

Burd L, Kerbeshian J (1985) Hyperlexia and a variant of hypergraphia. Perceptual and Motor Skills 60: 940–2.

Cambier J, Masson C, Benammou S, Robine B (1988) La graphomanie, activité graphique compulsive manifestation d'un gliome fronto-calleux. Revue Neurologique (Paris) 144: 158–64.

Frisoni G, Scuratti A, Bianchetti A, Trabucchi M (1993) Hypergraphia and brain damage. Journal of Neurology, Neurosurgery, and Psychiatry 56: 576–7.

Gil R, Neau JP, Aubert I, Fabre C, Agbo C, Tantot AM (1995) Graphomimie anosognosique: variété particulière d'hypergraphie au cours d'un infarctus sylvien droit. Revue Neurologique (Paris) 151: 198–201.

Hermann B, Whitman S, Wyler A, Richey E, Dells J (1988) The neurological, psychosocial and demographic correlates of hypergraphia in patients with epilepsy. Journal of Neurology, Neurosurgery, and Psychiatry 51: 203–8.

Imamura T, Yamadori A, Tsuburaya K (1992) Hypergraphia associated with a brain tumour of the right cerebral hemisphere. Journal of Neurology, Neurosurgery, and Psychiatry 55: 25–7.

Jancar J, Kettle L (1984) Hypergraphia and mental handicap. Journal of Mental Deficiency Research 28: 151–8.

Joseph A (1986) A hypergraphic syndrome of automatic writing, affective disorder, and temporal lobe epilepsy in two patients. Journal of Clinical Psychiatry 47: 255–7.

Kanemoto K, Akamatsu T, Itagaki Y, Nishitani H (1990) Early onset multiple sclerosis with hypergraphia and Klüver-Bucy syndrome: a case report. Neurological Medicine (Tokyo) 32: 301–3.

Lhermitte F (1983) Utilization behaviour and its relation to lesions of the frontal lobes. Brain 106: 237–55.

Ludwig A (1994) Mental illness and creative activity in female writers. American Journal of Psychiatry 151: 1650–6.

Manuila A, Manuila L, Nicole M, Lambert H (1970) Dictionnaire Français de Médecine et de Biologie. Paris: Masson.

Okamura T, Motomura N, Asaba H, Sakai T, Fukai M, Mori E, Yamadori A (1989) Hypergraphia in temporal lobe epilepsy, compared with stroke of the right cerebral hemisphere. Japanese Journal of Psychiatry and Neurology 43: 524–5.

Okamura T, Fukai M, Yamadori A, Hidari M, Asaba H, Sakai T (1993) A clinical study of hypergraphia in epilepsy. Journal of Neurology, Neurosurgery, and Psychiatry 56: 556–9.

Perkins M (1994) Repetitiveness in language disorders: a new analytical procedure. Clinical Linguistics and Phonetics 8: 321–36.

Pick A (1924) On the pathology of echographia. Brain 47: 417–29.

Roberts J, Robertson M, Trimble M (1982) The lateralizing significance of hypergraphia in temporal lobe epilepsy. Journal of Neurology, Neurosurgery, and Psychiatry 45: 131–8.

Trimble M (1986) Hypergraphia. In: Trimble M, Bolwig T (Eds) Aspects of epilepsy and psychiatry. London: John Wiley and Sons Ltd, pp 75–87.

Van Vugt P, Paquier P, Kees L, Cras P (1996a) Compulsive writing behavior in a demented alcoholic patient with frontal lobe hypoperfusion. Journal of the International Neuropsychological Society 2: 197.

Van Vugt P, Paquier P, Kees L, Cras P (1996b) Increased writing activity in neurological conditions: a review and clinical study. Journal of Neurology, Neurosurgery, and Psychiatry 61: 510–14.

Waxman S, Geschwind N (1975) The interictal behavior syndrome of temporal lobe epilepsy. Archives of General Psychiatry 32: 1580–6.

Waxman S, Geschwind N (1974) Hypergraphia in temporal lobe epilepsy. Neurology 24: 629–37.

Yamadori A, Mori E, Tabuchi M, Kudo Y, Mitani Y (1986) Hypergraphia: a right hemisphere syndrome. Journal of Neurology, Neurosurgery, and Psychiatry 49: 1160–4.

Note

1 This research was supported by the Provincie Antwerpen and by the Research Fund of the Antwerp University (UIA). We wish to thank Yvan de Smet for reviewing the manuscript and Michel Isacson for his kind bibliographical support.

Chapter 33
Sentence Comprehension Deficit in Alzheimer's Disease

MARK LEIKIN AND JUDITH AHARON-PERETZ

Alzheimer's disease (AD) is marked by a progressive decline in verbal communication, with fluent, spontaneous speech deteriorating from impaired naming and comprehension to a Wernicke's-aphasia-like impairment (Cummings, Benson, Hill and Read, 1985; Murdoch, Chenery, Wilks and Boyle, 1987). Anomia, diminished word comprehension, and impaired word-generation abilities comprise the first and most distinctive features of language breakdown in AD. To date, only a few studies have evaluated sentence comprehension in AD, and the results are still controversial (e.g., Rochon, Waters and Caplan, 1994). Theoretically, a loss of sentence comprehension can be caused by an inability to comprehend the information content of different types of words (lexical and grammatical semantics), by syntactic impairment or by non-language deficit such as damage to pragmatic comprehension or working memory. The aim of the present study was twofold: (a) to evaluate language impairment in Hebrew-speaking AD patients, as no such study has yet been conducted; (b) to test sentence comprehension deficits in AD patients.

Method

Participants

Thirty-three AD patients and 16 age-matched normal controls (age 66;4±5;3 years, education 12;1±4;1 years) participated in the study. SDAT patients fulfilled criteria for the clinical diagnosis of probable Alzheimer's disease according to the DST IV and NINCDS-ADRDA. They scored four or less on the Hachinski ischemia scale and 10 or less on the Hamilton Depression rating scale. The patients were divided according to the MMSE into two groups: 15 mild SDAT patients

(SDATm, MMSE 20–26, age 70;2±7;1, education 11;2±3;6) (the ADm group) and 18 severe SDAT patients (SDATs, MMSE 9-19, age 69;9± 6;1, education 13;5±3;7) (the ADs group). All subjects were right handed. Hebrew was their dominant language for more than 50 years.

Procedure

Language ability testing was performed with the Hebrew translation of the Western Aphasia Battery (WAB) (Kertesz, 1982) and the 'Rambam language evaluation' battery (RLE). RLE was used for further evaluation of auditory word and sentence comprehension and naming abilities as follows:

Comprehension tasks

1. Semantic judgment: 23 orally presented declarative sentences (semantically correct or incorrect) conveying different types of grammatical meanings such as locative, temporal, or causal (e.g. 'The horse is smaller than the dog'). The subject had to indicate whether the sentence was correct or not.
2. Sentence comprehension: (a) 12 instrumental constructions (e.g. 'with the pencil, point to the key'); (b) 12 attributive constructions (e.g. 'the mother of the daughter'); (c) 12 logicogrammatical (following Luria, 1966) constructions (e.g. 'a circle under a triangle'). In (b) and (c), the subject had to point to the appropriate picture.
3. Comprehension of commands: 16 sentences, such as 'raise your hand' or 'if it is raining now, give me your hand.'
4. Word meaning comprehension requested an explanation of the meaning of five orally presented words (e.g. 'glasses').

Naming tasks

1. Naming to confrontation: 33 line drawings of objects.
2. Naming from definition: 23 orally presented descriptions such as 'pair of lenses in a frame helping the eyesight.'
3. Production of antonyms: 60 orally presented words.
4. Production of synonyms: 20 words.
5. Word generation task: required to name as many members of the semantic category (e.g. 'Food' and 'Animals') as possible in one minute.

Statistical analysis included protected unpaired t-tests, using the SAS MULTTEST procedure (SAS Institute, version 6.11, running under UNIX).

Results

The performance of patients and controls on the WAB and on the RLE is depicted in Tables 33.1a (means and SD) and 33.1b (p values).

Table 33.1a. Performance of AD patients and controls on WAB and RLE (means and SD)

	ADm (n = 15)	ADs (n = 18)	Controls (n = 16)
WAB			
Spontaneous speech	17.53±2.06	19.16±1.15	19.8±0.34
Speech content	8.33±1.2	9.3±0.7	9.8±0.34
Speech fluency	9.2±1.08	9.77±0.54	10.00±0.0
Yes/no questions	53.40±3.6	56±2.52	57.00±0.0
Word recognition (total)	51.20±4.7	53.2±1.56	54.00±0.0
*Single words	46.2±4.31	47.66±0.97	48.00±0.00
Sequential commands	51.26±16.98	63.55±8.9	78.43±3.01
Comprehension (total)	155.86±21.86	172.83±10.70	189.43±3.01
Repetition (total)	58.73±17.52	69.94±11.57	75.50±1.15
**Repetition (2-5 words)	5.53±2.09	6.44±1.33	7.00±0.0
**Repetition (6-9 words)	0.4±0.8	1.16±0.9	1.8±0.4
Object naming	39.93±13.92	50.88±6.33	59.43±1.2
Word fluency	8.20±5.01	11.38±4.23	17.31±4.04
Naming (total)	64.53±21.11	81.72±7.2	96.75±3.8
RLE			
Semantic judgment	17.40±3.62	20.50±2.22	21.87±1.20
Instrumental const.	3.33±1.44	4.94±1.05	5.68±0.60
Attributive const.	5.0±1.36	5.83±0.38	5.93±0.25
Logicogrammatical const.	5.46±3.48	8.77±3.57	13.50±1.5
Commands	7.26±4.74	11.16±3.46	16.68±1.19
Word meaning	4.13±1.76	4.77±0.64	4.81±0.40
Naming (objects)	20,0±7.06	24.88±49	31.81±1.68
Naming (definitions)	8.73±5.9	14.22±3.97	21.31±1.53
Naming (antonyms)	42.53±13.1	53.55±5.4	58.75±1.29
Naming (synonyms)	6.46±5.02	10.22±4.64	17.62±2.7
Word fluency	8.2±5.01	11.38±4.23	17.31±4.04

Compared to the controls, the AD patients showed significantly worse results in almost all tasks. The impairment of AD patients in certain tasks involving sentence comprehension (e.g., sequence commands) and naming (e.g., RLE's confrontation naming) was already evident in the ADm group. Patients also displayed dissimilar impairments in different language abilities. AD patients were impaired with regard to

Table 33.1b. Performance of AD patients and controls on WAB and RLE (p-MULTITEST Values)

Variable	AD vs Controls		ADm vs Controls		ADs vs ADm	
	Raw p	Adj p	Raw p	Adj p	Raw p	Adj p
WAB						
Spontaneous speech	0.0003	0.0105	0.0670	0.4510	0.0006	0.0197
Speech content	0.0002	0.0084	0.0567	0.4385	0.0006	0.0202
Speech fluency	0.0091	0.1579	0.1746	0.5386	0.0096	0.1701
Yes/no questions	0.0022	0.0551	0.1268	0.5386	0.0025	0.0598
Word recognition (total)	0.0221	0.2764	0.2275	0.5957	0.0193	0.2599
*Single words	0.0802	0.4510	0.3471	0.6815	0.0469	0.4385
Sequential commands	0.0001	0.0001	0.0001	0.0052	0.0012	0.0327
Comprehension (total)	0.0001	0.0001	0.0005	0.0182	0.0005	0.0177
Repetition (total)	0.0019	0.0467	0.0918	0.4553	0.0051	0.1119
**Repetition (2-5 words)	0.0118	0.1849	0.1296	0.5386	0.0360	0.3752
**Repetition (6-9 words)	0.0001	0.0001	0.0085	0.1579	0.0030	0.0682
Object naming	0.0001	0.0013	0.0030	0.0682	0.0003	0.0127
Word fluency	0.0001	0.0001	0.0002	0.0066	0.0226	0.2809
Naming (total)	0.0001	0.0001	0.0006	0.0197	0.0002	0.0066
RLE						
Semantic judgment	0.0002	0.0076	0.0589	0.4385	0.0005	0.0177
Instrumental const.	0.0001	0.0003	0.0256	0.2976	0.0001	0.0021
Attributive const.	0.0191	0.2592	0.3532	0.6815	0.0023	0.0571
Logicogrammatical const.	0.0001	0.0001	0.0001	0.0009	0.0015	0.0366
Commands	0.0001	0.0031	0.0110	0.1817	0.0082	0.1579
Word meaning	0.1413	0.5386	0.4626	0.6815	0.0467	0.4385
Naming (objects)	0.0001	0.0001	0.0001	0.0041	0.0038	0.0837
Naming (definitions)	0.0001	0.0018	0.0331	0.3528	0.0001	0.0057
Naming (antonyms)	0.0001	0.0001	0.0001	0.0001	0.0075	0.1579
Naming (synonyms)	0.0005	0.0171	0.0660	0.4510	0.0013	0.0340
Word fluency	0.0001	0.0001	0.0002	0.0066	0.0226	0.2809

spontaneous speech. Although 'speech fluency' was relatively preserved in both groups, 'information content' deteriorated significantly only among the ADs patients, who were impaired even in comparison with ADm patients. Comprehension (total results of WAB) was reduced in both groups. Rescoring the results of the WAB word-recognition task, which also includes word-combinations (e.g. 'right shoulder') without grammatical constructions (designated by * in Tables 33.1a and 33.1b) revealed that both groups of patients were not impaired with regard to single-word comprehension. These results were in line with the results of word meaning comprehension in RLE. The predominant difficulties were manifested in sentence comprehension. The deficit was evident when patients were tested on the WAB sequence commands task and even more so on the RLE sentence-comprehension tasks. The impairment was evident even among ADm on 'sequence commands' (WAB), comprehension of logicogrammatical constructions, and oral commands (RLE), and it further deteriorated among ADs on almost all sentence comprehension tasks.

In naming abilities, AD patients were significantly impaired on all naming and word generation tasks as expected. In confrontation naming (as well as in naming for definition and antonym production), however, there were no significant differences between ADm and ADs patients. In contrast, the difficulties in word generation and synonym production tasks already had a pronounced character in the ADm group and did not deteriorate more significantly in ADs. Repetition became impaired as a function of sentence length (designated by ** in Tables 33.1a and 33.1b) but only among ADs.

AD patient scores on the WAB Aphasia Quotient (AQ) are shown in Table 33.2.

Table 33.2. Mean results of AD patients on the Western Aphasia Battery and data regarding transcortical sensory aphasis (TSA) and anomic aphasia (AA) (Kertesz, 1982*)

Groups	Fluency	Comprehension	Repetition	Naming	AQ
ADs (n=15)	9.2	7.8	5.9	4.5	72
ADm (n=18)	9.8	8.7	7	5	82
TSA*	5–10	0–6.9	8–10	0–9	59.6
AA*	5–10	7–10	7–10	0–9	83.3

Discussion

Language impairments in Hebrew-speaking Alzheimer patients closely resemble those described for English-speaking patients. Our results regarding spontaneous speech, naming, and word generation are also similar to those found in other languages (Cummings et al. 1985; Murdoch et al. 1987). The division of the patients into mild and severe groups enabled us to inspect selectively the different components of language deterioration in correlation with cognitive loss. Word generation appeared to be selectively affected by the disease process and had already been impaired in the ADm patients; 'single word comprehension', on the other hand, remained intact even in the ADs group. In contrast, some other language abilities (e.g. confrontation naming and sentence comprehension) deteriorated in the course of the disease.

The character of the impairments in the different components of AD patients' language ability allows us to discuss them as a definite clinical syndrome. Generally, the relatively isolated impairment in naming in the early stage of AD is described (Cummings et al. 1985; Murdoch et al. 1987; Sandson, Obler and Albert, 1987) as corresponding with that seen in anomic aphasia. The changes, including mild to moderately impaired auditory comprehension, that are found as the disease progresses resemble those found in Wernicke's aphasia (in the presence of a repetition deficit) or transcortical-sensory aphasia (when repetition is preserved). Our AD patients (mild and severe alike), however, performed better than those with anomic and transcortical-sensory aphasia on 'speech fluency' and comprehension (especially word comprehension), and worse on repetition (Table 33.2). This emphasis on language impairment in Alzheimer's disease cannot be classified in terms of an existent aphasia classification. An analysis of the comprehension deficit reveals that word comprehension is intact but that sentence comprehension is damaged even for word combinations, similar to the 'semantic aphasia' first described by Head (1926). Head defined an aphasia in which patients were unable to recognize simultaneously all the elements within a sentence. Later, Luria (1966) described semantic aphasia as a language impairment with fluent, syntactically correct but semantically empty conversational speech, anomia and impaired comprehension of grammatical relations (prepositions of place and time, reversed constructions, etc.) yet mostly relating the preserved comprehension of conversational speech, single words, and simple phrases. This clinical picture of semantic aphasia fully conforms with the results obtained from our Alzheimer's patients. It is interesting to note, too, that some authors (e.g. Luria, 1966) have related the syndrome of semantic aphasia to the posterior parietal-temporo-occipital region. This area was recently demonstrated to be affected in Alzheimer's patients (Jagust, 1994).

The mechanism of language deterioration in AD patients has been addressed by several researchers. Some (e.g. Martin and Fedio, 1983; Nebes, 1989) believe that the language difficulties of AD, particularly impairments in naming and word comprehension, reflect disturbances of lexical semantic processing; others have hypothesized that patients with AD suffer from an impairment in retrieving semantic knowledge. Our results regarding intact word comprehension and the knowledge of word meanings question the role of 'semantic system degeneration' as the exclusive factor in language impairment and point, at least partially, to an alternative explanation. This is that AD patients suffer from an inability to retrieve or access the desired word.

As to sentence comprehension, some writers (e.g. Rochon, Waters and Caplan, 1994) claim that AD patients' ability to understand syntactic constructions is impaired, whereas others (e.g. Smith, Murdoch and Chenery, 1989) suggest that this ability is preserved. Sentence comprehension can become impaired as a result of several processes, the most important of them being the following: (a) a loss of single-word comprehension (which was not evident in our study); (b) impairment in the 'system of grammatical meanings'; (c) impairment in syntax comprehension; and (d) a working memory-type deficit, in which comprehension deterioration is secondary to the inability to analyse 'on-line' the various components of the sentence. If this is the case, it can be predicted that patients will become impaired as the amount of information necessary to be kept in mind increases, without any correlation with the information conveyed by the sentence. The fact that AD patients' impairment in the repetition of long sentences only indicates that loss of working memory contributes to comprehension impairment.

Syntactic ability is believed to be preserved in Alzheimer's disease as AD patients usually evince fluent, grammatically correct, spontaneous speech. Evidence of preserved syntactic processing ability for production, however, does not hold for comprehension. Our patients showed impairment on almost all sentence comprehension tasks although the sentences did not include more than two propositions and three thematic roles. Similarly, the number of thematic roles was not found to be responsible for AD patients' sentence comprehension impairments (Rochon et al. 1994). Accordingly, syntactic complexity should not be held responsible for the deficit in the case of our AD patients. In contrast, comprehension of the logicogrammatical constructions was significantly reduced, even in the ADm patients, and resembled the deficit in 'semantic aphasia'. It is thus the ability to grasp grammatical meaning that appears to be predominantly affected. In this context, a two-component view may be proposed to account for the clinical picture of language breakdown in Alzheimer patients: it is the result of the intersection of impairments in language mechanisms (e.g. retrieval disorders and an inability to grasp grammatical meanings) and extra-linguistic impairments (e.g. attention resources deficit).

References

Cummings JL, Benson DF, Hill MA, Read S (1985) Aphasia in dementia of the Alzheimer type. Neurology 35: 394–97.

Head H (1926) Aphasia and Kindred Disorders of Speech. New York: Maxmillian.

Jagust WJ (1994) Functional imaging in dementia: an overview. Journal of Clinical Psychiatry 55: 5–11.

Kertesz A (1982) Western Aphasia Battery. New York: Grune & Stratton.

Luria AR (1966) Higher Cortical Functions in Man. New York: Basic Books.

Martin A, Fedio P (1983) Word production and comprehension in Alzheimer's disease: the breakdown of semantic knowledge. Brain and Language 19: 124–41.

Murdoch BE, Chenery HJ, Wilks V, Boyle R (1987) Language disorders in dementia of the Alzheimer type. Brain and Language 31: 122–37.

Nebes RD (1989) Semantic memory in Alzheimer's disease. Psychological Bulletin 106: 377–94.

Rochon E, Waters CS, Caplan D (1994) Sentence comprehension in patients with Alzheimer's disease. Brain and Language 46: 329–49.

Sandson J, Obler LK, Albert ML (1987) Language changes in healthy aging and dementia. In Rosenberg S (Ed) Advances in applied psycholinguistics. New York: Cambridge University Press, pp. 264–92.

Smith SR, Murdoch BE, Chenery NJ (1989) Semantic abilities in dementia of the Alzheimer type. 1. Lexical semantics. Brain and Language 36: 314–24.

Chapter 34
Linguistic Analysis of Spontaneous, Conversational Speech in Probable Alzheimer's Disease: a Comparison with Normal Older Adults

ROMOLA S. BUCKS, SAMEER SINGH, JOANNE M. CUERDEN AND GORDON K. WILCOCK

Introduction

Dementia is characterized by the breakdown of intellectual and communicative functioning accompanied by personality change (APA, 1987). Communication disorders are a common feature of dementia (Bayles, Kaszniak and Tomoeda, 1987), being present in 88–95% of sufferers. They are particularly pronounced in probable Alzheimer's disease (AD) (Alzheimer, 1907). Cummings, Benson, Hill and Read (1985) estimate that nearly all AD sufferers experience language impairment, the principle features of which are word-finding deficits, paraphasias, circumlocution, and comprehension impairments (Appell, Kertesz and Fisman, 1982; Irigaray, 1973; Hodges, Salmon and Butters, 1991) plus impairments in discourse, which worsen over the course of the disease (Ulatowska and Chapman, 1991). Phonemic and syntactic processes, however, have been shown to remain relatively intact (Hodges, Salmon and Butters, 1991; Kertesz, Appell and Fisman, 1986; Appell, Kertesz and Fisman, 1982).

Current assessments

Current assessments for the evaluation of expressive language deficits in AD have often been borrowed from aphasia research. In part this is because of the similarities between AD patients' productions and

Wernicke's or transcortical sensory aphasics (Obler and Albert, 1981). In mild AD, however, the deficits exhibited by AD patients have been likened to anomic aphasia (Appell, Kertesz and Fisman,1982). However, whilst aphasic patients generally exhibit effortful, telegrammatic, and asyntactic speech, AD patients usually have intact syntax (Appell, Kertesz and Fisman, 1982; Kempler and Zelinski, 1994).

One problem with borrowing techniques is that differences in the pattern of brain damage may make aphasia an inappropriate model for AD. For example, aphasia assessments can sometimes be insensitive to the communication deficits experienced by Alzheimer's sufferers and observed by their families in normal conversational situations – a criticism also levelled at these same tests when used with aphasic subjects. High scores on structured tests do not necessarily imply that the subject has no language difficulties. In the milder stages of dementia, a sufferer may be able to compensate for early language breakdown by substituting a synonym or non-word, by reformulating a sentence or by simplifying sentences – something that all normal individuals do on occasion.

Likewise, low scores on aphasia tests may misrepresent the true level of deficit present because the tests are 'unnatural'. Some common but unnatural ways of assessing language function in AD are confrontation naming, single word production, or generation of words beginning with a certain letter (verbal fluency) (Sabat, 1994). Finally, many tasks are extremely stressful and this can potentially reduce the quality of responses. Taking these criticisms into account, therefore, a more sensitive and naturalistic approach is required.

Why spontaneous speech?

There are both clinical and statistical reasons for focusing on spontaneous speech in the assessment of aphasia in AD. Clinically, evaluation of spontaneous speech represents a more ecologically valid method of assessing sufferers. As such it should be less stressful and could be used with more severe patients who would not tolerate formal testing. In addition, changes in spontaneous speech are often reported by families, suggesting that these may be sensitive markers of impairment. Previous researchers have found deficits in qualitative aspects of AD sufferers' conversation using discourse techniques (De Santi, Koenig, Obler and Goldberger, 1994). Finally, spontaneous conversation may well be supported by relatively intact social skills that should facilitate each patient's ability to be assessed.

Statistically, linguistic analysis of spontaneous speech allows both quantitative and objective analysis of patients' performance. This is because there is a good range of measures available for analysing aspects of speech including structural, syntactic, semantic and physical measures. Selected measures can be combined to form an index of performance, so offering wide variability in scoring which may help discrimination between normal and abnormal performance.

The study

A pilot study was conducted using a new technique for linguistic analysis developed for use with aphasic patients (Singh, 1995). The technique required interviewing and transcription of spontaneous speech in the context of a conversation. Subjects were given a semi-structured interview that was recorded on tape using a microphone. This interview lasted between 20 and 45 minutes, usually longer for patients. The length of interview varied in order to allow at least 1000 words of each subject's conversation to be transcribed. Only words spoken by the subjects were transcribed using a series of transcription guidelines (available from the author).

Eight patients were recruited from the Bristol Memory Disorders Clinic who had a diagnosis of probable Alzheimer's disease (DSM-III-R and NINCDS-ADRDA diagnostic criteria were used – American Psychiatric Association, 1987; McKhann, Drachman, Folstein, Katzman, Price and Stadlan, 1984). Four were women, four men, with a mean age of 67;8 years (range 57–77, sd 6.2) and an illness duration of between 31–70 months. On the Mini-Mental-State (MMSE, a general measure of cognitive impairment, Folstein and Folstein, 1975) AD subjects scored a mean of 15 out of 30 points (range 3–24, sd 6.8). The data for 16 age- and education-matched normal elderly people were also recorded. None of them was complaining of any difficulties with language or memory (all scored > 25 on the MMSE). Normal controls had a mean age of 61.8 years (range 51–79, sd 7.7) and there were seven males and nine females.

Linguistic measures

A total of eight linguistic measures were used, all word-frequency based and therefore capable of being combined to form a final index of performance. These were pronoun rate, noun rate, adjective rate and verb rate per hundred words, counted using the Oxford Concordance Programme (OCP; Hockey and Martin, 1988). Noun rate (N-rate) is a simple measure of ability to use nouns thought to be sensitive to word-finding difficulties. Pronoun rate (P-rate) contrasts well with N-rate. Adjective rate (A-rate) has not been used in most studies involving spontaneous speech and therefore seemed important in characterizing the 'colour' of subject's speech. Verb rate (V-rate) reflects the flow of speech. Three lexical richness measures were used. These were Type Token Ratio (TTR), Brunet's Index (W), and Honore's statistic (R).

TTR represents the ratio of total vocabulary (V) to the overall text length (N). This correlates positively with the length of text sampled, hence the importance of keeping the sample size constant. TTR was calculated for the whole transcription.

In Brunet's Index (Brunet, 1978), W quantifies lexical richness without being sensitive to text length.

The equation is $W = N^{V(-.165)}$, where N is the text length and V is the vocabulary used by the subject. The lower the value, the richer the speech.

Honore's statistic (Honore, 1979) establishes the number of words used only once by the subject [V(1)] as a proportion of the total number of words used. The higher the value of R, the richer the vocabulary used.

The equation is $R = 100 \log N / (1 - V(1)/V)$.

Finally a measure called CSU-rate (per 100 words) was calculated. This characterizes the subject's ability to form noun and verb phrases (clause-like semantic units) so giving an indication of the flow of speech. This does not use the linguistic definition of a clause. This definition could cause problems in aphasic or demented speech as clauses are commonly left unfinished. Normal speakers can cluster as many as 20 words together in a single CSU. CSU-rate is calculated by counting the number of words in each CSU. The lower the CSU-rate the better the performance. CSUs have boundaries at conjunction words such as 'but, since, so, because'. For example, 'I went to the market where I met my friend / but I didn't have any money / and he had to pay for me'. This shows three CSUs of 10, six and seven words in length. Repetitions were not included, nor were attempts to rephrase a sentence during speech. E.g. 'I [I, I, I] went to the market / and [buy no] bought a chicken' represents two CSUs of five and four words each.

Results

For AD subjects, neither MMSE nor duration of illness correlated significantly with any of the eight linguistic measures. This may have been a result of the small sample sizes, since some of the correlation coefficients reached 0.6 or above, suggesting these measures may indeed be sensitive to cognitive impairment (see Table 34.1.). For normal control subjects, age did not predict linguistic performance (all coefficients > 0.3).

Table 34.1 Correlations, for AD subjects only, of MMSE, age and Duration of illness, with the eight linguistic variables.

N=8	MMSE	Age (years)	Duration of illness (months)
N - rate	0.68	0.48	0.51
CSU - rate	−0.63	0.40	−0.06
R	0.42	0.19	0.26
V - rate	0.42	−0.07	−0.24
A - rate	−0.32	0.06	−0.33
W	−0.31	−0.70	−0.41
P - rate	0.22	−0.17	−0.58
TTR	0.16	0.66	0.44

All non-significant

AD = Alzheimer's disease; MMSE = Mini-Mental-State Examination

Mann-Whitney U tests were used to compare the performance of the AD and normal subjects on each linguistic variable and demonstrated significant differences on all measures (N-rate, P-rate, Honore's R, Brunet's W and TTR (all $p < 0.01$) A-rate and V-rate (both $p < 0.05$)) except the CSU-rate (see Table 34.2).

AD subjects had higher mean P-rate, A-rate and V-rate scores, but lower N-rate scores than normal controls. Looking at the use of pronouns revealed a trend towards higher use of 'I' by AD subjects than by normal controls. The three lexical richness measures showed the expected pattern of richer speech in normal controls. Mean CSU-rates did not differ, however, suggesting that whilst there were clear differences between AD and normal elderly subjects in lexical items and lexical richness, AD subjects did not differ significantly in their ability to form noun and verb phrases. This was an unexpected finding.

Discriminant analysis

Linear discriminant analysis was carried out to establish how well the eight measures predicted group membership. Figure 34.1. shows a plot of the discriminant function scores for the groups. Discrimination was excellent at 100%. The most important measures for discriminating between AD and normal subjects were N-rate, P-rate and Brunet's Index (W). A-rate, V-rate and CSU-rate were the least important. AD subjects generally had positive scores on the function, whilst normal controls had negative scores (AD, mean 3.18, sd 1.3; normal, mean −1.59, sd 0.8).

Even using cross-validation (see Fu, 1994) to avoid circularity in the discriminant analysis, the discrimination between the two groups was still good at 87.5% correct (cross-validation generates the discriminant function using $n-1$ subjects and then tests the remaining subject for

Table 34.2 *Linguistic measures for AD and normal elderly control subjects, descriptive statistics*

Measure Subjects	Mean	Std. dev.	Min.	Max.
N - rate				
AD	9.17	1.98	6.89	13.04
NC	15.91##	2.09	11.12	19.11
P - rate				
AD	23.72	4.10	14.29	27.12
NC	15.81##	1.82	13.19	19.03
A - rate				
AD	10.50	3.14	5.64	15.13
NC	7.23#	1.37	5.14	11.28
V - rate				
AD	25.23	5.77	15.04	30.52
NC	21.00#	2.46	16.63	27.36
TTR				
AD	0.26	0.04	0.22	0.33
NC	0.32##	0.02	0.29	0.35
CSU - rate				
AD	15.57	1.42	13.53	17.29
NC	15.19	2.17	10.97	17.94
W				
AD	15.77	0.91	14.58	16.90
NC	14.35##	0.31	13.75	14.79
R				
AD	1380.84	128.09	1140.89	1516.86
NC	1613.81##	136.56	1401.62	1863.65

Mann-Whitney U Test comparing AD with NC subjects: #$p<0.05$, ## $p<0.01$.
AD = Alzheimer's disease; NC=normal elderly control subjects

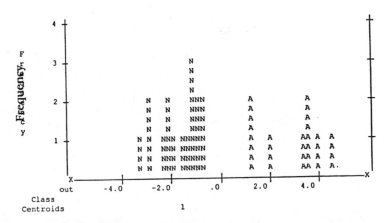

Figure 34.1. Stacked histogram of the canonical discriminant function. AD subjects are represented by As, normal elderly controls by Ns. A stack of four Ns or As represents a single subject

group membership. The process is repeated for all *n* subjects and the percentage of correct classifications calculated).

Discussion

This pilot study has demonstrated that there are significant, objectively measurable differences in the spontaneous speech of AD and normal elderly subjects. As anticipated, normal subjects produced lexically richer speech than demented subjects. AD subjects also produced higher mean adjective, verb and pronoun rates than normal subjects; a finding which is in direct contrast to Irigaray (1973) who showed reduced adjective and verb rates in AD. AD subjects also used more pronouns than normal subjects with a trend to using 'I' more often – a finding supported by Kempler and Zelinski (1994).

Further work is necessary to explore additional measures of linguistic competence that may add to the sensitivity of the technique. These could include perseveration or repetitions, the number of uncompleted clauses or words, attempts to generate a word, the use of default or meaningless words or of morphemes or mispronunciations. All are characteristic of AD speech and may prove powerful measures.

Once these techniques have been established they lend themselves to a range of uses. It has been suggested that AD can be divided into subtypes: early (young) onset versus late onset (older). A number of authors maintain that early-onset AD is characterized by more severe language deficits than late-onset AD (Becker, Huff, Nebes, Holland and Boller, 1988; Selnes, Carson and Rovner, 1988), whereas Bayles (1991) maintains the opposite, and other authors have found no relationship between language impairment and age at onset (Cummings et al. 1985; Grady, Haxby and Horwitz, 1987). This debate would benefit from the use of more objective, quantitative measures of spontaneous speech such as those used in this pilot study (Sevush, Leve and Brickman, 1993). Longitudinal studies of changes in normal ageing speech as well as studies of the progression from normal to dementing speech become possible, as does study of the progression of speech decline in dementias of all types. Indeed, if the technique is sensitive to decline (as suggested by the good correlations with MMSE scores) then it may also be sensitive to improvement with treatment. Finally, with advances in computer technology it may be possible to devise a speech recognition programme that would allow clinicians to use such analyses as the basis of clinical tools. Clearly, before the method can be taken this far such factors as test-retest reliability and the effect of the interviewer, premorbid ability, education and gender must be established. Further work has already been conducted analysing the physical characteristics of AD speech using, for example, speech rate, pause length and locution time (Singh, Bucks and Cuerden, in press).

References

Alzheimer A (1907) Of a particular disease of the cerebral cortex. Zentralblatt vur Nervenheilkunde und Psychiatrie 30: 177–9.

American Psychiatric Association (1987) Diagnostic and Statistical Manual of Mental Disorders – Revised, Washington, DC: APA.

Appell J, Kertesz A, and Fisman M (1982) A study of language functioning in Alzheimer patients. Brain and Language 17: 73–91.

Bayles KA (1991) Age at onset of Alzheimer's disease: Relation to language dysfunction. Archives of Neurology 48: 155–9.

Bayles KA, Kaszniak AW, and Tomoeda CK (1987) Communication and cognition in normal aging and dementia. Boston, MA, US: College-Hill Press/Little, Brown & Co.

Becker JT, Huff FJ, Nebes RD, Holland AL, and Boller F (1988) Neuropsychological function in Alzheimer's disease: pattern of impairment and rates of progression. Archives of Neurology 45: 263–8.

Brunét E (1978) Le Vocabulaire de Jean Giraudoux. Structure et Evolution. Genève: Slatkine.

Cummings JL, Benson DF, Hill MA and Read S (1985) Aphasia in dementia of the Alzheimer type. Neurology 29: 315–23.

De Santi S, Koenig L, Obler LK, and Goldberger J (1994) Cohesive devices and conversational discourse in Alzheimer's disease. In Bloom RL, Obler LK, De Santi S, and Ehrlich JS (Eds) Discourse Aanalysis and Applications: Studies in Adult Clinical Populations. Hillsdale, NJ, US: Lawrence Erlbaum Associates, p. 201–15.

Folstein MF and Folstein SE (1975) Mini-Mental State. A practical method for grading the cognitive state of patients for the clinician. Journal of Psychiatric Research 12: 189–98.

Fu L (1994) Neural Networks in Computer Intelligence. Singapore: McGraw-Hill.

Grady CL, Haxby JV, Horwitz B (1987) Neuropsychological and cerebral metabolic function in early vs. late onset dementia of the Alzheimer type. Neuropsychologia 25: 807–16.

Hockey S and Martin J (1988) OCP – User's Manual. Oxford: Oxford University Computing Service.

Hodges JR, Salmon DP, and Butters N (1991) The nature of the naming deficit in Alzheimer's and Huntington's disease. Brain 114: 1547–58.

Honoré A (1979) Some simple measures of richness of vocabulary, Association of Literary and Linguistic Computing Bulletin 7: 172–7.

Irigaray L (1973) Le Language des Dements. The Hague: Mouton.

Kempler D and Zelinski EM (1994) Language in dementia and normal aging. In Huppert FA, Brayne C and O'Connor DW (Eds) Dementia and Normal Ageing. Cambridge: Cambridge University Press.

Kertesz A, Appell J, Fisman M (1986) The dissolution of language in Alzheimer's disease. Canadian Journal of Neurological Sciences 13: 415–18.

McKhann G, Drachman D, Folstein MF, Katzman R, Price D, Stadlan EM (1984) Clinical diagnosis of Alzheimer's disease: Report of the NINCDS-ADRDA Work Group under the auspices of Department of Health and Human Services Task Force on Alzheimer's Disease. Neurology 34: 939–44.

Obler LK, and Albert ML (1981) Language in the elderly aphasic and in the dementing patient. In Sarno MT (Ed), Acquired Aphasia. New York: Academic Press.

Sabat SR (1994) Language function in Alzheimer's disease: a critical review of selected literature. Language and Communication 14: 331–51.

Selnes OA, Carson K, Rovner B (1988) Language dysfunction in early and late-onset possible Alzheimer's disease. Neurology 38: 1053–6.

Sevush S, Leve N and Brickman A (1993) Age at disease onset and pattern of cognitive impairment in probable Alzheimer's disease. Journal of Neuropsychiatry and Clinical Neurosciences 5: 66–72.

Singh S (1995) Computational linguistics for analysing conversation in speech and language disorders. Proceedings of the Third International Conference on Statistical Analysis of Textual Data, Rome, 11–13 December, 1995.

Singh S, Bucks RS, Cuerden J (in press) Speech analysis of Alzheimer's patients as an indicator of patient performance. Submitted to Brain and Language.

Ulatowska HK, and Chapman SB (1991) Discourse studies. In Lubinski R (Ed), Dementia and Communication. Philadelphia: BD Decker, pp. 115–32.

PHONOLOGY

Chapter 35
Segmental Errors in Aphasia as (Psycho) linguistic Evidence of the Nature of Phonological Representations

JEAN-LUC NESPOULOUS

From the very outset of aphasiology, the main (if not only) goal of clinicians – mainly neurologists at the time – has been to identify in language performance (e.g. word and sentence production) the superficial locus and nature of aphasic errors in an almost exclusively descriptive way (labelled 'clinical symptomatology'). Within such a 'first generation' approach, segmental errors were thus characterized in such gross categories as omissions, additions, substitutions and displacements.

In what follows, we will try to show how 'second generation' neuropsychologists, starting with Roman Jakobson in the 1930s, managed to go beyond the simple characterization of pathological surface manifestation (here at the segmental level) to attempt to capture their underlying determinants. These neuropsychologists constantly resorted:

- first, to formal models of linguistic structure (i.e to 'competence models' accounting in an abstract (and static, non-functional) way for the 'structural architecture' of a given natural language and, hopefully, of linguistic universals present in all languages);
- second, to psycholinguistic models of language processing (i.e to 'performance models' accounting for the 'functional architecture' of lexico-phonological computations necessary for the actual dynamic (and, hopefully, 'on-line') production of canonical strings of phonemes and sounds at the output level).

Indeed, it was the valuable contribution of Roman Jakobson to draw aphasiology away from the mere surface description of symptoms and to provide the first interpretations of aphasics' language disturbances in a linguistically motivated way. As far as segmental errors were concerned, he was thus able to interpret the nature of phonemic paraphasias by resorting to such linguistic theoretical constructs as features and markedness. Through these features it was possible to understand, for instance, the preferential tendencies often observed (on the paradigmatic axis) in phonemic substitutions. This was something that his predecessors, clinicians of the first generation, could not do. In the same way, although with less sophistication, consonantal omissions – particularly in clusters – were interpreted as simplification of so-called 'syntagmatic' patterns and some displacements of segments were interpreted as assimilations such as the ones that the philologists had been observing for years in diachronic studies.

In this paper, we will try to address the following issues and questions:

1. From Prague School phonology to modern non-linear phonological models, what is the (psycho)linguistic relevance of such constructs as 'feature', 'markedness', 'syllabic structure' etc. for the definition of the phonological representations that seem to be at play in aphasics' deviant oral performances?
2. We will also address the problem of the 'transfer' (can it be 'total' or only 'partial'?) of such originally linguistic constructs into processing models of lexical-phonological information, which will lead us to the crucial question of determining:
(a) what has to be actively computed whenever a lexical-phonological representation must be constructed? Aphasic segmental errors are clearly of interest here, as 'external evidence' for building up the functional architecture of phonological processes (even in normals); versus
(b) what, in the patient's performance, has to do not with the direct consequence of some specific processes supposed to be at fault but rather with the 'automatic' coming into play of 'repair strategies' – whatever the causal factor(s) of the patient's deviant performance:
• strategies that are governed by structural constraints that are part and parcel of the abstract, intrinsic properties of the speaker's 'passive' phonological system, knowledge and competence;
• strategies that are governed, in other terms, by a kind of inertia of the linguistic system enshrined in the speaking subject's mind and, no doubt, brain.

As can be gathered from the above, we will thus try to capture at one and the same time:

1. the representational level and/or the 'processing units' supposed to be at fault in a given patient on the basis of what we think we know about the functional architecture of lexical-phonological processing;

2. the structural, linguistic constraints which, whatever the source of the deficit in a given patient, may account for at least part of the deviant surface manifestations he or she produces.

This means that we consider pathological surface performance (and maybe also so-called 'performance errors' in normals) as the potential coalescence of at least three factors that we can label. These are positive factors (what is still functioning in the patient's lexical-phonological processor), negative factors (what is at fault in phonological processing) and adaptive (palliative?) strategies – whether consciously called up or not – whose aim is to repair damage done to target canonical linguistic representations in order to pass the message through.

This also means that pathological performance can, of course, be constrained by at least three types of parameters:

1. It can first be constrained by abstract structural properties of the language spoken by the patient. Violations of structural canonicity are thus assumed not to be random: they are predictable on the basis of our knowledge of the intrinsic structure of the language. Hence the use of linguistic theory in aphasiology!
2. Pathological performance can also be constrained by procedural factors concerning the way the above-mentioned abstract structures are actively processed by the human mind. We refer here, for instance, to those mnesic and attentional processes that underlie on-line language processing. Hence, the importance of psycholinguistic models of language processing. Now, since a psycholinguistic model has to process linguistic structures, one may wonder what procedural, psycholinguistic models would be like without strictly defined linguistic structures! In other words, if it is indeed possible for a linguist to have no interest in performance models, it is utterly impossible for a psycholinguist to disregard the daily more and more sophisticated models of language structure provided by modern linguistics (although this does not, of course, mean that he is going to buy them all).
3. Pathological surface manifestations are also partly conditioned by the eventual coming into play of adaptive strategies, be they natural and spontaneous or consciously devised by patients and/or their therapists. Here again, psycholinguistics has its say, together with modern pragmatics.

Hence – and if we agree with such an approach – our aim is clearly to try to disentangle the three above-mentioned types of factors and parameters for a better understanding of language disturbances – here segmental errors – in aphasia and, hopefully, in other contexts.

Distinctive features and the generation of segmental errors

From the pioneering work of Alajouanine, Ombredane and Durand (1939) substitutions of segments are ideal for assessing the paradigmatic similarity – in Jakobson's terms – between both segments involved. Moreover, the first phonological theory, that of Trubetzkoy, relied upon features in its characterization of the structural properties of a phonological system.

From the works of several aphasiologists, including the work of Sheila Blumstein (1973) and our own, it clearly follows that segments involved in substitutions very often share all their distinctive features but one. In other words, erroneous productions, in such cases, are close approximations to the target and we have shown that patients with arthric, phonetic problems – such as Broca's aphasics – evidence such a tendency more often than other aphasic patients (i.e. patients without phonetic disturbances). We are thus left with three possibilities to account for the former patients' deviant output, as stated in an old paper of ours:

- either the patient has adequately computed the abstract phonological representation of, say, a word and he or she has only been in trouble when coming to its phonetic, motor implementation at a more peripheral level;
- or the patient has had problems at the abstract phonological level itself;
- or the patient has had problems at both levels.

It is far from easy to choose between these three hypotheses.

Let us take a first example: voicing errors (e.g. : /b, d, g/ → /p, t, k/). Such errors can indeed be considered as the consequence of a phonetic implementation problem when the timing characteristics of speech sounds uttered by the patient are completely abnormal and do not represent the appropriate timing characteristics for either phonetic category (voiced or voiceless). This does not mean, though, that Broca's aphasics, who produce a lot of voicing errors (cf. infra), do not have phonological problems as well. Indeed, how could we account for such errors as place of articulation alterations (p → t or p → k)? How could we account for assimilation errors and for metatheses – which, moreover, can occur across word boundaries? Such errors clearly indicate that phonological planning – i.e. computation that, at an abstract level, leads to the building-up of phonemic strings – is often at fault, even in those patients who show evidence of phonetic problems.

We have seen in the above that similarity of features tended to constrain the production of segmental errors in aphasia, although it may do so differently from one patient to another. Indeed, if such a 'similarity effect' can be found in all patients, it tends to be more apparent (and more stable – we will come back to this in a moment) in patients with speech output problems who can thus be considered, in classical terms, as having a 'phonetic' problem, than in patients without a phonetic problem, who would thus be affected at a more abstract level. MacNeilage generally labels this level 'premotor' but we will call it 'phonological' or 'phonemic'.

If part of the story of a patient with so-called Broca's aphasia can be understood at this point, the story is still unclear for patients with so-called 'conduction aphasia' who also produce a lot of phonemic substitutions at Interphonemic Distance (ID) 1 in the absence, this time, of phonetic problems. A closer, qualitative look at consonantal substitutions is thus necessary if we want to know whether the causal factors behind those segmental errors are partially or totally identical in both cases or not.

Our work suggests that substitution patterns are indeed different when one distinguishes those patients with phonetic problems (i.e. Broca's aphasics) from those patients without phonetic problems (i.e. conduction aphasics). Two basic tendencies seem to characterize the former patients' segmental errors:

- Voiced segments tend to be replaced by their unvoiced equivalents. Is this a phonetic implementation problem?
- Unvoiced segments, when involved in a substitution, tend to be replaced by segments whose place of articulation is different. Is this a phonological planning problem?

Such a preferential substitution pattern cannot be found in patients with conduction aphasia, even if the latter keep on producing a lot of substitutions at ID 1. Broca's aphasics' substitutions thus seem to be more strictly constrained than those of conduction aphasics, which leads one to assume that an important difference indeed exists in the basic underlying causality or determinism of segmental errors generated by the two groups of patients. This does not, of course, mean that they are totally different (we must not forget that all error types found in Broca's aphasics can be found in patients with conduction aphasia and vice versa). After all, the only difference between both error patterns may only be the stability of those that are generated by Broca's aphasics versus the relative variability of those generated by conduction aphasics.

Now, with respect to markedness, if the absence of coherence and stability in conduction aphasics' errors makes it clear that no 'marked-

ness effect' plays a role in the pathogenesis of these patients' deviations, it does not follow from the presence of coherence and stability
in Broca's aphasics' errors that the preferential deviations of the latter
are the outcome of an abstract, phonological, 'markedness effect'. Even
if their coherent deviation patterns can be interpreted as 'simplification
strategies', as originally claimed by Roman Jakobson, the need to resort
to phonological markedness to account for such a simplification
process remains to be assessed. As already mentioned, other alternatives do exist to grasp their deficit, such as the simplification of
phonetic (or motor) patterns in speech production or the reduction of
articulatory gestures. If an interpretation of the pathogenesis of Broca's
aphasics' errors were set forth in terms of markedness, one would need
to specify which of the above-mentioned definitions of markedness one
would resort to. In other words, if there were some 'markedness effect'
at stake in the genesis of the errors characteristic of Broca's aphasia,
would such an effect be interpreted as deriving from abstract structural properties of the phonological system, as accounted for by linguists,
or would it derive more directly – as we think – from phonetic implementation? The latter does seem to be the case at least in the voicing
errors we mentioned earlier.

As a concluding remark on this first point, we will thus claim that:

- abstract, and thus phonological featural components of phonemes
  do constrain segmental errors in all patients;
- such constraints appear to be strengthened when the patients
  have more peripheral problems at the 'phonetic implementation'
  level;
- there is no clear-cut abstract, phonological 'markedness effect' in
  aphasic patients' segmental errors. When researchers thought that
  they had evidence for the existence of such an effect, this evidence
  was (a) either insignificant (Blumstein, 1973, for conduction
  aphasics) or (b) to be reinterpreted in phonetic terms.

So far we have dealt only with substitutions of segments and one may
legitimately wonder about other 'classical' error types mentioned in the
aphasiological literature: displacements, additions and deletions of segments.

Displacements and context-sensitive segmental errors

On the basis of the data available to us (in French), we were able to
show that:

- even though segmental errors with a contextual contamination effect were present in patients with and patients without phonetic disturbances, they were more frequently found in the latter type, in so-called 'conduction aphasics'.
- as far as displacements and 'exchange errors', in Merrill Garrett's terms, are concerned, we were able to show that they were particularly frequent in patients without phonetic impairment.

This evidence suggests a more 'central' deficit in the latter type of patients. In other words, these patients seem to have planning problems with phonemic strings just before resorting to phonetic implementation routines that seem, in their turn, to be impaired (maybe together with phonological planning) in the other type of patients.

In all cases of displacement errors – assimilations and exchange errors – phonological constraints come into play in that no illegal, uncanonical string of phonemes is generated by the patient, at least when one takes into account only oral production. Even though we have not yet mentioned syllabic structure as a determining factor in error generation, 'phonotactic constraints', as we used to say in older days, are not violated. (We have just specified that we were talking about oral production, because, in written production, it is very clear that highly illegal letter strings can be observed in aphasia (e.g. CH → HC), which seems to indicate that oral production is probably more constrained by phonology than written production, in which one can observe letter strings that would be unpronounceable orally.)

Let us now move on to another type of error commonly found in aphasic patients' segmental errors, namely additions. These provide an opportunity to bring in the notion of syllable or syllabic structure.

Segmental additions and syllabic structure

The birth of the notion of 'syllable' within phonological theory is fairly recent and such a notion has clearly evolved for the last 15 years or so. There exists nowadays a consensus in representing a syllable as a hierarchical structure whose superior node dominates two constituents: the onset and the rhyme. The 'onset' corresponds schematically to the different consonants that precede the vocalic nucleus; the 'rhyme' corresponds, at the segmental level, to the vocalic nucleus and the following consonants.

The appearance of the syllable in phonological theory is closely linked to the development of a non-linear conception of phonological representations. Such representations are thus described as tri-dimensional objects with (a) the 'syllabic plane' and (b) the 'segmental plane' being linked together by (c) the 'skeleton'. In some theories, the 'skeleton' is characterized as a 'CV-type' sequence (Clements and Keyser, 1983) whereas, in others, it is only a series of 'X's corresponding to 'positions' or 'time units' without phonological content.

What about the notion of syllable within the context of aphasiology? Its importance and relevance were first questioned, mainly on the basis of the rarity of performance errors involving whole syllables of the /bato/ → /toba/ type. Errors involving whole syllables are very rare in normal speaking subjects (Fromkin, 1973). The 'processing unit' involved in phonological errors is clearly the phoneme but what we have just said does not mean that syllable structure does not play any significant role in the generation of segmental errors. On the contrary, we now have evidence that, even though the syllable is not very often manipulated as a processing unit of its own, syllabic structure, within and across words, does constrain the types of segmental errors made by a patient, or even by a normal speaking-subject.

Let us now look at some addition errors. Blumstein (1978) shows that consonantal additions are found in three particular contexts:

- in word-onsets within words beginning with a vowel: /abylas/ → /babylas/;
- between two vocalic segments: /neo/ → /neno/;
- within the context of a non-branching onset, which is thus transformed into a branching onset: /pyblik/ → /plyblik/.

The first two examples clearly evidence a tendency to replace a 'marked' syllabic structure with an 'unmarked' one of the classical 'CV' type, if we believe in the markedness scales put forward by such authors as Kaye and Lowenstamm (1984).

The last example, on the contrary, is difficult to interpret in terms of a 'syllabic markedness effect' since the patient generates a syllabic structure that is more complex than its target. Nevertheless, Valdois (1990) elegantly showed that the creation of branching onsets happens almost exclusively in words that already have a branching onset. If all this is correct, it clearly indicates that syllabic structure does constrain the segmental errors that interest us here.

The substitution phenomena mentioned earlier are relevant to the issue of syllabic constraints upon segmental errors. Blumstein (1978) notes that consonantal substitution errors occur more often in singletons (i.e. in non-branching consonantal onsets) than in consonantal clusters (77% as opposed to 22%). It is fairly easy to understand why. Phonemes that are potential candidates for substitution – on the paradigmatic axis as Jakobson would have put it – are definitely more numerous in a non-branching consonantal structure than in a branch-

ing one. In other words there are no specific structural syllabic constraints in the former case, whereas there are in the latter. On that matter, Valdois went even further: she assessed the vulnerability of both
consonants involved in consonantal clusters. She did so because she
was convinced that (a) the onset-rhyme distinction was not sufficient to
characterize syllabic structure and (b) because she thought that both
consonants present in a cluster might not have the same representational weight, and thus that they would not be accessible in the same
way for production. She thus showed:

- that clusters of the 'S + consonant' type behaved differently when
  compared to other types of consonantal clusters;
- that C2 (i.e. the second consonant of a cluster) was preferentially
  modified (i.e. omitted, mainly) when the error involved a cluster of
  the 'obstruent-liquid' type (tR → t);
- that C1 was more frequently modified when appearing in other
  types of consonantal clusters;
- that such errors did not specifically affect certain types of segments.

She also showed:

- that consonantal additions mainly appeared in the C2 position, the
  initial consonant (or C1) always being an obstruent in such cases (p,
  t, k . . .);
- that additions in the C1 position always occurred when C2 was a
  liquid (R → tR);

She thus corroborated, at least partly, the findings of Stemberger (1984)
and of Stemberger and Treiman (1986) on segmental errors observed
in normal-speaking subjects. These authors indeed advocated – on the
basis of an activation model – that the level of activation of C1 was
higher than that of C2, singletons being considered as occupying a
'strong' C1 position. (They thus explained why segment additions were
more frequent in the C2 position.) Now, on the basis of aphasic data,
Valdois legitimately pointed out that, when C1 is a liquid, segment addition often leads to the relegation of C1 in C2 position, since a consonantal cluster of the obstruent + liquid type is produced by the patient,
which again shows that the story is more complicated than originally
expected by Stemberger. Valdois, on the basis of phonological models
put forward by Kaye and Lowenstamm (1984), tried to explain such an
apparent contradiction between Stemberger's findings and her own by
advocating the existence of an interacting effect between the segmental
level and the syllabic level, but clearly further studies are needed in
order to clarify the nature of such an interaction.

On the basis of the data that we have just reported, it thus appears:

- that the notion of syllable is definitely necessary for the interpretation of aphasic errors;
- that such errors are strongly constrained, at least in some cases, by the syllabic structure of the lexical item to be produced, which means that a 'syllabic coding' of information is certainly necessary in production models;
- that both segmental and syllabic levels are autonomous, even if the existence of a certain type of interaction between them is certain to be considered seriously and specified in future research;
- that non-linear phonological models of linguistic structure allow us to go further than linear models in the characterization of aphasic segmental errors.

Of course, other pieces of evidence documenting the importance of syllable structure in the pattern of phonological errors could be sought, in the literature on 'performance errors' in normal-speaking subjects (cf. *supra*), or in the literature on aphasia. One more example from the latter is that the occurrence of assimilation errors across word boundaries. As clearly stated by Blumstein (1990), 'such assimilation errors preserve syllable structure relations between the contaminating and assimilated phoneme. If the contaminating phoneme is in the onset, so is the assimilated phoneme; if the contaminating phoneme is in the coda, so is the assimilated phoneme.' These observations indicate that 'syllable structure must be represented in the lexical structure of words and must be marked as such when lexical items are accessed and organized in some type of a planning buffer for sentence production. Otherwise, such syllabic constraints would not emerge across word boundaries.'

To conclude, we will go back to the notion of 'repair strategy' that we mentioned in our introduction. This is a type of strategy that might be a consequence of the 'inertia of the phonological system' and which would come into play (automatically?) in error generation when a particular patient – consciously or not – tries to overcome a specific problem with the production of some phonological structures and representations. If our approach is correct, the 'surface manifestation' finally produced by the patient would thus be the consequence equally of the phonological deficit from which the patient is suffering and of the intrinsic strategic properties inherent to the structure of the phonological system enshrined in the patient's mind and (probably) brain.

In order to exemplify what the notion of 'repair strategy' is about (Paradis, 1988) we will resort to old data gathered by ourselves and published in 1984 in 'Advances in Neurology'.

In this paper, whose aim was to document the existence of a 'markedness effect' in the aphasic production of consonantal clusters (i.e. CCV sequences being replaced by CV sequences far more often than the reverse) we found that such a tendency was only clearly present in patients with a phonetic impairment (Broca's aphasics) and that it was absent in patients without such an impairment (conduction aphasics) but we did not resort at the time to any of the new advances in phonological theory that we have just mentioned.

If we re-examine, with more modern tools, the error patterns of the four patients who were frequently destroying clusters, we observe:

- that one of them (Broca 3) is resorting to syncope (or deletion) of the second consonant of a cluster in 88% of the cases and that he is resorting to epenthesis (or vocalic addition in between C1 and C2) in the remaining 12% of the cases (this patient clearly corresponds to the most impaired subject of the four on classical clinical criteria);
- that a second patient (Broca 4) who is the only patient with phonetic impairment to produce cluster creations (45.7%) together with cluster destruction (54.3%) resorts more frequently to epentheses than to syncopes (71% as opposed to 29%);
- that the other two patients (Broca 1 and 2) resort to epentheses more often than to syncopes but at a lesser (although statistically significant) degree than the previous patient: 62% versus 38% in Broca 1; 58% versus 42% in Broca 2.

Such data suggest:

(a) that, linguistically speaking and as clearly stated by Béland in her doctoral dissertation (1985), both epenthesis and syncope indeed are equivalent 'repair strategies' available (considering the structural phonological properties of a language such as French) to a speaking subject who is having difficulties with the production of consonant clusters. Interestingly enough, Broca 2 resorts to both strategies – epenthesis and syncope – at different moments on the same lexical items, which is certainly a clear indication of the equivalence of both strategies.

(b) that, psycholinguistically speaking, it is quite possible for a patient to resort to one of the two equivalent strategies more frequently than to another (again whether consciously or not).

If our interpretation is correct it indicates that the characterization of segmental error patterns in terms of segment addition or deletion, at least in the cases mentioned above, must be more accurately accounted for in terms of the coming into play of 'repair strategies' that are predictable from the structural properties of the natural language spoken by the patient (and maybe predictable from universal structural properties of phonological systems) than in the terms provided by any 'error generation model' we can think of.

As Sheila Blumstein remarked:

The pattern of deficits (in aphasia) indicates a structural richness to the phonological representation of words. In particular, the data are consistent with theories in which features are primitives in phonological representation. The nature of the feature errors that occur, however, suggests that there is internal structure to the organization of phonemic features. Moreover, lexical entries must not only contain features but also syllable structure representations. The aphasic data thus disconfirm those phonological theories in which the minimal unit of sound structure is the segment those theories in which features are represented as undifferentiated bundles and those theories in which lexical entries are represented solely in terms of a linear organization of segments and features.

References

Alajouanine T, Ombredane A, Durand M (1939) Le Syndrome de Désintégration Phonétique dans l'Aphasie. Paris: Masson.

Béland R (1985) Contraintes Syllabiques sur les Erreurs Phonologiques dans l'Aphasie. Thèse pour le Doctorat, Université de Montréal.

Béland R (1990) Vowel epenthesis in aphasia. In Nespoulous J- L, Villiard P (Eds) Morphology, Phonology and Aphasia. New York: Springer Verlag, pp. 235–52.

Blumstein S (1973) A Phonological Investigation of Aphasic Speech. The Hague: Mouton.

Blumstein S (1978) Segment structure and the syllable in aphasia. In Bell A, Hooper J (Eds) Syllables and Segments. Amsterdam: North Holland, pp. 189–200.

Clements G (1990) The role of the sonority cycle in core syllabification. In Kingston J, Beckman M (Eds) Papers from the First Conference in Laboratory Phonology. Cambridge and New York: Cambridge University Press, pp. 283–333.

Clements G, Keyser S (1983) CV Phonology: a Generative Theory of the Syllable. Linguistic Inquiry Monographs, 9. Cambridge MA: The MIT Press.

Fromkin V (1973) Speech Errors as Linguistic Evidence. The Hague: Mouton.

Halle M, Vergnaud J (1987) An Essay on Stress. Current Studies in Linguistics 15. Cambridge MA: The MIT Press.

Jakobson R (1942) Kindersprache, Aphasie und allgemeine Lautgesetze. Uppsala Univ. Arsskr 9.

Kaye J, Lowenstamm J (1984) De la syllabicité. In Dell F, Hirst D, Vergnaud J (Eds) Forme Sonore du Language. Paris: Hermann, pp. 123–61.

Paradis C (1988) On constraints and repair strategies. The Linguistic Review 6(1): 71–97.

Stemberger J (1984) Structural errors in normal and agrammatic speech. Cognitive Neuropsychology 1: 281–313.

Stemberger J, Treiman R (1986) The internal structure of consonantal cluster. Journal of Memory and Language 25: 163–80.

Valdois S (1990) Internal structure of two consonant clusters. In Nespoulous J-L, Villiard P (Eds) Morphology, Phonology and Aphasia. New York: Springer Verlag, pp. 253–69.

Note

This paper is based on previous work and publications by the author and his collaborators. Part of it can also be found (a) in the volume edited by Y Lebrun (1997) From the Brain to the Mouth; Acquired Dysarthria and Dysfluency in Adults, Dordrecht, Kluwer Academic Publishers, and (b) in the volume edited by R Bastiaanse and E Visch-Brink (in press) Proceedings of the Groningen symposium on Clinical Linguistics, Svets and Zeitlinger.

Chapter 36
Is there a Link between Phonemic Paraphasias and Loanword Adaptations?[1]

RENÉE BÉLAND AND CAROLE PARADIS

In this longitudinal case study, we compare the syllabic paraphasias (i.e. the phonemic errors affecting the syllabic structure) produced by a primary progressive aphasic (PPA) patient with the syllabic adaptations in loanwords. We will show that the paraphasias are phonologically principled and thus highly predictable, which implies that the basic phonological component is impaired in this PPA case. More specifically, we show that the strategies to which the patient resorts to modify a form are very similar to those applied by normal speakers of different languages when they adapt borrowings. The study is based on the theory of constraints and repair strategies (TCRS) of Paradis (1988, 1995a, 1995b). According to this model, the phonology of a language results from principles and parameter settings. 'Principles' describe what is common to all languages, whereas 'parameter settings' concern the differences among languages. Some languages possess a given combination of features (i.e. a segment or class of segments) or (syllabic) structure, whereas others do not, thus excluding the segment / class of segments or structure from their inventories. For instance, we see in (1) that the interdental fricatives θ and ð are allowed in English, but not in French.

(1) Parameter: Interdental fricatives? Settings: English: Yes

French: No (constraint)

This raises the question of what happens to 'foreign' combinations/structures in loans? They are adapted (salvaged) in the vast majority of cases. In Quebec French, the interdental in English thrill yields a stop (thrill [θɹɪl] → [tɾɪl]), not deletion. The same thing occurs to 'foreign' syllabic structures. Consider Fula, which disallows branching onsets. French *classe* [klas] is ill-formed in Fula, and must therefore be adapted. As shown in (2), it is indeed realized as [kalas], i.e. with an epenthetic vowel between the two consonants of the branching onset, not *kas, with deletion of one of the two consonants.

(2) French (Fr.) *classe* [klas]'class' → Fula (F.) [kalas]

Why does segment preservation have the edge over segment deletion? A form like [kas] would also have complied with the constraint against branching onsets in Fula. According to TCRS, (favoured) preservation and (disfavoured) deletion is due to the combined effects of the preservation and threshold principles, enunciated in (3) and (4), respectively:

(3) Preservation principle:
    Segmental information is maximally preserved within the limits of the threshold principle.

(4) Threshold principle:
    a) All languages have a tolerance threshold to segment preservation.
    b) This threshold constitutes a limit to the number of steps (repairs) that are allowed by a language within a constraint domain (a slightly modified version of the Paradis and LaCharité (1997) threshold principle).

The threshold principle stipulates that a problematic segment/structure requiring too many repairs (i.e. phonological operations) to be adapted is not protected by the preservation principle (i.e. it can be deleted). In other words, the threshold principle decides when a repair is too costly. For instance, the adaptation of French *biscuit* /biskɥi/ 'cookie' in Fula is problematic because the second onset contains two malformations: (a) a branching onset *kɥ (note that Fula does not allow diphthongs with rising sonority either), and (b) the labio-coronal glide, *ɥ, impermissible in Fula. Both adaptation and deletion of *ɥ are attested in Fula, as shown in (5) and (6), respectively. In (5), *ɥ is adapted (to ω), as opposed to being deleted, because its adaptation requires only one step: deletion of the articulator coronal, which yields the labio-velar *w* (cf. Paradis, 1995a, 1995b and Paradis and LaCharité, 1997 for details). Note that the forms preceded by an asterisk in (5) correspond to the forms that would have been obtained if the borrowings had undergone segment deletion.

(5) Segment adaptation: no violation of the threshold principle

French			Fula		gloss
de l'huile	[dœlɥil]	→	dilwil	*dilil	oil
minuit	[minɥi]	→	minwi	*mini	midnight

These examples contain no syllabic problems since no onset or coda is required to branch. In French *de l'huile* [dœlyil] 'oil', for instance, which yields Fula [dilwil], the first *l* is syllabified into the coda of the first syllable (*dil*), and the glide, into the onset of the next syllable (*wil*). Compare now the examples in (5) with those in (6), where segment deletion occurs.

(6) Loss of a consonant: violations of the threshold principle

French			Fula		Gloss
biscuit	[biskɥi]	→	biski	*biskuwi	biscuit
cuivre	[kɥivr]	→	kiri	*kuwiri	copper

Segment deletion applies in (6) because segment preservation would have required more than two repairs – the threshold established by Fula with respect to the threshold principle – within the domain of the unsyllabifiable sequence. By contrast with the first *l* in French *de l'huile*, k in French [biskɥi] cannot be syllabified into the coda of the first syllable in Fula, since this syllable already has a coda consonant, *s*, and since Fula disallows branching codas. The sequence skɥ in [biskɥi] is thus unsyllabifiable as is. To adapt the structure, a nucleus (N) would have to be inserted in a first stage (*[biskNɥi]). In a second stage, the epenthetic nucleus would have to be filled with segmental material (in Fula, this is generally accomplished by spreading an adjacent vowel or glide, e.g. *[biskuɥi]). Finally, in a third stage, the ill-formed consonant *ɥ itself would have to be adapted (here to *w*), as in (5). This three-step alternative is rejected. The Fula output biski displays a segment loss instead, i.e. that of ɥ. The same is true of [kɥivr], which underwent two segment deletions (that of ɥ and *v*) for the same reasons. In other words, the segment ɥ is adapted in (5) because only one repair is required, whereas the same segment is deleted in (6) because its adaptation would have required more than two repairs, the limit imposed by Fula on multi-step adaptation.

Hypotheses

(7) Hypothesis 1. Well-formed stimuli in the patient's native language become problematic for the patient since they violate her or his constraints, just as loanwords are problematic for speakers of a borrowing language when the loanwords contain segments or structures that are prohibited in the borrowing language. We thus expect loanword adaptations and paraphasias to be very similar.

(8) Hypothesis 2. In phonemic (including syllabic) paraphasias as well as in borrowings, adaptation or insertion of a segment is preferred to segment deletion.

(9) Hypothesis 3. The threshold principle entails that (normal or aphasic) speakers have a 'tolerance threshold' to complex repair. We predict that the patient's tolerance threshold will be lowered with the progression of the deficit. We therefore expect a malformation in the later stages to trigger segment deletion more frequently than in earlier stages.

Patient: H.C. is a university educated right-handed female and a native speaker of French. She developed a progressive language impairment at the age of 58 years. H.C. fulfilled the criteria proposed by Mesulam and Weintraub (1992) to identify a PPA clinical syndrome. We have collected 638 syllabic paraphasias produced by the patient during the last three years of a five-year illness progression. We distinguished four periods corresponding to the patient's rehabilitation programme:

(10) The four periods of testing: (a) March 1989 to November 1989 (nine months), (b) February 1990 to November 1990 (ten months), (c) January 1991 to October 1991 (ten months), and (d) January 1992 to August 1992 (eight months).

For the sake of comparison between the different contexts, data collected during the first 19 months are collapsed. We will refer to this period as Phase 1 (early stage of the illness progression). Data collected during the last 18 months are also collapsed, and will be referred to as Phase 2 (late stage). We have compared the syllabic errors produced by the patient with syllabic adaptations in French loanwords in different borrowing languages with respect to the six syllabic contexts in (11).

(11) The six syllabic contexts: (a) branching onsets (e.g. *place* /plas/ 'place'); (b) branching codas (e.g. *contre* /kɔtr / 'against'); (c) simple codas (e.g. patte /pat/ 'paw'); (d) diphthongs (e.g. *boisson* / bwasɔ̃/ 'drink'); (e) hiatus (e.g. *mosaïque* /mozaik/ 'mosaic'); and (f) word-initial empty onsets (e.g. *ambassade*/ ɑ̄basad/ 'embassy').

Borrowing data: The loanword data include three corpora of borrowings listed in (12):

(12) The three corpora of borrowings are: French borrowings in (a) Moroccan Arabic, (b) Kinyarwanda, and (c) Fula.

Table 36.1 Distribution of syllabic adaptations (segment insertions), non-adaptations and segment deletions in the six tested contexts for French borrowings in Kinyarwanda, Fula and Moroccan Arabic.

	Kinyarwanda		Fula		Moroccan Arabic		Total	
1- Branching Onsets	432		160				592	
Adaptations (Insertions)	417	96.53%	126	78.75%			543	91.72%
Non-adaptations	12	2.78%	33	20.63%			45	7.60%
Deletions	3	0.69%	1	0.62%			4	0.68%
2- Branching Codas	153		110				263	
Adaptations (Insertions)	134	87.58%	83	75.45%			217	82.51%
Non-adaptations	5	3.27%	18	16.36%			23	8.75%
Deletions	14	9.15%	9	8.18%			23	8.75%
3- Codas	1520						1520	
Adaptations (Insertions)	1492	98.16%					1492	98.16%
Non-adaptations	5	0.33%					5	0.33%
Deletions	23	1.51%					23	1.51%
4- Diphthongs	266						266	
Adaptations (Insertions)	248	93.23%					248	93.23%
Non-adaptations	4	1.50%					4	1.50%
Deletions	14	5.26%					14	5.26%
5- Hiatus	43		11		44		98	
Adaptations (Insertions)	41	95.35%	8	72.73%	31	70.45%	80	81.63%
Non-adaptations	0	0%	2	18.18%	0	0%	2	2.04%
Deletions	2	4.65%	1	9.09%	13	29.55%	16	16.33%
6- Word-Initial Empty Onsets					178		178	
Adaptations (Insertions)					104	58.43%	104	58.43%
Non-adaptations					5	2.81%	5	2.81%

Table 36.1 (cont.)

	Kinyarwanda	Fula	Moroccan Arabic		Total	
Deletions			69	38.76%	69	38.76%
Word-Initial						
Empty Onsets						
a) ≤ 3 syllables			154			
Adaptations (Insertions)			96	62.33%		
Non-adaptations			5	3.24%		
Deletions			53	34.42%		
b) ≥ 4 syllables			24			
Adaptations (Insertions)			8	33.33%		
Non-adaptations			0	0%		
Deletions			16	66.67%		

These three loanword corpora comprise a total of 2917 syllabic malfor-ma-tions from the point of view of the borrowing language. Loanwords were collected from dictionaries, lexicons and other existing corpora of borrowings and each was tested with three informants. Table 36.1 shows that the effect of the preservation principle is uniform through all syllabic contexts and corpora: segment preservation is overwhelm-ingly preferred to segment deletion. The only context in which segment preservation is not as strong as in the other contexts is that of word-ini-tial empty onsets in Moroccan Arabic. This is attributed to the fact that there is also a constraint on word length in Moroccan Arabic, a point that will be addressed later.

Comparison between patient data and borrowing data

For each context, we compare the syllabic paraphasias produced by the patient to the syllabic adaptations in French loans. According to (8), segment insertion should be preferred over segment deletion in the patient's errors as well as in borrowings. In all the above contexts we therefore expect to find more segment insertions than deletions, at least in Phase 1. Following (9), the patient's tolerance threshold will be lowered with the progression of the deficit. We therefore expect to find more segment deletions than insertions in Phase 2.

Results

Examples of syllabic adaptations in loanwords, and examples of syl-labic paraphasias collected during Phase 1 and 2 for each of the six con-texts are reported in Table 36.2.

1. Branching onset: French branching onsets in loans must be adapted in languages that prohibit such syllabic constituent. The adaptation generally consists in a V (vowel) insertion between the two conson-ants (13). As seen in (14), the strategy adopted by the patient in Phase 1 is identical.
2. Branching coda: As shown in (15), the adaptation of French branch-ing codas in Fula consists in a V insertion, exactly like the syllabic errors (Phase 1) in (16).
3. Simple coda: French codas in borrowings must be adapted to con-form to the constraint against codas in Kinyarwanda. The adaptation consists in a V insertion after the problematic consonant (17). Again, this adaptation is identical to the repair strategy applied by the patient in Phase 1 to handle a coda consonant (18).
4. Diphthong: The adaptation of French diphthongs in Kinyarwanda consists in a C (consonant) insertion between the two vowel-like

Table 36.2. Examples of syllabic adaptations in French borrowings and syllabic errors produced by the patient in the six syllabic contexts tested (Fr. = French, F. = =Fula, K. = Kinyarwanda, MA = Moroccan Arabic, V = vowel, C = consonant)

1 – Branching onset
(13) Adaptations (V insertion) in French borrowings
Fr. *place* [plas] 'place' → F. [palas]
Fr. *briquet* [brikɛ] 'briquet' → K. [ßurice]
(14) V insertions produced by the patient
Fr. *citron* [sitrɔ̃] 'lemon' → patient [siterɔ̃]
Fr. *crabe* [krab] 'crab' → patient [karab]
2 – Branching coda
(15) Adaptations (V insertion) in French borrowings
Fr. *contre* [kɔ̃tr] 'against' → F. [kɔntɔr]
Fr. *filtre* [filtr] 'filter' → F. [filtir]
(16) V insertions produced by the patient
Fr. *meuble* [mœbl] 'furniture' → patient [mœbly]
Fr. *parc* [park] 'park' → patient [parkə]
3– Simple coda
(17) Adaptations (V insertion) in French borrowings
Fr. *mine* [min] 'mine' → K. [mini]
Fr. *docteur* /[dɔktœr] 'doctor' → K. [dojiteeri]
(18) V insertions produced by the patient
Fr. *fougère* /[fuʒɛr] 'fern' → patient [fuʒɛrə]
Fr. *bol* [bɔl] 'bowl' → patient [bɔlə]
4 – Diphthong
(19) Adaptations (C insertion) in French borrowings
Fr. *boîte* /[bwat] 'box' → K. [ßuwaati]
Fr. *lieutenant* [ljøtnã] 'lieutenant' → K. [rijetona]
(20) Examples of C insertions produced by the patient
Fr. *fouet* /[fwɛ] 'whip' → patient [fulɛ]
Fr. *piéton* [pjetɔ̃] 'pedestrian' → patient [pitetɔ̃]
5 – Hiatus
(21) Adaptations (C insertion) in French borrowings
Fr. *mosaïque* [mozaik] 'mosaic' → MA [møzaiik]
Fr. *Noël* /[nɔɛl] 'Christmas' → MA [nɔwʉl]
(22) Examples of C insertions produced by the patient
Fr. *véhicule* [veikyl] 'vehicle' → patient [fetil]
Fr. *jouer* [ʒue] 'to play' → patient [ʒuwe]
6 – Word-initial empty onset
(23) Adaptations (C insertion) in French borrowings
Fr. *ambassade* /[ãbasad] 'embassy' → MA [lambaṣad] or [ʔambaṣad]
Fr. *amérique* [amerik] 'America' → MA [ʔemirika]
(24) Examples of C insertions produced by the patient
Fr. *hache* [aʃ] 'axe' → patient [waʃ]
Fr. *université* /[yniversite] 'university/' → patient [nyniversite]

segments of the diphthong, thus forming two syllables instead of one (19). The same strategy was applied by the patient in examples with a diphthong (20).

5. Hiatus context: French hiatus in loans are adapted in Moroccan Arabic by the insertion of an onset consonant between the two vowels (21). The patient also inserts a consonant in the same context in both phases (22).

6. Word-initial empty onset: French word-initial empty onsets in loans are adapted in Moroccan Arabic by a C insertion before the vowel (23). The same strategy is applied by the patient in the same context (24).

The syllabic errors produced by the patient are very similar to the syllabic adaptations found in borrowings, thus confirming hypothesis 2. According to hypothesis 3, we expect a contrastive error pattern for Phase 1 and 2: more insertions than omissions in Phase 1 with the reverse pattern in Phase 2. The distribution of segment insertions and deletions collected during Phase 1 and 2 in the six contexts is given in Table 36.3. Results obtained in four contexts (branching onset, branching coda, simple coda and diphthong) confirm hypothesis 3. In the other two contexts (word-initial empty onset and hiatus), the patient produced more insertions than deletions in Phase 2. A possible explana-

Table 36.3. Distribution of error types in the six syllabic contexts tested during both phases and level of significance of the Chi-Square (χ^2) test for the difference in the proportion of error types collected in Phase 1 versus Phase 2.

Context	Phase	V insertions	C deletions	χ^2
branching onset	1	19 (54.3%)	16 (45.7%)	
	2	4 (7.8%)	47 (92.1%)	**
branching coda	1	40 (62.5%)	24 (37.5%)	
	2	1 (16.7%)	5 (83.3%)	n.s.
simple coda	1	103 (68.7%)	47 (31.3%)	
	2	29 (39.7%)	44 (60.3%)	**

Context	Phase	C insertions	V deletions	χ^2
diphthong	1	21 (51.2%)	20 (48.8%)	
	2	10 (20%)	40 (80%)	*
hiatus	1	8 (47%)	9 (53%)	
	2	45 (83.3%)	9 (16.6%)	*
word-initial empty onset	1	21 (70%)	9 (30%)	
	2	40 (59.7%)	27 (40.3%)	n.s.

Note: ** indicates $p<0.001$, * indicates $p<0.01$, n.s. indicates not significant ($p>0.05$).

tion could be that what was inserted here is a consonant, and that C insertion is less costly than V insertion in those contexts. Vowel insertion necessarily results in the addition of a whole syllable whereas it is rarely the case for C insertion. The only context in which C insertion results in the addition of a syllable is the diphthong context. For example, *fouet* [fωɛ] 'whip' is a monosyllabic word. Insertion of a consonant between the two nucleus parts of the diphthong results in a bisyllabic word (e.g. *fouet* [fωɛ] 'whip' → [fulɛ]). We thus reasonably predict that in this context, contrary to the word-initial empty onset and hiatus contexts, C insertions will be less frequent in Phase 2 than in Phase 1. As expected, in this context, the patient produced more C insertions than. As expected, in this context, the patient produced more C insertions than V deletions in Phase 1, whereas V deletions were more frequent than C insertions in Phase 2 (see Table 36.3). This shows that the patient complied with the preservation principle until late in the evolution of the disease as long as it did not entail the addition of a syllable, that is, word lengthening. This is consistent with the word lengthening effect found in Moroccan Arabic. As indicated in Table 36.1, adaptations in the word-initial empty onset context are sensitive to the number of syllables in the word. If the number of syllables of the word is ≤ 3, adaptation by insertion is more frequent than deletion. If the number of syllables is ≥ 4, the opposite pattern is observed.

Conclusion

From these results, we conclude that the syllabic paraphasias produced by our patient, like the syllabic adaptations in loanwords, are phonologically principled, and thus predictable. One point of difference between the syllabic adaptations and the syllabic paraphasias produced by our patient is that, in loanword adaptations, insertion is always overwhelmingly favoured over deletion. Analysis of the patient data revealed that insertion is generally favoured over deletion in the early stages but this is not true in all contexts in the late stages. There are two possible interpretations for this evolution pattern:

(a) with the progression of the illness there is a decline in the power of the preservation principle or, as we suggested;
(b) the patient's tolerance threshold to multi-step repair is lowered because of the procedural weight involved in a complex repair.

The reason why we favour the second interpretation is that the patient's performance varied according to the phonological contexts. Only the second interpretation accounts for the results obtained in all six contexts.

References

Mesulam MM, Weintraub, S (1992) Primary Progressive Aphasia: Sharpening the focus on a clinical syndrome. In Boller F, Forette F, Khachaturian Z, Poncet M, Christen Y (Eds) Heterogeneity of Alzheimer's Disease. Berlin: Springer-Verlag, pp 43–66.

Paradis C (1988) On Constraints and Repairs Strategies. The Linguistic Review 6(1): 71–97.

Paradis C (1995a) Derivational constraints in phonology: Evidence from loanwords and implications. In Proceedings of the 31st Chicago Linguistic Society Meeting. Chicago: Chicago Linguistic Society, pp 360–74.

Paradis C (1995b) The Inadequacy of Faithfulness and Filters in Loanword Adaptation. In Durand J and Laks B (Eds) Current Trends in Phonology: Models and Methods. Salford: University of Salford Publications, pp. 509–34.

Paradis C, LaCharité D (1997) Preservation and Minimality in Loanword Adaptation. Journal of Linguistics 33: 1.

Note

1   This research was supported by the MRC Program grant PG-28, by the FRSQ grants # 952342 and # 952291, by the SSHRC grants # 410-92-0015, # 410-90-0575 and # 410-94-1296 and by the FCAR grants # 96CE0176, # 90-NC-0383 and 95-ER-2305. The first author was supported by a Chercheur Boursier award from the FRSQ (Québec).

PROSODY

Chapter 37
The Cortical Processing of Affective Speech Prosody: a DC-Potential Study[1]

HANS PIHAN, ECKART ALTENMÜLLER,
INGO HERTRICH AND HERMANN ACKERMANN

The intonation of verbal utterances is important in conveying information about speakers' emotional states. Usually, these speech components are referred to as 'affective prosody' (for a review see Ackermann, Hertrich and Ziegler, 1993). Pitch, loudness and segment durations of spoken sentences contribute to perceived emotional tone (Bergmann, Goldbeck and Scherer, 1988). So far, clinical as well as experimental studies have yielded conflicting data on the role of the two cerebral hemispheres for the processing of emotional prosody (Gainotti, 1989; Heilman, Bowers and Valenstein, 1993). Patients with damage to the right hemisphere (RH) have been reported to be more impaired than subjects with left-sided lesion on tasks requiring the identification of affective-prosodic speech modulation (Tucker, Watson and Heilman, 1977; Weintraub, Mesulam and Kramer, 1981). It has been suggested that disorders associated with RH lesions reflect not only a perceptual disturbance but also a reduced ability to activate specialized representations of non-verbal communicative expressions (Blonder, Bowers and Heilman, 1991). Other studies, however, found similar performance by patients with unilateral damage to either hemisphere when asked to recognize emotional intonation (Schlanger, Schlanger and Gerstmann, 1976; Van Lancker and Sidtis, 1992) and indicated a rather bilateral representation of affective speech components.

Experimental studies in normal subjects provided further insight into lateralization of emotional processing. A left ear/right hemisphere advantage was obtained in dichotic listening tasks requiring the detection of speakers' mood while recall of verbal aspects of the same stimuli was lateralized to the right ear/left hemisphere (e.g. Ley and Bryden, 1982). However, inferences about the manner in which cognitive and emotional processing is represented in the two hemispheres remained necessarily indirect.

Functional imaging provides an alternative in this regard. The present study used recordings of DC-potentials from scalp electrodes. This approach has been shown to be valuable for identifying the language-dominant hemisphere (Altenmüller, Kriechbaum, Helber, Moini, Dichgans and Petersen, 1993) and for assessing hemisphere differences during the processing of tonal melodies (Altenmüller, 1986).

Assuming that the RH stores representations of all affective speech categories, a significantly lateralized electrophysiological signal must be expected during tasks requiring discrimination of various emotional intonations. By applying pairs of test sentences, which were systematically varied either in the temporal or in the pitch domain, we tried to clarify whether the activation of RH emotional categories is linked to the processing of two defined acoustic parameters.

Evaluation of a speaker's emotional state from his or her voice naturally takes place during verbal communication, e.g. while the speaker produces sentences. Rather than single words, the present study thus used pairs of sentences for the evaluation of emotional tone. In short, the paired stimuli represented variants of the same emotional category, differing in expressiveness. As a control, utterances with neutral tone were included. Subjects were asked, first, to recognize the emotional category (neutral or sad or happy) and, second, to indicate the stimulus that sounded more expressive, in the case of happy or sad utterances, or excited, in instances of neutral sentences.

A professional actress produced four different declarative sentences (Figure 37.1) with either neutral, happy or sad intonation. The resulting 12 utterances contained evenly distributed accents in order to avoid

*   Sie wollte seh'n, was das Leben im Süden bieten kann.
    (She wanted to see what life in the South could give her.)

*   Er kam spät am Abend und ging früh am Morgen.
    (He came late at night and left early in the morning.)

*   Sie gab nach, und verflogen war der ganze Unmut.
    (She gave in and all annoyance vanished.)

*   Er sprach mit langen Sätzen, und niemand hörte zu.
    (He spoke in winded sentences and nobody listened.)

Figure 37.1. Test sentences used in the present study: vowels of stressed syllables are typed in bold letters (English translation in parenthesis).

focal effects of pitch or time parameter variation. Propositional content was compatible with each of the three prosodic modulations considered. In order to create a perceptual task that is controlled with respect to the acoustic structure of the stimulus, resynthesized variants of the twelve original utterances were considered as test stimuli. In line with psychoacoustic standards, the pitch-contours of the original utterances were extended or reduced relative to the sentence-final F0-level being kept constant (Ladd, Silverman, Tolkmitt, Bergmann and Scherer, 1985). Three stimuli differing in F0-range were resynthesized from each of the 12 spoken sentences by means of commercially available software (LPC Parameter Manipulation/Synthesis Program of the Computerized Speech Lab CSL 4300; Kay Elemetrics, USA). The duration of the vowels of stressed syllables was also varied in each original utterance. This was achieved by either cutting out or doubling single periods of the acoustic signal. Two certified speech pathologists as well as the authors verified that the resynthesized stimuli had natural sound. At perceptual evaluation, the pitch- and time-manipulated variants of happy and sad utterances differed in the degree of perceived intensity of the respective emotion. In contrast, the respective neutral sentences sounded more-or-less excited. A block of 48 stimulus pairs was created and presented twice in regular order and twice in reversed order (the individual time course is displayed in Figure 37.2). At the end of each trial the subjects had to specify the emotional category of each pair (happy, sad or neutral) and to indicate the sentence (first or second) which showed stronger expression of the perceived emotion (happier, sadder or more excited). Under forced choice conditions answers were considered as 'correct' if the sentence with broader F0-range or shorter syllable duration was recognized as 'more expressive'. In sadly intoned pairs the utterance with longer syllable duration was expected to be labelled as 'sadder'.

Cortical aspects of sustained mental activity are typically reflected by DC-components of the EEG signal (for a description see Rockstroh, Elbert, Canavan, Lutzenberger and Birbaumer, 1989). DC-potentials were recorded from the scalp by 28 non-polarizable AgCl-electrodes (impedance below 10 kOhms). Signals were amplified and digitized using Neuroscan software and hardware (NeuroScan Inc., USA). Electrodes were positioned according to the Jasper 10/20 system (Jasper, 1957) using unipolar leads with linked mastoid-electrodes as a reference. The electrooculogram was simultaneously assessed by means of additional diagonal bipolar recordings between nasion and the anterior zygomatic arch. For further data processing, only trials without artifacts were accepted. Generally, between 10 and 20 trials per condition and subject were averaged and analysed relating the mean amplitude of the two presentation periods to a baseline taken from a 1.5 s pre-stimulus period (Figure 37.2).

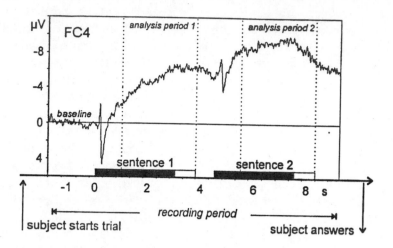

Figure 37.2. Time course of a single trial and corresponding averaged DC-potential as obtained at electrode position FC4. Values of mean activation within analysis periods 1+2 constituted the basis for data normalization and statistical evaluation. Evoked potentials within the first second of stimulus presentation were expected to contain unspecific responses to activation and orientation and were, therefore, not included. The variable end of each utterance lies within the light part of the grey bar. A declination of potential amplitudes within this period was typically observed at central regions.

In order to evaluate amplitude and distribution effects by an ANOVA, all values were normalized according to the standards proposed by McCarthy and Wood (1985). Emotional category (happy, sad, neutral), acoustic parameter (F0, syllable duration) and presentation period (first/second sentence) were taken as independent variables, the values at 26 electrode positions constituted the dependent variables. Lateralization and local amplitude differences were assessed by contrast analysis. Sixteen right-handed healthy students (eight males, eight females; age 19–34 years) from the University of Tübingen participated in the present study. Handedness was assessed by means of the Edinburgh Inventory (Oldfield, 1971). None of the subjects was familiar with the aims of the research work.

As a rule, subjects consistently recognized the emotional category (neutral versus sad versus happy) of a given pair of test sentences. In other words, they correctly identified the affective state of the original spoken utterance. A few sentences with a happy or sad tone were categorized as instances of neutral intonation. The evaluation of expres-

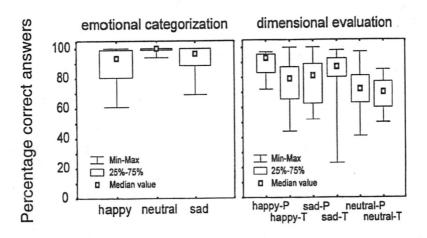

Figure 37.3. Overall view on percentage numbers of correct answers in the 'emotional categorization' task (left panel) and the 'dimensional evaluation' task (right panel). The suffixes 'P' and 'T' indicate F0 (pitch) and duration (time) varied stimuli.

siveness within a given emotional category yielded less consistent results. Obviously, subjects used different concepts for the evaluation of expressiveness or changed their strategy during the experiment (Figure 37.3).

Three major findings emerged from the statistical analysis of DC-potentials. First, mean amplitudes of presentation period 1 and 2 were significantly lateralized towards the RH at frontal, central, temporal and parietal electrode positions as revealed by contrast analysis (Figure 37.4 a and Table 37.1 – left part). Second, the processing of sentences with happy or sad intonation, irrespective of whether syllable durations or F0-range had been manipulated, as well as the discrimination of pitch varied neutral utterances, yielded no significant differences in amplitudes or distributions of DC-potentials (Figure 37.4 a). Third, a significant two-way interaction emerged between acoustic parameter and emotional category with respect to amplitude differences ($p < 0.0098$), which could be largely attributed to low activation elicited by time varied neutral sentences, mainly over the RH (Figure 37.4 b). When compared to their F0-varied counterparts, contrast analysis revealed significant differences in potential amplitude ($p < 0.001$) and distribution ($p < 0.001$). Details are outlined in Figures 37.4 b,c and Tables 37.1 – right part.

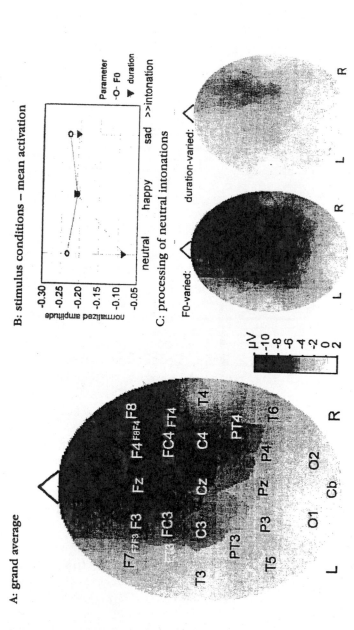

Figure 37.4. a : Grand average data plotted into a black-and-white map with grey levels representing mean amplitude values of the second presentation period. The interelectrode values of the matrix were computed by a linear algorithm taking into account the nearest four electrode values (Buchsbaum, Coppola, Rigal, Cappelletti, King and Johnson, 1982). Highest amplitude values were recorded at right-frontal and right-central electrode positions. Levels of significance for RH lateralization, as shown in Table.37.1, were obtained from contrast analysis. b: Plot of normalized amplitudes of all six stimulus conditions. Only neutrally intoned sentences differed significantly with respect to potentials' amplitudes ($p<0.001$) and distribution ($p<0.001$) as revealed by contrast analysis. c: Average data map obtained during the processing of F0 and duration varied pairs of sentences (second presentation period). Significance levels of topographic amplitude differences are shown in Table 37.1.

Table 37.1.

grand average: RH lateralization: significance level (p<0...)			neutral stim. conditions: LH comparison		neutral stim. conditions: RH comparison	
electrodes	1. sentence	2. sentence	electrodes	level of signific.	electrodes	level of signific.
F7, F7F3, F3 – F4, F8F4, F8	0.000026	0.000001	F7, F7F3, F3	p<0.240322	F8, F8F4, F4	p<0.000251
FC3, C3 – FC4, C4	0.000001	0.000001	C3, FC3	p<0.000089	C4, FC4	p<0.000015
P3, PT3 – PT4, P4	0.000001	0.000001	P3, PT3	p<0.001639	P4, PT4	p<0.000162
T3, T5 – T4, T6	0.000001	0.000001	T3, T5	p<0.231270	T4, T6	p<0.001361

The present study revealed a very similar distribution of recorded DC potentials, in terms of a significantly lateralized activation towards the RH, during the processing both of utterances with sad or happy tone. The RH thus seems to participate equally in the recognition of positive and negative emotions in normal subjects. This contrasts with occasional observations of 'depressive-catastrophic' reactions during temporary pharmacological inactivation (Wada test) of the left hemisphere (LH) and in-patients with LH lesions. Affection of the contralateral side yielded, in contrast, 'euphoric-maniacal' states (Heilman, Bowers and Valenstein, 1993).

A possible interpretation of such laterality effects suggests that the left hemisphere mediates 'positive' emotions, whereas the right counterpart, in contrast, supports 'negative' feelings, As an alternative, a depressive mood might occur as a reactive state in case of abrupt speech loss.

Linguistic processing primarily depends upon the LH. In the presence of simultaneous decoding both of the propositional content and the emotional tone of verbal utterances, lateralization effects may be masked. These suggestions could explain the conflicting data reported in the literature with respect to the perception of affective prosody. The present study comprised altogether 192 successive pairs of utterances. The propostitional content of this corpus of test stimuli was derived from only four different sentences. Under these conditions, the semantic load of the administered task can be considered minimal. A significantly lateralized activation of the cortex might therefore have emerged.

An unexpected finding was that neutral sentences with variation of pitch yielded a right-hemisphere activation pattern as well. Since the subjects correctly identified the latter items as neutral utterances, the observed lateralization effects during the processing of pitch-manipulated sentences, thus, cannot simply be accounted for by an RH activation of stored emotional representations. However, psychoacoustic studies revealed that a broad F0-range of neutrally intonated utterances is perceived as a speaker's high arousal (Bergmann, Goldbeck and Scherer, 1988). In consideration of these findings, the evaluation of sensory information as performed by the RH might extend beyond specific emotions such as joy and sadness to a broader range of speakers' inner states and feelings. Neutral sentences with variation of syllable durations yielded a significant decrease of activation predominantly over RH areas when compared to their pitch-varied counterparts. Conceivably, duration information in neutrally intoned sentences is not equally potent in mediating arousal states and, therefore, fails to activate corresponding RH representations.

References

Ackermann H, Hertrich I, Ziegler W (1993) Prosodische Störungen bei neurologischen Erkrankungen - eine Literaturübersicht. Fortschritte der Neurologie und Psychiatric 61: 241–53.

Altenmüller E (1986) Hirnelektrische Korrelate der cerebralen Musikverarbeitung beim Menschen. European Archives of Psychiatry and Neurological Sciences 235: 342–54.

Altenmüller E, Kriechbaum W, Helber U, Moini S, Dichgans J, Petersen D (1993) Cortical DC-potentials in identification of the language-dominant hemisphere: linguistic and clinical aspects. Acta Neurochirurgica 56: 20–33.

Bergmann G, Goldbeck T, Scherer KR (1988) Emotionale Eindruckswirkung von prosodischen Sprechmerkmalen. Zeitschrift für experimentelle und angewandte Psychologie 35: 167–200.

Blonder LX, Bowers D, Heilman KM (1991) The role of the right hemisphere in emotional communication. Brain 114: 1115–27.

Buchsbaum MS, Coppola R, Rigal F, Cappelletti J, King C, Johnson J (1982) A new system for gray-level surface distribution maps of electrical activity. Electroencephalography and Clinical Neurophysiology 53: 237–42.

Gainotti G (1989) Disorders of emotions and affect in patients with unilateral brain damage. In Boller F, Grafman J (Eds) Handbook of Neuropsychology Vol 3. Amsterdam: Elsevier, pp 345-361.

Heilman KM, Bowers D, Valenstein E (1993) Emotional disorders associated with neurological diseases. In Heilman KM, Valenstein E (Eds) Clinical Neuropsychology. New York: Oxford University Press, pp 461–97.

Jasper HH (1957) Report of the Committee on Methods of Clinical Examination in Electroencephalography. Electroencephalography and Clinical Neurophysiology 10: 370–5.

Ladd DR, Silverman KEA, Tolkmitt F, Bergmann G, Scherer KR (1985) Evidence for the independent function of intonation contour type, voice quality, and F0 range in signaling speaker affect. Journal of the Acoustical Society of America 78: 435–44.

Ley RG, Bryden MP (1982) A dissociation of right and left hemisphere effects for recognizing emotional tone and verbal content. Brain and Cognition 1: 3–9.

McCarthy G, Wood CC (1985) Scalp distribution of event-related potentials: an ambiguity associated with analysis of variance models. Electroencephalography and Clinical Neurophysiology 62: 203–8.

Oldfield RC (1971) The assessment and analysis of handedness: the Edinburgh inventory. Neuropsychologia 9: 97–113.

Rockstroh B, Elbert T, Canavan A, Lutzenberger W, Birbaumer N (1989) Slow Cortical Potentials and Behaviour. München: Urban and Schwarzenberg.

Schlanger BB, Schlanger P, Gerstmann LJ (1976) The perception of emotionally toned sentences by right-hemisphere damaged and aphasic subjects. Brain and Language 3: 396–403.

Tucker DM, Watson RD, Heilman KM (1977) Discrimination and evocation of affectively intonated speech in patients with right parietal disease. Neurology 27: 947–50.

Van Lancker D, Sidtis JJ (1992) The identification of affective-prosodic stimuli by left- and right-hemisphere-damaged subjects: all errors are not created equal. Journal of Speech and Hearing Research 35: 963–70.

Weintraub S, Mesulam MM, Kramer L (1981) Disturbances in prosody. Archives of Neurology 38: 742–4.

Note

1   This study was supported by the German Research Foundation (SFB 307; B8: Altenmüller, B10: Ackermann/Daum) and the Graduiertenkolleg Neurobiologie, University of Tübingen. A more comprehensive report of this study was published in Neuroreport 8(3): 623–27.

Chapter 38
Processing of Emotional Prosodic Information in Patients with Unilateral Brain Lesions

ANDREA GEIGENBERGER AND WOLFRAM ZIEGLER

Introduction

Studies concerning interhemispheric localization of emotional processing in normals and brain-damaged patients reach diverging and even contradictory results. A majority of investigations described evidence for the superiority or even the overall dominance (Blonder and Heilman, 1991; Ross, 1993) of the right hemisphere for functions of emotional expression and emotional comprehension, independent of the valence of an emotion category or a particular communication channel. Other authors reported results implying bilateral processing of emotional information, both hemispheres having equivalent or complementary functions (Gainotti, Caltagirone and Zoccolotti, 1993; Cancelliere and Kertesz, 1990).

Some authors assume a specialization of the left hemisphere for positive emotions and of the right hemisphere for negative emotions (Sackheim, Greenberg, Weiman, Gur, Hungerbuhler and Geschwind, 1982). These findings, however, were disconfirmed by other studies (Gainotti, 1989).

A communication-channel-specific impairment in the processing of emotional information in brain-damaged patients is discussed by several authors (Borod, 1992; Breitenstein, 1995).

The topic of the present study is the comprehension of emotional prosodic information in patients with unilateral cerebrovascular lesions. We wanted to assess the evidence of receptive emotional aprosodia in right and left hemisphere-damaged patients and to look for differences between these groups. To evaluate dissociations between different communication channels in the processing of emotional information we moreover tested the comprehension of emotional facial expression. The question of a dissociation between emotional and non-emotional prosodic processing was investigated using a focus recognition task.

Methods

Comprehension of emotional prosody

The materials were constructed from an emotionally ambiguous test phrase (*Say that again. I can't believe it. What a day.*) (Tischer, 1993). This phrase was spoken by female and male actors posing the following emotion categories: anger, fear, sadness, happiness, tenderness, desire. Two realizations for each of the six emotion categories were selected, one by a female and one by a male speaker.

Test items were presented binaurally. Each utterance was repeated three times in a randomized order, resulting in a total of 36 items. Subjects were required to judge each stimulus on a continuous interval scale. The whole procedure was repeated three times with different scales representing three emotional dimensions, i.e.

- Valence (person feels bad — good)
- Potency (person feels weak — strong)
- Activation (person is calm — activated)

Rating scales were presented graphically on the computer screen. The ratings were transformed to a scale of 0–100.

Comprehension of emotional facial expression

The materials consisted of 24 photographs of emotional faces (Ekman, 1976) representing fear, anger, sadness and happiness, each category being posed by three male and three female actors. The photographs were presented in a randomized order, and subjects were requested to score them on the dimension scales as above.

Comprehension of linguistic prosody

The material consisted of 10 focus-ambiguous test sentences, each of which could carry four different focus markings, i.e. person, action, time, place. The test sentences were spoken three times, each with a different focus marking, by a trained female speaker, resulting in a set of 30 test items.

Test items were presented binaurally in a randomized order. Subjects were instructed to rate each test sentence on a computer-presented four-point nominal scale representing the four possible focus markings.

The sample of this preliminary investigation contained a group of 17 patients with right cerebrovascular brain-damage, three females and 14 males, aged 21 to 59 (mean 55), and a group of 14 patients with left cerebrovascular brain-damage, four females and 10 males, aged 30 to 71 (mean 47). The aphasic patients contained in the latter group had only mild, if any, comprehension deficits.

The control group consisted of 30 neurologically healthy adults. Normals and patients were matched for age, education and gender. The subjects of all experimental groups were right-handed native speakers of German.

Results

Comprehension of emotional prosody and emotional facial expression

A first analysis of the data showed a considerable between- and within-subject variation of judgements in each group of participants.

Ratings on the valence scale were most consistent for all emotion categories. Consistency on the activation and the potency scales depended on the stimulus category to be rated. Ratings on the activation scale were the most variable for each of the three experimental groups.

Stimuli whose ratings scattered over more than 90% of a scale in the normals were excluded from further data analysis for that particular scale.

Figures 38.1 and 38.2 show the ratings of the three experimental groups for each of the remaining items on the valence scale. For each of the two presentation modalities, the RHD group showed considerable deviation from the normals and a high intra- and intersubject variance on most of the items.

Ratings of the LHD group were substantially less variable for both communication channels and showed less deviation from the normal median on most of the items.

Collapsing the data across stimuli for positive and negative valence separately emphasizes the differences between the three groups. In particular, the RHD group deviated considerably from the LHD and the normal group on the stimuli expressing positive valence. This was true for both the prosody (Figure 38.3) and, to a lesser extent, the facial expression stimuli (Figure 38.4).

Prosody–valence

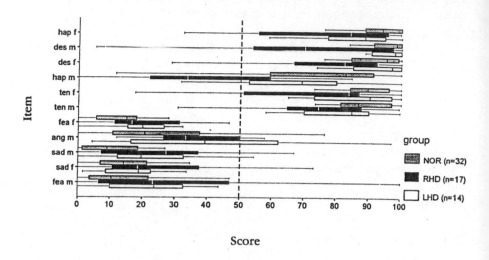

Figure 38.1. Processing of emotional prosodic information: ratings for selected stimuli on the valence scale (hap: happiness, des: desire, ten: tenderness, fea: fear, ang: anger, sad: sadness; m: male speaker, f: female speaker).

Facial expression–valence

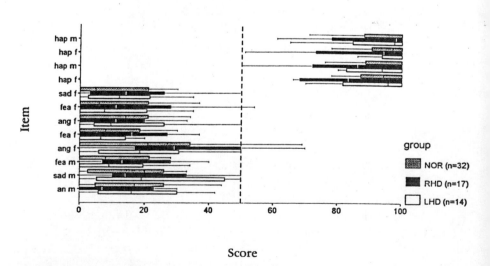

Figure 38.2. Processing of emotional facial expression: ratings for selected stimuli on the valence scale (hap: happiness, fea: fear, ang: anger, sad: sadness; m: male actor, f: female actor).

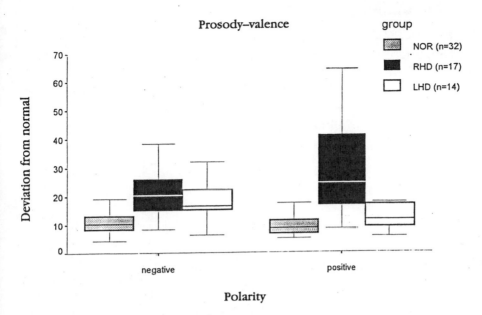

Figure 38.3. Processing of emotional prosodic information: deviation from normal rating for data collapsed across stimuli for positive and negative valence separately.

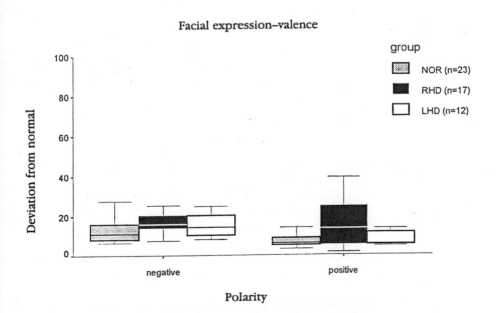

Figure 38.4. Processing of emotional facial expression: deviation from normal rating for data collapsed across stimuli for positive and negative valence separately.

Comprehension of linguistic prosody

Normals made almost no errors in the recognition of focus. Both patient groups were impaired, but LHD patients were significantly worse than RHD patients (Figure 38.5). It could be made clear by control tasks that the LHD patients had no problem understanding the wording of the test sentences or in performing categorizations. The data obtained for the LHD group therefore point to a specific comprehension deficit for the prosodic marking of focus.

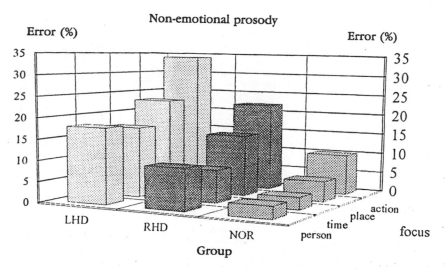

Figure 38.5. Processing of non-emotional prosodic information: errors of the three experimental groups on the focus recognition task.

Relationship between tasks

There was a high correlation between the emotional prosody task and the emotional facial expression task in the valence ($r = 0.67$) and the potency dimensions ($r = 0.67$), indicating that the impairment was independent of the respective communication channel, acoustic or visual (see Figure 38.6 for the valence dimension).

No significant correlation was found between the processing of non-emotional and emotional prosodic information.

Conclusion

Compared to the normals and the LHD group, RHD patients were impaired in processing visually and acoustically based emotional information. The two channels were highly correlated, suggesting a channel-independent processing deficit after right hemisphere-damage.

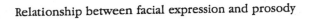

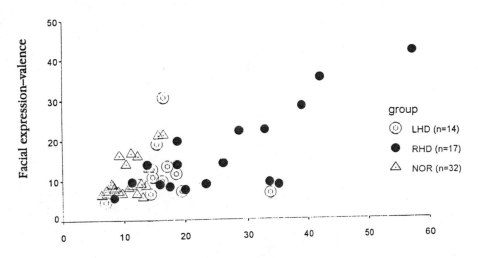

Figure 38.6. Correlation between the processing of acoustically and visually presented emotional information.

For the two patient groups there was a double dissociation between emotional and non-emotional conditions in the processing of prosodic information. The RHD group was considerably impaired on the emotional, the LHD group on the non-emotional tasks.

No evidence for a dominance of the right hemisphere in processing negative emotions or the left hemisphere in processing positive emotions was found in this study.

References

Blonder LX, Heilman KM (1991) The role of the right hemisphere in emotional communication. Brain 1: 1115–27.

Borod JC (1992) Interhemispheric and intrahemispheric control of emotion: a focus on unilateral brain-damage. Journal of Consulting and Clinical Psychology 60: 339–48.

Breitenstein C (1995) Affektverarbeitung nach kortikaler und subkortikaler Hirnschädigung: Die Tübinger Affekt Batterie. Unpublished Inaugural Dissertation, Tübingen.

Cancelliere AEB, Kertesz A (1990) Lesion localization in acquired deficits of emotional expression and comprehension. Brain and Cognition 13: 171–81.

Ekman P (1976) Pictures of Facial Affect. Pola Alto: Consulting Psychologists Press Inc.

Gainotti G, Caltagirone C, Zoccolotti P (1993) Left/right and cortical/subcortical dichotomies in the neuropsychological study of human emotions. Cognition and Emotion 7 (1): 71–93.

Gainotti G (1989) The meaning of emotional disturbances resulting from unilateral brain injury. In Gainotti G, Caltagirone C (Eds) Emotions and the Dual Brain. Heidelberg: Springer.

Ross ED (1993) Nonverbal aspects of language. Behavioural Neurology 11 (1): 9–23.

Sackheim HA, Greenberg MS, Weiman AL, Gur RC, Hungerbuhler JP, Geschwind N (1982) Hemispheric asymmetry in the expression of positive and negative emotions. Archives of Neurology 39: 210–18.

Tischer B (1993) Die vokale Kommunikation von Gefühlen. Weinheim: Psychologie Verlags Union.

Chapter 39
Patterns of Prosodic Disability in a Person with a Non-Fluent Aphasia

SUE PEPPÉ, KAREN BRYAN, JANE MAXIM AND
BILL WELLS

Introduction

Apart from problems such as word-finding, agrammatism and phonemic paraphasias, many subjects with aphasia 'sound odd', which may be the result of disordered or impaired prosody.

Many studies have demonstrated impairment in specific phonetic aspects of prosody such as pitch-range and volume (Blumstein, 1973; Kent and Rosenbek, 1982; Danly and Shapiro, 1982; Hird and Kirsner, 1993; Ouellette and Baum, 1994; Samuel, Couillet, Louis-Dreyfus, Azouvi, Roubeau, Bakchine and Bussel, 1996). Other studies demonstrate that subjects with aphasia have impaired ability in performing linguistic tasks normally effected through prosody (Schlanger, Schlanger and Gerstman, 1976; Tucker, Watson and Heilman, 1977; Bryan, 1989; Vance, 1994).

Prosodic impairment has been characterized (Monrad-Krohn, 1963; Crystal, 1982; Brewster, 1989) in broad categories, such as dysprosody (phonetic-prosodic impairment) and prosodic disability (functional or phonological impairment affecting linguistic organization). One widely used assessment of prosodic ability is the PROP ('PROfile of Prosody') devised by Crystal (1982) and largely used with children; this allows for a broadly phonetic characterization of a sample of a subject's conversation, indicating what prosodic 'rules' are being transgressed and thus making the speech sound odd. Several other tests of prosody have been devised, using either natural or elicited speech; and some testing of prosody is included as part of assessments of specific disorders such as tests of dysarthria and right-hemisphere disability (Enderby, 1983; Bryan, 1995).

Tests of aphasia such as the Western Aphasia Battery (WAB: Kertesz, 1980) and Psycholinguistic Assessments of Language Processing in Aphasia (PALPA: Kay, Lesser and Coltheart, 1992) provide only incidental insights into prosodic aspects of language.

One particular drawback of PROP and other prosody tests is that the relationship between phonetic-prosodic impairment and the ability to convey meanings is not clear. Ill-formed prosody (where prosodic rules are transgressed) on the part of subjects with aphasia can cause delay in understanding by conversational partners, which is undesirable; but it could also lead to misunderstandings. Thus it would be advantageous to know whether, in addition to sounding odd, a person's ability to convey meanings with prosodic features is impaired.

Another disadvantage of most existing prosody tests is that no testing of a subject's comprehension of prosody is carried out. Any relationship between reception and production in prosody is not clear but in some circumstances deficits in the one could affect the other. Equally, we were interested in exploring the possibility of dissociations between deficits in different elements of prosody.

We have devised a new prosody test to take account of these considerations, and the study outlined below describes the performance of one subject with aphasia and the possible implications of the test results for communication and rehabilitation. The investigation was carried out to see how the prosodic performance of this person with non-fluent aphasia compared with control subjects without impairment, looking particularly at:

- his or her understanding (reception) of prosody;
- syntactic, semantic and segmental phonetic aspects of his language, to see whether the subject's abilities in these areas were associated with his or her prosodic abilities or dissociated from them;
- his or her prosodic expression (production).

Subject

The subject is RD, a man of 64 who had a stroke caused by an infarction in the left middle cerebral artery three years before the investigation described here. The stroke left him with a non-fluent aphasia and a pervasive articulatory dyspraxia. In conversation, RD gave the impression that his understanding was of a high level, perhaps completely unimpaired, and that production was his only significant problem. Psychometric testing shows no impairment of his memory or problem-solving abilities.

Method

It was decided to administer a prosodic assessment procedure to find out whether these impressions would be borne out by the subject's performance in a test environment where the function of his utterances was determinable and could be compared with the form of what he actually said, and where his understanding could be similarly verified.

Procedure

RD was tested on the PEPS (Profiling Elements of Prosodic Systems: Peppé, in preparation) procedure, which looks at the reception and production of nine different elements of prosody: loudness, length, pitch, pitch-range, glide-presence, glide-direction, silence, rhythm and accent. Table 39.1 gives a summary of the form of these elements and the communicative functions of each that were selected as the basis for tasks in the procedure (based on Crystal, 1969):

Table 39.1. Profiling Elements of Prosodic Systems

Elements	Phonetic form	Communicative function
Loudness	presence of energy in speech	need for loud/quiet speech
Length	speech-rate; relative length of syllables	briskness/'relaxedness'
Pitch	relative pitch-height of syllables	affirm/request repetition
Range	width of on-syllable pitch-movement	surprise/no surprise
Glide	direction of on-syllable pitch-movement	question/statement
Silence	breaks in speech	certainty/hesitancy
Rhythm	rhythmicality of speech	said repeatedly/first time
Level	presence/absence of on-syllable pitch-movement	information-chunking
Accent	presence of stress on syllables	focal point of utterance

Each element was tested for reception and production, at a functional and at a formal level. Examples of this four-way testing in one element (Glide) are shown in Table 39.2.

The procedure was specifically designed to tap the prosodic skills of unimpaired speakers but also to be usable with clients showing a variety of speech disorders. It has been used to profile prosody in fluent and non-fluent aphasia and in Parkinson's disease. PEPS has been standardized on 90 unimpaired adult speakers. Using these data, lower limits to the range of normal prosodic abilities have been set at two standard deviations below the mean scores on the tasks for each element. The assessment of RD's prosodic ability, to be presented below, is therefore compared with the abilities of unimpaired speakers.

Table 39.2. Examples of tasks for Glide

Form reception	Form production
Same or different?	*Imitate what you hear:*
fòur fóur (different)	À (falling)
éight éight (same)	É (rising)

Function reception	Function production
Questioning or stating?	*Sound either questioning or stating:*
Mónday	2 o'clock
Tùesday	10.30

Reception

In Figure 39.1, RD's scores for understanding prosodic meaning (prosodic 'function reception') as conveyed by each element are shown in the white columns on the right; the lower limits of normal ability are shown as the grey columns in the middle, and the mean scores of the unimpaired speakers are the dark columns on the left.

Function reception

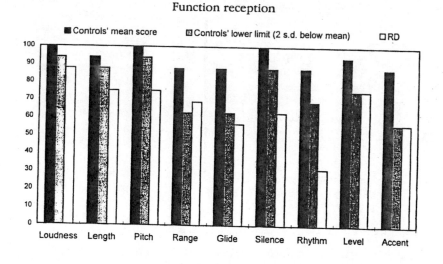

Figure 39.1. Percentage of correct responses to the 'function reception' tasks of PEPS.

It can be seen from Figure 39.1 that RD's scores were, in general, below the lower limit of normal ability. In six out of the nine tasks he scored below the lower limit for normal controls. In one task, 'range', he was above the lower limit; in the 'level' and 'accent' tasks he scored at the lower limit, and in the 'loudness' and 'glide' tasks he was one standard deviation below the lower limit and in 'length' two standard deviations below. He was three to five standard deviations below the lower limit in the remaining tasks ('pitch', 'silence', 'rhythm').

The next question was to decide whether his difficulties with understanding prosodic meaning were caused by reduced ability to process the cues accurately at a phonetic level. Figure 39.2 shows his scores on the form reception tasks. In six out of nine elements, he scored within normal limits. In the 'loudness' task he scored above the mean, and in five other tasks ('length', 'pitch', 'glide', 'silence', 'level') he scored at or above the lower limit; in only one task ('range') did he score both well below the mean (more than four standard deviations) and lower than in the function task. The overall picture in prosodic form reception is of scores only just below those of normal controls.

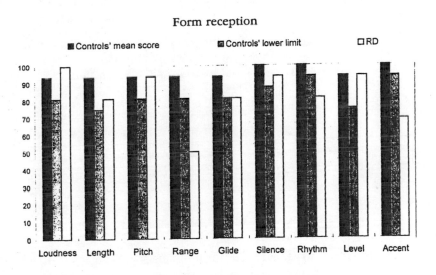

Figure 39.2. Percentage of correct responses to the 'form reception' tasks of PEPS.

Tests of other aspects of language: syntax, semantics and segmental phonetics

RD also underwent a series of other language tests to see how he performed on tasks specifically looking at his understanding of meanings of words and at his ability to perceive segmental phonetic distinctions. These were selected tests from PALPA (Psycholinguistic Assessment of Language Processing in Aphasia: Kay, Lesser and Coltheart, 1992) and the WAB (Western Aphasia Battery: Kertesz, 1980), and his results are presented in Figure 39.3.

The first two tasks shown on the chart were same-different judgement tests of segmental phonetic discrimination: PALPA 15 concerns vowel distinctions, i.e. whether two words rhyme or not (e.g. card-ward) PALPA 2 deals with consonantal differences (e.g. bed-bet). The remaining four tests explore:

1. the auditory input lexicon: PALPA 5 uses word/non-word judgements (e.g. dunkey, foaster);
2. aspects of the syntactic and semantic system: PALPA 58 concerns locative relations (e.g. which of four pictures best represents such phrases as 'boxes beside buckets', 'square above circle')
3. PALPA 49 concerns synonym judgments (e.g. story-tale, tool-crowd); and
4. 'real world' meaning: the WAB comprehension test.

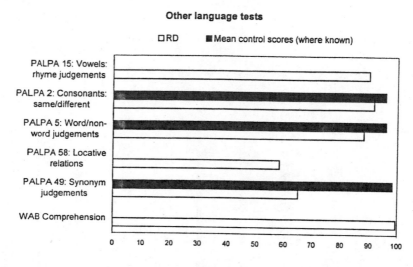

Figure 39.3. RD's scores on selected language tasks (PALPA and WAB).

RD's results in the two segmental phonetic tasks paralleled his results on the PEPS form reception tasks in that they were not significantly lower than normal controls: the mean score for unimpaired subjects on the consonantal task is 96%; RD scored 92% on that task and (90%) on the rhyme task. The other four tests show a mixed picture, and merit closer analysis.

In the WAB comprehension test RD scored almost 100%. The yes-no questions were simple ones relating to himself and his knowledge of the world (e.g. *Are you a man? Is this Toronto?*); auditory word recognition concerned names of common objects (mugs and matches), and the sequential commands involved pointing to common objects. This score reveals an important aspect of his conversational ability in that he appears to be very well able to make use of pragmatic and circumstantial detail. In the test for distinguishing words from non-words, non-word status was in many of the cases determined by one phoneme only (as in the examples given, 'foaster' and 'dunkey'). This task, in which he scored 88%, can therefore to some extent be classed with the tests of segmental phonetic discrimination discussed above, in which he scored similarly well. In the tasks on synonym judgements and locative relations RD scored below normal limits: this highlights his difficulty with linguistic meaning.

The pattern of results suggests that RD has specific deficits in linguistic comprehension, in syntactic and semantic (although not pragmatic) aspects. These deficits are unlikely to be compensated for by prosody since he has deficits in the functional comprehension of prosody (as shown in Figure 39.1), and the converse is also true: misunderstandings caused by his difficulty with functional comprehension of prosody are unlikely to be elucidated by reference to the syntax or semantics of an utterance.

Production

The PEPS production tasks sought to establish the likelihood of RD being misunderstood rather than providing a measure of general intelligibility. His production presents a more complex picture than his reception skills, without the same dissociation between function and form. Figure 39.4 shows his scores on function production tasks.

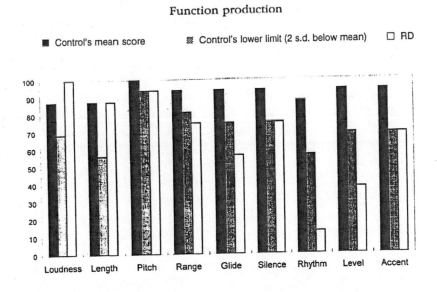

Figure 39.4. Percentage of correct responses to the 'function production' tasks of PEPS.

He scored at or above the mean in the 'loudness' and 'length' tasks, and at the lower limit in the 'pitch', 'silence' and 'accent' tasks. He scored below the lower limit of normal controls in 'range', 'glide', 'level' and 'rhythm': in 'rhythm' his score was three standard deviations below the lower limit. Figure 39.5 shows his results on form production tasks.

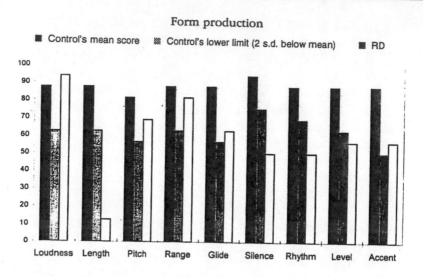

Figure 39.5. Percentage of correct responses to the 'form production' tasks of PEPS.

He scored at or above the mean in tasks for 'loudness', 'pitch', 'range', 'glide' and 'accent', and below the mean for 'level', 'rhythm', 'silence' and 'length'. There is no simple parallel to the finding of high scores on form tasks and low scores on function tasks in reception. What can, however, be observed in both modes (form and function) is that, with the exception of his 'length' score, he tended to score higher in the monosyllabic tasks shown on the left in the bar chart. Tasks are displayed in the order in which they were presented, but fatigue does not account for the apparent deterioration in performance, since the assessment was conducted in three separate sessions. The order of tasks represents the complexity of the elements: the first five can be produced on single syllables, the last four involve the production of polysyllabic utterances. All the form production tasks for the first five elements required monosyllabic replies except in the case of 'length', where the task investigated whether lengthening occurred at the end of the subject's polysyllabic utterances; subjects had to copy short phrases that they heard on tape, such as 'more and more', 'on and on', to see whether the item in end position was lengthened. This task highlighted RD's marked tendency towards syllable-timing, which is a characteristic of non-English languages, English being 'stress-timed' (Pike, 1946). A correlation between RD's scores and the number of syllables needed in the responses to each task found a high inverse relationship; the function task for 'rhythm' required five or six syllables. On tasks requiring monosyllabic responses, however, he managed quite well; an example is the function production task for 'length' where there were monosyllabic names to say, such as 'Di', 'Lee' and 'Jay' and these were said in either a hurried, brisk way or in an unhurried, relaxed way, using more or less length on a single syllable. His difficulties therefore could be related to the functional processing load of longer utterances.

The functional consequence of RD's problem with increasing utterance-length manifests itself in such tasks as the one for 'accent'. Here he had to say a sequence such as 'HA7' (this being being part of a postcode), placing the focus on the 'A'. The first two examples in Figure 39.6. show how controls produced prosody; the third is RD's version.

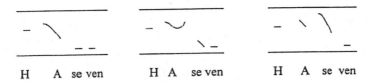

| H | A | se ven | | H | A | se ven | | H | A | se ven |

Figure 39.6. Realization of the utterance 'HA 7' (stress on 'A') by two controls (left and middle) and by RD (right).

Controls produced either a primary accent (falling glide) on the 'A' with 'seven' de-stressed, or a default accent pattern with a falling glide on the 'seven' and but extra stress on the 'A'. RD had initially all the right prosodic factors in play on the right letter but the balance was upset on subsequent tokens. His version tends to give the impression that he made a mistake initially in emphasizing the 'A' and wished to correct it by placing even greater prominence on the 'seven'. Thus the focus of his utterance is not clear. A summary of RD's prosody is shown in Fig. 39.7.

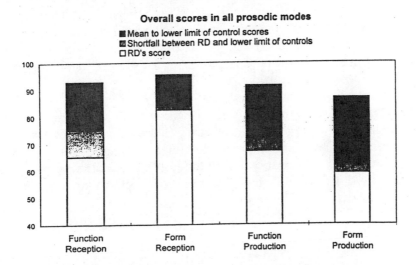

Figure 39.7. Overall scores in all prosodic modes of RD in relation to the normal controls.

It can be seen that the main deficit is in prosodic function reception – in the understanding of prosodic meaning – and that form reception is the least affected. His production scores show some overall deficit.

Conclusions

The assessment of RD's prosodic skills using the PEPS procedure led to the following conclusions.

On the input side:

There is significant deficit in prosodic function.
There is dissociation between form and function, which suggests that functional problems with prosody cannot be accounted for by phonetic level deficit.
The deficit is paralleled by semantic and syntactic deficits.
RD's deficit involves a number of elements that are affected in reception, production, form and function.
On any given element his performance varies; his deficits are not constant across all elements, nor is there one element with a specific deficit such that it is affected in reception, production, form and function.

On the output side:

There is no overall pattern of deficit for form and function.
Dissociations between form and function in individual elements show the effect of utterance-length: prosody deteriorates with utterance-length, presumably as a consequence of the greater processing load.
The conclusions have some implications for the management of RD's aphasia.
It cannot be assumed that RD understands the meaning of prosodic features, even though he may appear to do so in conversation.
In order to assess prosody adequately there is a need to look at several features in context, and extended utterances cause extra problems. Requiring RD to produce extended utterances is likely to induce prosodic difficulty that may give rise to communication breakdown with conversational partners.

References

Blumstein S (1973) A phonological investigation of aphasic speech. The Hague: Mouton.

Brewster K (1989) The assessment of prosody. In Grundy K (Ed) Linguistics In Clinical Practice. 1st edn. London: Taylor & Francis, pp. 169–81.

Bryan K (1989) Language prosody and the right hemisphere. Aphasiology 3(4): 285–99.

Bryan K (1995) The Right Hemisphere Language Battery. London: Whurr.

Crystal D (1969) Prosodic systems and intonation in English.

Crystal D (1982) Profiling Linguistic Disability. London: Edward Arnold.

Danly M, Shapiro B (1982) Speech prosody in Broca's aphasia. Brain and Language 16: 171–91.

Enderby P (1983) The Frenchay Dysarthria Assessment. San Diego: College Hill Press.

Hird K, Kirsner K (1993) Disprosody following acquired neurogenic impairment. Brain and Language 45: 46–60.

Kay J, Lesser R, Coltheart M (1992) Psycholinguistic Assessments of Language Processing in Aphasia (PALPA). Hove: Lawrence Erlbaum.

Kent RD, Rosenbek JC (1982) Prosodic disturbance and neurologic lesion. Brain and Language 15, 259–92.

Kertesz, A (1980) Western Aphasia Battery. University Of Western Ontario.

Monrad-Krohn, GH (1963) The third element of speech: prosody and its disorders. In Halpern L (Ed) Problems in Dynamic Neurology. Jerusalem: Hebrew University Press.

Ouellette GP, Baum SR (1994) Acoustic analysis of prosodic cues in left- and right-hemisphere-damaged patients. Aphasiology 8(3): 257–83.

Peppé SJE (In preparation) Profiling elements of prosodic systems.

Pike KL (1946) The Intonation of American English. Michigan: Ann Arbor, p 35.

Samuel C, Couillet J, Louis-Dreyfus A, Azouvi P, Roubeau B, Bakchine S, Bussel B (1996) Dysprosody after severe closed head injury. European Journal of Neurology 3, supplement 2.

Schlanger BB, Schlanger P, Gerstman LJ (1976), The perception of emotionally-toned sentences in right-hemisphere damaged and aphasic subjects. Brain and Language 3: 396–404.

Tucker DM, Watson RT, Heilman KM, (1977). Discrimination and evocation of affectively intoned speech in patients with right parietal disease. Neurology, 27: 947–50.

Vance J (1994) Prosodic deviation in dysarthria. European Journal of Communication Disorders 29: 6–76.

Chapter 40
Affective Prosody in Patients with Parkinson's Disease

CATERINA BREITENSTEIN, IRENE DAUM AND
HERMANN ACKERMANN

Recent research on the neuropsychological correlates of emotional processing

Several investigations during the last decade could not support the widely accepted notion of right-hemisphere dominance in the identification and expression (Cancelliere and Kertesz, 1990; Hornak, Rolls and Wade, 1996; Stone, Nisenson, Eliassen and Gazzaniga, 1996; Van Lancker and Sidtis, 1992, 1993) of facial emotions as well as affective prosody. Recent results show that patients with cortical lesions who had additional damage to the basal ganglia and/or the anterior temporal lobes (Cancelliere and Kertesz, 1990) presented the most pronounced deficits, independent of the lesion side. Further evidence for the important role of the basal ganglia in emotional functions is provided by studies describing prosodic and facial comprehension/expression disorders in patients with Parkinson's disease (PD): Scott, Caird and Williams (1984) reported impaired performance in the identification of facial emotions and affective prosody as well as deficits in the vocal production of anger (as measured by subjective ratings of judges) in PD patients in (presumably) more advanced stages of the disease. Convergent evidence was reported by Jacobs, Shuren, Bowers and Heilman (1995) who showed reduced performance by PD patients (also presumably in more advanced stages of the disease) in the discrimination of facial emotions (identification performance was not directly examined in this study). For PD patients in early stages of the disease, performance in the expression of affective prosody (subjective ratings by experts) was impaired whereas the identification of facial emotions and affective prosody was preserved (Blonder, Gur and Gur, 1989). Few studies analysing acoustic correlates of the clinically observed 'flat speech' of PD patients indicated reduced variability of fundamental frequency in small patient samples (Darkins, Fromkin and Benson, 1988; Flint, Black, Campbell-Taylor Gailey and Levinton, 1992; Pitcairn, Clemie, Gray and Pentland, 1990).

In the earliest stage of Parkinson's disease, the pathophysiological processes are generally limited to subcortical structures (substantia nigra and basal ganglia), whereas during the later course of the disease functionally related neuroanatomical structures (especially the frontal lobes) are involved (Owen, James, Leigh, Summers, Marsden, Quinn, Lange and Robbins, 1992). Dysfunction of the direct neuroanatomical connections between the striatum and the limbic system/frontal cortex could explain the observed deficits in responding to emotional stimuli of patients with PD in more advanced stages of the disease (Heimer, Switzer and Van Hoesen, 1982). According to Jacobs, Shuren, Bowers and Heilman (1995) the literature supports the important role of fronto-striatal circuitry in the identification of non-verbal emotional cues ('visual habits').

In a previous study a standardized measure of emotional perception and affective prosodic expression (Tübingen Affect Battery) was developed (Breitenstein, Daum, Ackermann, Lütgehetmann and Müller 1996) and administered to four groups of patients with focal cortical lesions and two groups of patients with dysfunction of the basal ganglia (PD patients) in another study. The findings implied involvement of the fronto-striatal circuitry in emotional processing as only patients with PD in more advanced stages of the disease as well as patients with focal damage to the (right) frontal lobe differed significantly from controls in the identification of facial expressions and affective prosody (Breitenstein, Daum and Ackermann, 1997a).

A controlled study of emotional processing in Parkinson's disease

The present study aimed to investigate further the contribution of the basal ganglia loop to the expression of affective prosody by comparing the performance of PD patients in early and more advanced stages of the disease to normal control subjects.

We tested seven patients in the early stages of PD, seven patients in the more advanced stages and 12 normal control subjects with comparable age, sex, and IQ. This research design therefore allows some degree of estimation of the differential contribution of purely subcortical and cortical brain structures to the production of affective prosody. All patients were medicated at the time of testing (a standard combination of levodopa, D2-agonist, and MAO-B inhibitor), none of the patients had undergone surgical treatment for Parkinson's disease (details of clinical and demographic patient characteristics are provided in Breitenstein et al., 1997a).

A short audiometric examination (testing frequencies between 500–8000 Hz) as well as a neuropsychological screening battery were administered to all subjects to control for general performance deficits (basic intellectual functioning, attention span, mood) which might influence the affective processing test performance. Patient groups and healthy control subjects did not differ in any of the neuropsychological background variables or in hearing ability (see Breitenstein et al., 1997a).

The expressive tasks consisted of a 'posed' and a 'free' condition. In the 'posed' condition, all subjects had to repeat one sentence five times each with different emotional intonations (happy, angry, frightened, sad, neutral). All model sentences were recorded by a professional actress and presented to the subjects on a tape recorder (interstimulus interval of 4s). For the 'free' condition, all subjects had to read one sentence (presented to them on a piece of paper) with five different affective intonations.

All sentences were recorded using a portable digital tape player. Acoustic analyses (Computerized Speechlab 4300; Kay Elemetrics Corp., USA) were performed to extract fundamental frequency (FO), a 'variation coefficient' (defined as FO-variability divided by mean FO to control for sex differences) and speech duration (in seconds).

The results revealed significantly reduced variation coefficients for PD-I and/or PD-II patients compared to healthy controls in angry, sad, happy, and neutral intonations (see Figure 40.1). In the free condition, group differences were found for 'neutral' and 'happy' sentences (for details concerning the procedure and results see Breitenstein, Daum, Hertrich and Ackermann, 1997b). Patients both in early and more advanced stages presented with significantly lower variation coefficients compared to normal controls. No group differences were found for

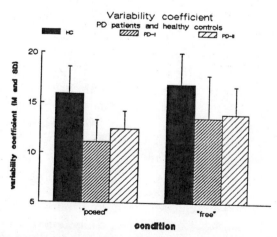

Figure 40.1. Variability of fundamental frequency (variation coefficient: mean and standard deviation) in the 'free' and 'posed' condition for patient and control groups (HC = healthy controls, PD = patients with Parkinson's disease: I = early stages, II = advanced stages).

mean F0 or speech duration, which might be due to small sample sizes. Separate analyses for male and female subjects in the parameter mean fundamental frequency could not be conducted at all for that reason.

In summary, the present findings indicate that patients both in early and more advanced stages of PD showed significantly lower variation coefficients in happy, angry, sad, and neutral intonations, which might contribute to the clinical impression of 'flat speech' in Parkinson's disease. Reduced F0-variability in neutral statements could be explained by a non-emotional disturbance in producing intonation patterns. As patients with PD, however, were impaired in the identification of affective intonations (see Breitenstein et al. 1997a), the present data support the inference of an affective prosodic deficit in patients with PD. The present study therefore provided more evidence for an involvement of the basal ganglia in emotional functions, especially in producing emotional speech intonations.

References

Blonder LX, Gur RE, Gur RC (1989) The effects of right and left hemiparkinsonism on prosody. Brain and Language 36: 193–207.

Breitenstein C, Daum I, Ackermann, Lütgehetmann R, Müller E (1996) Erfassung der Emotionswahrnehmung bei zentralnervösen Läsionen und Erkrankungen: Psychometrische Gütekriterien der 'Tübinger Affekt Batterie' [Assessment of deficits in emotional perception following cortical and subcortical brain damage: Psychometric properties of the Tübingen Affect Battery]. Neurologie and Rehabilitation 2: 93–101.

Breitenstein C, Daum I, Ackermann H (1997a) Affective processing following cortical and subcortical brain damage: contribution of the fronto-striatal circuitry. Submitted for publication.

Breitenstein C, Daum I, Hertrich I, Ackermann H (1997b) Acoustic correlates of flat emotional speech in patients with Parkinson's disease. Submitted for publication.

Cancelliere AEB, Kertesz A (1990) Lesion localization in acquired deficits of emotional expression and comprehension. Brain and Cognition 13: 133–47.

Darkins AW, Fromkin VA, Benson DF (1988) A characterization of the prosodic loss in Parkinson's disease. Brain and Language 34: 315–27.

Flint AJ, Black SE, Campbell-Taylor I, Gailey GF, Levinton C (1992) Acoustic analysis in the differentiation of Parkinson's disease and major depression. Journal of Psycholinguistic Research 21: 383–99.

Heimer L, Switzer RD, Van Hoesen GW (1982) Ventral striatum and ventral pallidum: components of the motor system? Trends in Neurosciences 5: 83–7.

Hornak J, Rolls ET, Wade D (1996) Face and voice expression identification in patients with emotional and behavioral changes following ventral frontal lobe damage. Neuropsychologia 34: 247–61.

Jacobs DH, Shuren J, Bowers D, Heilman KM (1995) Emotional facial imagery, perception, and expression in Parkinson's disease. Neurology 45: 1696–702.

Owen AM, James M, Leigh PN, Summers BA, Marsden CD, Quinn NP, Lange KW, Robbins TW (1992) Fronto-striatal cognitive deficits at different stages of Parkinson's disease. Brain 115: 1727–51.

Pitcairn TK, Clemie S, Gray JM, Pentland, B (1990) Impressions of Parkinson patients from their recorded voices. British Journal of Disorders of Communication 25: 85–92.

Scott S, Caird FI, Williams B (1984) Evidence for an apparent sensory speech disorder in Parkinson's disease. Journal of Neurology, Neurosurgery, and Psychiatry 47: 840–43.

Stone VE, Nisenson L, Eliassen JC, Gazzaniga MS (1996) Left hemisphere representations of emotional facial expressions. Neuropsychologia 34: 23–9.

Van Lancker D, Sidtis JJ (1992) The identification of affective-prosodic stimuli by left- and right-hemisphere-damaged subjects: all errors are not created equal. Journal of Speech and Hearing Research 35: 963–70.

Van Lancker D, Sidtis JJ (1993) Brain damage and prosody reconsidered: reply to Heilman. Journal of Speech and Hearing Research 36: 1191–2.

Chapter 41
Prosodic Characteristics of the Speech of Patients with Parkinson's Disease and Friedreich's Ataxia[1]

GUYLAINE LE DORZE AND JOHN RYALLS

Introduction

This study investigated how Parkinson's disease and Friedreich's ataxia affect the production of certain aspects of prosody by comparison with a group of normal speakers.

Acoustic studies are not conclusive about the alterations caused by these two diseases. Acoustic studies of the rate of speech of Parkinson's patients have described it as reduced (Weismer, 1984), more variable than normal (Canter, 1963), faster than normal (Illes, Metter, Hanson and Iritani, 1988) and essentially similar to that of normal speakers (Ackermann and Ziegler, 1991; Hertrich and Ackermann, 1993; Lethlean, Chenery and Murdoch, 1990). The fundamental frequency of male speakers with Parkinson's disease has generally been described as higher than normals (Canter, 1963; Illes et al. 1988; Ramig, Scherer, Titze and Ringel, 1988), and the few female speakers studied have been reported to have lower than normal fundamental frequency (Hertrich and Ackermann, 1993; Lethlean et al. 1990). Pitch ranges have been described as reduced compared to the normal range in males (Canter 1963) and in a female speaker (Lethlean et al. 1990). Lethlean et al. (1990) also report a greater than normal pitch range in one male patient.

Acoustic studies of the speech of Friedreich's ataxics are much fewer in number. Ackermann, Hertrich and Hehr (1995) report slower than normal diadochokinetic rates in Friedreich's ataxics and Gentil (1990) reports longer sentence durations. Fundamental frequency in sustained vowels appears to be variable in Friedreich's ataxic speakers (Gentil, 1990).

One important use of prosody in speech production is to distinguish questions from statements. In so-called rhetorical questions, a rising intonation at the end of the sentence is the relevant distinguishing feature (Lieberman, 1967). Such question–statement pairs offer a unique opportunity to investigate prosody independent from phonemic content. In a preliminary study, dysarthric speakers of various types were found to produce significantly less intonation difference than normal control subjects (Le Dorze, Ouellet and Ryalls, 1994). It is not known how various types of dysarthric speakers produce rhetorical questions.

Existing information about the prosodic alterations of Parkinson and Friedreich's ataxic speakers is inconclusive. The objectives of this study were to determine how the speech of speakers with Friedreich's ataxia and Parkinson's disease differs from that of normals on prosodic variables of: (a) rate, (b) mean fundamental frequency, and (c) intonation difference in rhetorical question–statement pairs.

Methodology

Subjects

All subjects were native speakers of French. They all gave their written consent to participate in the research project.

Ten patients with a diagnosis of Parkinson's disease were referred to us for this study. They were all under stable drug regimens for their Parkinson's disease. Mean age was 64.5 years and mean educational level was 14.6 years (see Table 41.1).

Table 41.1. Characteristics of subjects with Parkinson's disease and intelligibility ratings

Characteristics No.	Gender	Age	Education	Duration of illness	Intelligibility Speech	Reading
1P	M	46	15	19	3	2
2P	M	48	19	3	1.5	1
3P	M	63	20	10	5.5	3.5
4P	M	67	15	1	3	1
5P	M	71	12	1.5	4	1
6P	M	72	12	9	2	2
7P	M	89	11	2	3.5	2.5
8P	F	44	15	3	1	1
9P	F	72	15	7	n/a	1
10P	F	73	12	2	2	2

n/a not available

A group of 10 patients with a diagnosis of Friedreich's ataxia was also recruited from a rehabilitation centre known for treating such patients. Mean age was 35.1 years and mean educational level was 12.9 years for nine of these subjects (see Table 41.2).

Table 41.2. Characteristics of subjects with Friedreich's ataxia and intelligibility ratings

| Characteristics | | | | | Intelligibility | |
No.	Gender	Age	Education	Duration of illness	Speech	reading
1FA	M	27	17	14	6.5	5.5
2FA	M	27	16	20	4.5	4.5
3FA	M	33	19	27	5	3.5
4FA	M	39	7	24	3	2
5FA	M	43	15	31	2	2
6FA	F	30	12	17	4.5	3
7FA	F	31	17	23	7	5.5
8FA	F	35	11	29	5	5
9FA	F	36	15	29	2.5	n/a
10FA	F	50	n/a	42	3.5	3.5

n/a not available

Twenty neurologically normal individuals were paired with each participant from both patient groups on the basis of gender and age (± 5 years). The normal individuals, matched to the Parkinson's patients, had an average age of 64.3 years and an average of 14.8 years of education. Since Friedreich's ataxia occurs at a much younger age, a different group of normal subjects was recruited to compare with these patients. The 10 normal individuals matched to the Friedreich's ataxics had an average age of 34.8 years with an average of 18.8 years of education.

Dysarthric speakers were evaluated for overall severity of dysarthria on the basis of their speech intelligibility. Two speech-language pathologists, native speakers of French, listened to five minutes of tape-recorded spontaneous speech and reading of a standardized text. These judges were unaware of speakers' neurological condition and determined their scores independently. They employed a seven-point rating scale to determine overall intelligibility. The following statement: 'Speech is intelligible without effort on the part of the listener' was associated with a score of 1, while the score of 7 was associated with the statement 'Speech is unintelligible most of the time even with multiple listenings.'

Stimuli

A prosodic battery of 20 sentence pairs in the French language (40 sentences in all) was employed, as presented in Le Dorze, Lever, Ryalls and Brassard (1995). Each sentence was five to seven syllables in length and had a simple SVO (subject, verb, object) word order. Sentences were printed on to separate cards with the appropriate punctuation. Participants were instructed to read sentences in as natural a manner as possible, as if they were speaking to someone. Their productions were recorded directly on to diskettes using IBM's SpeechViewer program implemented on an IBM personal computer (model 30-386). The screen was turned away from the participants so that visual feedback would not influence their speech production. The resulting recordings then underwent more detailed analysis in the University laboratory to extract acoustic measures.

Measures

A measure of the average fundamental frequency for the sentence was taken. SpeechViewer automatically calculates this value once the sentence has been isolated by means of cursors. Cursor placement was guided both visually and auditorily.

Speech rate was calculated by taking the total number of syllables in that sentence and dividing by the overall duration of the sentence (in seconds).

Intonation was measured as the difference in Fo on the last syllable of the sentence between the question and statement versions. The last syllable was first isolated by means of cursors and SpeechViewer then displayed the fundamental frequency for this syllable. This value was used to determine the intonation difference.

Results

Rate

An analysis of variance revealed that the three groups differed significantly in terms of rate ($F_{(2, 37)} = 21.2$, $p < 0.001$). Ataxic speakers were slower than both normal and Parkinson speakers. See Table 41.3. There was an overall main effect of sentence type, with interrogatives (M = 4.4 [syll/s], SD = 0.9) produced at a significantly faster rate ($F_{(1, 37)} = 11.3$, $p < 0.01$) compared to declaratives (M = 4.2 [syll/s], SD = 0.9).

Fundamental frequency

Groups did not differ significantly in terms of Fo ($F_{(2, 37)} = 0.1$, $p > 0.05$). See Table 41.3. Fo values differed significantly as a function of sentence type ($F_{(1, 37)} = 39.1$, $p < 0.001$). Interrogatives were produced at a higher mean Fo level of 178 Hz (SD = 42), while declaratives were produced at a mean Fo of 156 Hz (SD = 39).

Intonation

An analysis of variance performed on intonation values revealed a significant effect for group ($F_{(2, 37)} = 7.1$, $p < 0.01$). Both ataxic and Parkinson speakers had less intonation difference than did normal speakers. See Table 41.3.

Table 41.3. Means and standard deviations for the variables of Rate, Fo, and Intonation in the three subject groups

	Ataxic (n = 10)	Parkinson (n = 10)	Normal (n = 20)
Rate	3.2 syll/s (0.7)	4.7 syll/s (0.7)	4.7 syll/s (0.7)
Fo	171 Hz (43)	169 Hz (40)	164 Hz (44)
Intonation values	44.9 Hz (30.0)	47.6 Hz (30.0)	77.9 Hz (23.2)

Intelligibility

Speakers with Parkinson's disease (M = 2.2) were judged to have better intelligibility than speakers with Friedreich's ataxia (M = 4.0) (t = -3.249, p<0.01). For speakers with Parkinson's disease, there were moderate-to-weak relationships between intelligibility and some of the prosody variables. The only statistically significant correlation was between intelligibility and rate of declaratives (r = 0.649; p<0.05). For speakers with Friedreich's ataxia, none of the correlations between intelligibility and prosodic variables were significant.

Discussion

To summarize the findings, speakers with Parkinson's disease demonstrated speech rates that were not significantly different from that of normal speakers, but higher speech rates were moderately correlated with lower intelligibility scores in this group of speakers. Speakers with Friedreich's ataxia had statistically slower speaking rates. In this last group, no relationship was revealed between prosodic variables and intelligibility. For both neurological groups, mean fundamental frequency was not significantly different from that of normals. However, intonation values were significantly reduced for both neurological groups.

Although both groups were comparable in their reduced intonation difference, ataxic individuals differed from Parkinson individuals in their significantly slower rate of speech in sentence production. These results may offer some preliminary evidence for a differential diagnosis based on acoustic speech measures.

It is important to emphasize that whereas prosody was clearly impaired in both clinical groups, these neurologically impaired speakers still retained certain aspects of normal prosody (i.e. in differentiating declaratives and interrogatives in terms of speech rate). This provides evidence of intact speech planning in the face of a disorder that affects speech performance. We believe that similar investigations with other neurological disorders can offer a better understanding of the processes by which the brain organizes speech and prosody, as well as the particular manner in which they are affected by various motor speech disorders.

References

Ackermann H, Hertrich I, Hehr T (1995) Oral diadochokinesis in neurological dysarthrias. Folia Phoniatrica and Logopaedica 47: 15–23.

Ackermann H, Ziegler W (1991) Articulatory deficits in Parkinsonian dysarthria: an acoustic analysis. Journal of Neurology, Neurosurgery, and Psychiatry 54: 1093–8.

Canter, GJ (1963) Speech characteristics of patients with Parkinson's disease: I. Intensity, pitch, and duration. Journal of Speech and Hearing Disorders 28: 221–9.

Gentil M (1990) Acoustic characteristics of speech in Friedreich's disease. Folia Phoniatrica 42: 125–34.

Hertrich I, Ackermann H (1993) Acoustic analysis of speech prosody in Huntington's and Parkinson's disease: A preliminary report. Clinical Linguistics and Phonetics 7: 285–97.

Illes J, Metter EJ, Hanson WR, Iritani S (1988) Language production in Parkinson's disease: Acoustic and linguistic considerations. Brain and Language 33: 146–60.

Le Dorze G, Lever N, Ryalls J, Brassard C (1995) Valeurs de certains paramètres prosodiques obtenues auprès de sujets francophones sans trouble de la communication. Folia Phoniatrica et Logopaedica 47: 39–47.

Le Dorze G, Ouellet L, Ryalls J (1994) Intonation and speech rate in dysarthric speech. Journal of Communication Disorders 27: 1–18.

Lethlean JB, Chenery HJ, Murdoch BE (1990) Disturbed respiratory and prosodic function in Parkinson's disease: A perceptual and instrumental analysis. Australian Journal of Human Communication Disorders 18: 83–97.

Lieberman P (1967) Intonation, Perception, and Language. Cambridge, MA: MIT Press.

Ramig LA, Scherer RC, Titze IR, Ringel SP (1988) Acoustic analysis of voices of patients with neurologic disease: Rationale and preliminary data. Annals of Otology, Rhinology, and Laryngology 97: 164–78.

Weismer G (1984) Articulatory characteristics of Parkinsonian dysarthria: Segmental and phrase-level timing, spirantization, and glottal-supraglottal coordination. In McNeil MR, Rosenbek JC, Aronson AE (Eds) The dysarthrias: Physiology, acoustics, perception, management. San Diego, CA: College Hill Press, pp. 101–30.

Note

1   We would like to express our gratitude to all the participants of this study and to Nancy Boulanger, Danielle Ratté and Christine Brassard. This research was supported, in part, by a grant from the Social Sciences and Humanities Research Council of Canada.

Neuromotor Speech Processes

Chapter 42
A Motor Skill Approach to Stuttering

WOUTER HULSTIJN AND PASCAL VAN LIESHOUT

Introduction

The view proposed in this paper is that stuttering must be seen as a disorder or a deficiency in the motor output of speech. This motor approach to stuttering has grown continuously during the last decade. One can easily verify this trend by reading the proceedings of the three conferences on speech motor control and stuttering that have been held in the last 10 years. The first book (Peters and Hulstijn, 1987) appeared at a time when emotional issues and learning theory approaches were on the way down, and when a new interest in the role of speech motor behaviour was initiated by Zimmermann (1980). The proceedings of the second conference (Peters, Hulstijn and Starkweather, 1991) made it clear that this interest in speech motor control had expanded and matured. In the third book (Hulstijn, Peters, Van Lieshout, 1997), which has arisen from the most recent conference held in 1996, this trend continued. It is one of the aims of this chapter to give an impression of the current state of stuttering research, based on the contributions to this third conference. However, we will do this from our own perspective. The second aim of this chapter is therefore to present a view on dysfluency that we have developed over the past 10 years. As such this chapter summarizes the extensive review given by Van Lieshout in his thesis (Van Lieshout, 1995; Chapter 1). In addition, this chapter is a strongly abbreviated version of the paper that we presented at the 1996 ICPLA Conference in Munich. Occasionally, we will refer to the full version (Hulstijn, and Van Lieshout, in press).

The motor programming model and theories on stuttering

Recent brain-imaging studies on stuttering are collected in Hulstijn, Peters and Van Lieshout (1997) and are summarized in Hulstijn and Van

Lieshout (in press). Together they show that the motor-systems particularly in the cortex and the cerebellum display extensive hyperactivity related to dysfluency. But they do not show what types of processing actually occur in these active areas. We need speech production models that are specific enough to detail the different stages that are involved and the type of processing that takes place in these stages. One of the most seminal models is the one given by Levelt (1989, 1992). Here we will focus only on the motor aspects of speech, called *articulation* in Levelt´s model. Table 42.1 details their stages and processes and combines them with dysfluency theories that localize the origin of stuttering in the specific process that are presented in the left part of the table.

Table 42.1. Motor programming processes and disfluency theories

Stages Processes	Disfluency theories	Authors
Motor Plan Assembly		
phonological encoding	error in phoneme selection covert repair hypothesis	Postma & Kolk (1993)
abstact motor planning	programming disorder	Peters et al. (1989)
Muscle Command Preparation		
retrieval of motor programmes	learning failure resulting in ineffective motor programmes	Kent, Kalveram & Natke Ludlow et al., McClean (all: 1997)
parameter setting/selection		
sensory afference reduced kinaesthetic acuity		De Nil (1994)
force control timing	higher neuromotor noise skill: speed-accuracy	Grosjean et al. (1997) Van Lieshout (1995)
initiation		
triggering	less reflex suppression prior to fluent speech	McClean (1997)
force discharge coordination	excessive EMG activity (see later)	Starkweather (1995)
Muscle command execution		
	defective or inefficient execution resulting in kinematic differences	many authors
feedback processing		
proprioceptive & kinesthetic auditory	defective propr. and kinest. feedback processing defective auditory feedback processing learning deficiency in 'audio-phonatoric coupling'	De Nil (1994) Neilson & Neilson (1987) Howell et al. (1987, Kalinowski et al. (1995) Kalveram & Natke (1997)

Motor plan assembly

If we start with the motor plan assembly stage, we see that the first process mentioned in Table 42.1 is phonological encoding. In this process the correct phonemes for a particular word are supposed to be selected. In the covert repair hypothesis, which is a well known recent theory to explain stuttering, proposed by Postma and Kolk (1993), it is assumed that individuals who stutter encounter more difficulties in the selection of the correct phoneme than controls. Speech is internally monitored and if errors in phoneme selection are encountered a speaker tries to correct these covertly. This covert repair is often too late resulting in a blocking of the system or a repetition of the wrongly selected phoneme until the correct next one is selected. It is our opinion that this theory goes quite a way in explaining the details of stuttering. However, our objections are, first, that the evidence that has been given in favour of this view can also be explained by motor processes at lower stages, and, second, that specific lower-level motor phenomena (see later), like the longer pre-speech EMG durations found in fluent speech of stuttering persons (Van Lieshout, Peters, Hulstijn and Starkweather, 1993) cannot be explained by this theory.

The second process in the motor plan assembly stage is called abstract motor planning (in Table 42.1) or phonetic encoding (by Levelt (1992)). It is a process in which phonological syllabic units are translated into motor plans, either by a retrieval from long-term motor storage or through an *ad hoc* assembling process. Such a plan is still rather abstract; it may, for example translate the 'p' in the word 'pub' to a plan for lip closing. The closing of the lips may involve movements of the upper lip, lower lip and jaw, but may also be performed with a stiff upper lip or even by only moving the jaw upwards. Therefore, the plan does not specify all movement details.

Our earlier work (Peters, Hulstijn and Starkweather, 1989) was undertaken to test whether stutterers have more problems in this planning or programming process – both terms are used interchangeably to denote the same process – than non-stuttering control subjects. In particular, the findings that dysfluencies occur at the beginning of words and most frequently at the beginning of long words, which can be viewed as long movement sequences, were strong arguments to test this programming hypothesis. This view, postulating that persons who stutter encounter more problems in programming, would predict that they will need more time to initiate a word, and that this group difference in reaction times will become larger for longer words. In our first study (Peters et al. 1989) the results were very promising, but in later testing, with more methodological refinements, the difference in reaction time between stuttering subjects and controls disappeared (Van

Lieshout, Hulstijn and Peters, 1996a, 1996b). We have not disproved the idea but we do not believe in it any more.

Muscle command preparation

The second stage in the motor production of speech is the muscle command preparation stage. In the process of phonetic encoding, described earlier, well-learned motor plans were retrieved from long-term motor memory. But what would be the result if these motor plans were not well learned? This idea, which explains stuttering as a learning failure resulting in inefficient plans, has been advanced by many authors. At the recent conference on speech motor production and fluency disorders it was proposed by Kent (1997), Kalveram (1997), Ludlow, Siren and Zikria (1997) and McClean (1997).

Following traditional motor control literature, a stored motor plan does not specify the muscle commands directly. It has to be adjusted to the specific demands of the situation. A motor plan can be seen as a computer subroutine that has to be supplied with values or parameters before it can actually run. The selection of the proper values for these parameters requires the processing of sensory information or sensory afference. One form of sensory afference is kinesthetic or proprioceptive information about the position or movement of the articulators. De Nil (1994) found that stuttering individuals are less accurate in their use of this sensory information. Their thresholds for reacting to small changes in propriocepsis were higher.

There is also evidence for a reduced ability in the precise regulation of forces related to stuttering. In a recent study by Grosjean, Van Galen et al. (1997), subjects had to press with their lips on a pressure transducer. No speech production was required. It was found that this pressure was less strong and much more inaccurate or variable in stuttering subjects compared to non-stuttering controls. This finding was explained by Grosjean et al. by assuming that stuttering was the result of a higher level of neuromotor noise, but at least we may conclude that force control is less accurate in persons who stutter. This is further supported by data obtained by Howell, Au-Yeung and Rustin (1997), who asked children to track a sinusoidal moving target with their lower lip. Stuttering children were less accurate in this task. Additional analyses revealed that this poor tracking performance did not result from a timing deficit but was caused by a larger motor variance. It must be emphasized that these results were obtained in non-speech tasks, refuting the idea that the nature of stuttering must be sought in the interconnection between motor and linguistic processes (as proposed, amongst others, by Ludlow et al. 1997). Very recently, Zelaznik, Smith, Franz and Ho (in press) reviewed research on non-speech motor performance in stuttering and presented an elegant study of bimanual finger movements. Their review and results led them to infer that individuals who stutter perform less well on these non-speech tasks but only if these tasks ask for the coordination of multiple effector systems and require precise spatiotemporal coupling.

Speed-accuracy trade-off

The conclusion that speech requires precise spatio-temporal coordination prompts us to make a small excursion to the topic of speed and accuracy in motor tasks. One of the basic laws in movement control is Fitts' law (Schmidt, 1988), which states that movement time is a simple function of two variables: the length of the movement trajectory and the required accuracy. The smaller the target is that has to be reached, the longer is the time taken to hit the target. When movements have to be made in a time shorter than the time predicted by Fitts' law, the error will be larger when the movement time is smaller. This inverse relation between speed and accuracy is 'known' or exploited by most individuals, when they trade-off speed against accuracy. Speech is a motor activity and as such it will obey Fitts' law. This simple conclusion has two implications. The first is that if subjects (who stutter) have problems with precise motor control (cf. Van Lieshout et al. 1996a; 1996b) they can increase accuracy by reducing movement speed. A longer time for speech execution has been repeatedly found for individuals who stutter (see Table 42.2). The second implication concerns the measurement of accuracy in speech. In research and diagnostic assessment, the time required for speech movements (or for speech sound production) is carefully registered but the accuracy of the movements is seldom determined. Acoustic measurements may give a clue, and judgments of listeners may give a hint (Franken, Boves, Peters and Webster 1995), but how well the specified targets for speech movements are hit cannot be exactly determined by these methods. Only careful kinematic analyses will reveal imprecisions.

Initiation

Initiation is the third stage of muscle command preparation listed in Table 42.1. After the retrieval of the correct motor pattern and after determining the right parameter values, the now concrete programme must be initiated. McClean (1997) discusses a distinct mechanism for initiation, involving recurrent-loops between motor cortex, cerebellar nuclei, and red nucleus. The triggering function associated with these recurrent loops may be impaired in speech disfluency. It was also shown by McClean (1996) that persons who stutter show less lip-muscle reflex suppression just prior to the onset of (fluent) speech compared to non-stutterers. This might be taken as a sign for abnormal sensory processing.

Initiation problems may also result from ineffective force discharge, as reflected in excessive EMG activity. This idea has been advanced by Starkweather (1995). The coordination of the many muscles within and between systems involved in speech may also be less optimal, resulting in initiation delays or dysfluencies. Coordination, however, is the subject of a separate part of this chapter, and will therefore be dealt with later.

Muscle command execution

A very large number of authors have pointed to defective or inefficient speech movement execution processes (see Van Lieshout, 1995, for an extensive review). Slowed and/or inaccurate movements may have a number of causes. The same factors that impede efficient planning and programming of muscle commands before the onset of speech may also obstruct the planning and programming of later units during execution of earlier segments. Sensory afference, which is needed for parameter selection, is also needed during or after movement as feedback. Defective proprioceptive and kinesthetic feedback processing has been suggested as a possible cause for stuttering by De Nil (1994) and Neilson and Neilson (1987). Others have focused on the role of auditory feedback in stuttering and fluency enhancement (Howell, El-Yaniv, and Powell, 1987; Kalinowski, Armson, Stuart, Hargrave, Sark and Mcleod, 1995; Kalveram, 1997; see also Van Lieshout, 1995).

Until now we have discussed only theories but we have not detailed the evidence for these theories. A detailed description of the multiple findings would take too much space here and would duplicate the elaborate survey of the findings given by Van Lieshout (1995). The many studies mentioned there, and those reviewed by Adams (Adams, 1985) are counted and summarized in Table 42.2. From this table, we may conclude that the results of studies on peak EMG, and on voice onset time are mixed, but that all the other variables that are listed show clear positive group differences.

Coordination

The previous discussion of dysfluency theories was based on the traditional programming conception of motor control. An alternative approach, which has become very influential in the past 10 years, is the dynamical perspective (see Kelso, 1995). It has resulted, amongst others, in a task-dynamic model (e.g. Saltzman, 1991) for skilled actions like speech. Built on this task-dynamic model Browman and Goldstein have worked out their well-known gestural phonology model (a recent and clear description of this theory can be found in Browman and Goldstein, 1997; a very short introduction is offered by Hulstijn and Van Lieshout, in press), which offers a powerful contemporary theory for speech production. One of the attractive features of this model is that the traditional distinction between phonemes and articulatory actions as two separate systems, has been transformed into one single system, which can be described at the macroscopic level as phonological units (called gestures) and at the microscopic level as coordinative structures (coupled movements of individual articulators).

Table 42.2. Group differences (stuttering versus control) on variables which might be related to motor control

Stage	finding	number of studies showing positive	/no effects
muscle force control			
	higher peak EMG	6	4
	longer EMG duration	5	–
initiation			
	longer simple reaction time		
	Adams (1985): before 1985	14	3
	after 1985	12	–
	delays in initiation of phonation and respiration	7	–
	longer voice onset time (VOT)	10	8
execution			
	slower speech rates and longer speech segment durations	11	–
	kinematics of articulatory movements:		
	– longer duration, lower amplitude and lower velocity	7	–
	– larger variability	5	–

Stuttering and 'discoordination'

Stuttering may be related to problems either in intergestural coordination or in intra-gesture coordination, i.e. at the level of coordinative structures. Most research has focused on the latter type of coordination, i.e., the coupling between articulatory movements within a gesture. We have presented examples of 'good' and 'bad' coordination in the gesture of lip closing earlier (see Hulstijn, and Van Lieshout, in press). The relative time at which peak velocity is reached is often selected as the most critical measure (see Alfonso, 1991; Hulstijn, Van Lieshout and Peters, 1991). In our examples, taken from a study by Van Lieshout, Alfonso, Hulstijn, and Peters (1994), the moments of peak velocity seemed to be closely aligned in time for the control speaker and dispersed over a long period for the stuttering subject. Other measures of discoordination that have been tested are the sequential patterning of the articulatory movements and whether the velocity profile is not bell-shaped but has multiple peaks.

In a recent study by Alfonso and Van Lieshout (1997), many measures of the movements of the three articulators involved in lip closure were compared, such as peak and relative displacement, and temporal stability and sequence pattern. Some differences between the group of stuttering individuals and the control group were found but they were not stable over sessions and they changed (for some subjects quite dramatically) over speech rate, which varied between slow, normal and fast. The most impressive finding was the large variability between subjects, between sessions and between speech rates.

Stability and flexibility

This variability constitutes a large problem for the measurement of discoordination. The implicit notion in dynamic models is that some invariant characteristics underlie normal speech production. These relatively stable attributes will not only characterize the nature of speech motor control but will also provide measures for abnormal movement execution (Alfonso and Van Lieshout, 1997). However, variability, like a coin, has two sides. The bad side is its instability. Viewed from that side, a large variation suggests a lack of control. However, the other side of variability is flexibility. A high amount of motor skill allows flexible adaptation if required by the circumstances, or if there are no specific reasons to repeat the movements exactly as before. Viewed from this side a stable movement pattern may be a sign of a lack of skill. Stability has turned into rigidity, into a non-flexible mode of control, used as a strategy to overcome coordination problems. Other strategies may be to freeze degrees of freedom, as when subjects perform lip closure (a three degrees of freedom movement) by stiffening the upper lip or by using only the lower lip or the jaw. The deliberate reduction of degrees of freedom is a strategy that is commonly used in the beginning phase of learning a new skill. This suggests that it might also be used when the skill is not sufficiently mastered or when the system creates unpredictable or 'noisy' output.

The idea that variability may have two meanings (instability and flexibility) and that stability has two interpretations (rigidity versus stable control) suggests that one has to devise methods to disentangle stability from rigidity, and flexibility from unpredictability. One way to do this might be to push the system very close to, or even over, its limits and thereby remove the freedom of deliberately choosing alternative modes of control. The highest possible speed that an individual may achieve can also be used to characterize the amount of skill (or fluency) of an individual subject (Hulstijn and Van Lieshout, 1995). One can also increase demands on flexibility by requiring sudden changes of an utterance. The effect of unexpected perturbations may reveal instability but these are only suggestions that have to be put to experimental test.

The measurement of relative phase

An additional possibility is to use another measure for coordination. A promising candidate, which has recently been advanced by Van Lieshout, Hulstijn, Alfonso and Peters (1997), is the measurement of continuous relative phase. This measure is illustrated in Figure 42.1.

The subject is repeating the utterance 'ipa', and he tries to increase speech rate. In the left part of the figure we see the regular repetitive movements of the upper and lower lips, moving in counter phase. The phase relation of these two signals is not measured only at lip closing but is estimated continuously (see Van Lieshout et al. 1997, for details) showing a more-or-less straight line until at about the middle of the figure this stable counterphase relation is disturbed. The subject has probably reached a certain limit forcing him to continue with increasing his speed but with reduced movement amplitude. It is interesting that this sudden 'discoordination' could not be detected by acoustical or perceptual methods.

In the experiments performed by Van Lieshout et al. (1997) subjects were asked to increase the rate at which they repeated non-word utterances like 'api' and 'ipa'. We emphasized in our instructions that accuracy must be maintained and should not be traded against speed. With this procedure many control speakers can be brought to a point where they lose their fluency. This loss of coupling stability is clearly revealed by the continuous estimate of relative phase.

Stuttering viewed as a deficiency in speech motor skill

Skill is a fundamental concept both in the programming approach and from a dynamic perspective. Learning a motor skill proceeds through stages from a cognitive stage to automatic performance or, according to the dynamic approach, from forming a coordinative structure (dis-

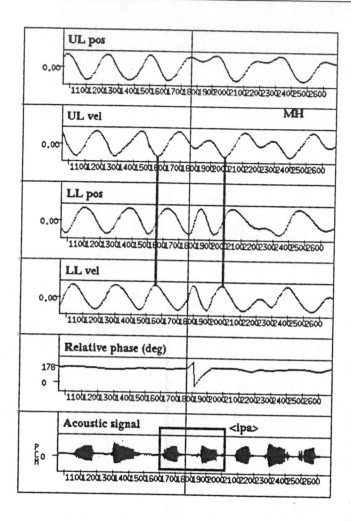

Figure 42.1. Illustration of the continuous measurement of relative phase. Upper lip (UL) and lower lip (LL) position and velocity signals are normalized and their phase is calculated. Only the difference between upper and lower lip phase (called 'relative' phase) is shown, as well as the acoustic signal. A normal speaker (MH) tries to increase the movement speed while repeatedly uttering the non-word 'ipa'. Just to the right of the long vertical marker in the middle of the figure, the lower lip position signal (LL pos) shows a fast full closure, but the upper lip (UL pos) seems unable to follow, which results in a sudden drop of stability in relative phase. Note the quick return to a stable coupling in the next cycles, but now with a different pattern of closing and opening movements for UL and LL.

covering how movement variables are related), to acquiring control (assigning values to the movement variables), and finally to reaching a skill (when the optimal values have been learned). Individuals may differ largely in the amount of speech motor skill that they have achieved or that they can ever reach. This might be seen as a continuum. We suppose that stuttering individuals compared to normal speakers are more toward the low end of a speech motor skill continuum. They reach the maximum movement rate – the rate at which one begins to show disfluencies – at a lower frequency than non-stuttering individuals. Every extra demand taxes their limited speech motor skill strongly and lowers their optimal frequency even more.

It might be added, that 'stuttering is an extremely nonlinear disorder', to quote Smith (1997: 144). Viewed from a dynamic perspective it can easily be understood that small changes in underlying factors can have a dramatic impact on the output of a system (Smith, 1997). Many of the variables that have long been known to affect stuttering frequency may have a motor component which may explain such a 'dramatic impact' on fluency. One of these variables is speech rate or, more precisely, movement rate. Movement rate has to be distinghuished from speech rate, because the latter is influenced to a large extent by pauses and steady state durations. The motor implications of this variable have been discussed in the previous section. Choral reading and singing, being conditions in which stuttering is reduced markedly, may also have strong motor implications (cf. Stager and Ludlow, 1993). Movement rate is usually lower in singing, less accurate articulation is required, and the external timing can provide an 'entrainment' signal which may enhance coordination. The latter would also hold for metronome pacing or another supply of an external rhythm, which enhance fluency. Masking noise and delayed or altered auditory feedback may derive their positive effects on fluency enhancement from the fact that the speaker is unable to hear his own voice with great precision and as a result begins to speak with less precise articulated movements and without much intonation. Other speech characteristics that affect fluency, such as loudness, stress, and duration, may have their effect on stuttering because they change the speech motor demands in terms of coordination, timing and accuracy. Emotional and motivational effects on speech fluency will influence the motor aspects of speech just as well as they influence motor performance in sport. Finally, the demonstrated effects of cognitive and attentional variables on stuttering frequency (e.g. Bosshardt, 1997) may also be explained by their effects on the motor aspects of the task.

A motor-skill approach has one serious disadvantage: it evades the problem of specifying which of the possible components of a motor skill is particularly vulnerable. It is still a family of approaches or theories. This, however, may also be its strength. Many authors have presented a multifactorial model. A few of them would feel seriously misunderstood if their theory were be characterized only by its position in the list of stages and processes given in Table 42.1. This holds strongly for McClean (1997) and Smith (1997), but it is also true for distinguished scholars in stuttering as Starkweather (1987) or Van Riper (1982). A multifactorial model may also help in explaining the very high intersubject variability between persons who stutter. It is quite likely that stuttering individuals will differ in the relative amount in which various skill components, like the learning of sequence patterns, force regulation, timing, initiation and availability or use of feedback, are affected. This suggests that assessment procedures should encompass all these components. We hope to have demonstrated that kinematic measures of accuracy and coordination might offer a valuable contribution to this assessment.

References

Adams MR (1985) Laryngeal onset and reaction time of stutterers. In Curlee RF, Perkins WH (Eds) Nature and Treatment of Stuttering: New Directions. San Diego: College-Hill Press, pp 89–104.

Alfonso PJ (1991) Implications of the concept underlying task-dynamic modeling on kinematic studies of stuttering. In Peters HFM, Hulstijn W, Starkweather CW (Eds) Speech Motor Control and Stuttering. Amsterdam: Elsevier Science Publishers, pp 79–100.

Alfonso PJ, Van Lieshout PHHM (1997) Spatial and temporal variability in obstruent gestural specification by stutterers and controls: Comparisons across sessions. In Hulstijn W, Peters HFM, Van Lieshout PHHM (Eds) Speech Production: Motor Control Brain Research and Fluency Disorders. Amsterdam: Elsevier Science, pp 151–60.

Bosshardt HG (1997) Mental effort and speech fluency. In Hulstijn W, Peters HFM, Van Lieshout PHHM (Eds) Speech Production: Motor Control Brain Research and Fluency Disorders. Amsterdam: Elsevier Science, pp 503–14.

Browman CE, Goldstein L (1997) The gestural phonology model. In Hulstijn W, Peters HFM, Van Lieshout PHHM (Eds) Speech Production: Motor Control Brain Research and Fluency Disorders. Amsterdam: Elsevier Science Publishers, pp 57–72.

De Nil LF (1994) The role of oral sensory feedback in the coordination of articulatory movements in adults who stutter. Journal of Fluency Disorders 19: 169–70.

Franken MC, Boves L, Peters HFM, Webster RL (1995) Perceptual rating instrument for speech evaluation of stuttering treatment. Journal of Speech and Hearing Research 38: 280–88.

Grosjean M, Van Galen GP, De Jong P, Van Lieshout PHHM, Hulstijn W (1997) Is stuttering caused by failing neuromuscular force control? In Hulstijn W, Peters HFM, Van Lieshout PHHM (Eds) Speech Production: Motor Control Brain Research and Fluency Disorders. Amsterdam: Elsevier Science, pp 197–204.

Howell P, El-Yaniv N, Powell DJ (1987) Factors affecting fluency in stutterers when speaking under altered auditory feedback. In HFM Peters and W Hulstijn (Eds) Speech Motor Dynamics in Stuttering. Wien: Springer, pp 361–9.

Howell P, Au-Yeung J, Rustin L (1997) Clock and motor variances in lip-tracking: A comparison between children who stutter and those who do not. In Hulstijn W, Peters HFM, Van Lieshout PHHM (Eds) Speech Production: Motor Control Brain Research and Fluency Disorders. Amsterdam: Elsevier Science, pp 573–8.

Hulstijn W, Van Lieshout PHHM, Peters HFM (1991) On the measurement of coordination. In Peters HFM, Hulstijn W, Starkweather CW (Eds) Speech Motor Control and Stuttering. Amsterdam: Elsevier Science Publishers, pp 211–30.

Hulstijn W, Van Lieshout PHHM (1995) Motor coordination in speech. In Starkweather CW, Peters HFM (Eds) Stuttering: Proceedings of the First World Congress on Fluency Disorders. The International Fluency Association, University Press Nijmegen, The Netherlands, pp 3–5.

Hulstijn W, Peters HFM, Van Lieshout PHHM (1997) (Eds) Speech Production: Motor Control Brain Research and Fluency Disorders. Amsterdam: Elsevier Science.

Hulstijn W, Van Lieshout PHHM (in press) Speech Motor Production and Dysfluency. Nijmegen Institute for Cognition and Information (NICI), Internal Report, 97–102.

Kalinowski J, Armson J, Stuart A, Hargrave S, Sark S, Macleod J (1995) Effect of alterations in auditory feedback on stuttering frequency during fast and normal speech rates. In Starkweather CW, Peters HFM (Eds) Stuttering: Proceedings of the First World Congress on Fluency Disorders. The International Fluency Association, University Press Nijmegen, The Netherlands, pp 51–55.

Kalveram KT, Natke U (1997) Stuttering and misguided learning of articulation and phonation or why it is extremely difficult to measure the physical properties of limbs. In Hulstijn W, Peters HFM, Van Lieshout PHHM (Eds) Speech Production: Motor Control Brain Research and Fluency Disorders. Amsterdam: Elsevier Science, pp 89–98.

Kelso JAS (1995) Dynamic Patterns: the Self-Organization of Brain and Behavior. Cambridge MA: MIT Press.

Kent RD (1997) Speech motor models and developments in neurophysiological science: new perspectives. In Hulstijn W, Peters HFM, Van Lieshout PHHM (Eds) Speech Production: Motor Control Brain Research and Fluency Disorders. Amsterdam: Elsevier Science, pp 13–36.

Levelt WJM (1989) Speaking: From Intention to Articulation. Cambridge MA: MIT Press.

Levelt WJM (1992) Accessing words in speech production: Stages Processes and Representation. Cognition 42: 1–22.

Ludlow CL, Siren K, Zikria M (1997) Speech production learning in adults with chronic developmental stuttering. In Hulstijn W, Peters HFM, Van Lieshout PHHM (Eds) Speech Production: Motor Control Brain Research and Fluency Disorders. Amsterdam: Elsevier Science, pp 221–30.

McClean MD (1997) Functional components of the motor system: an approach to understanding the mechanisms of speech disfluency. In Hulstijn W, Peters HFM, Van Lieshout PHHM (Eds) Speech Production: Motor Control Brain Research and Fluency Disorders. Amsterdam: Elsevier Science, pp 99–118.

Neilson MD, Neilson PD (1987) Speech motor control and stuttering: A computational model of adaptive sensory-motor processing. Speech Communication 6: 325–33.

Peters HFM, Hulstijn W (Eds) (1987) Speech Motor Dynamics in Stuttering. Wien: Springer Verlag.

Peters HFM, Hulstijn W, Starkweather CW (1989) Acoustic and physiological reaction times of stutterers and nonstutterers. Journal of Speech and Hearing Research 32: 668–80.

Peters HFM, Hulstijn W, Starkweather CW (Eds) (1991) Speech Motor Control and Stuttering. Amsterdam: Elsevier Science.

Postma A, Kolk H (1993) The covert repair hypothesis: Prearticulatory repair processes in normal and stuttered disfluencies. Journal of Speech and Hearing Research 36: 472–87.

Saltzman E (1991) The task-dynamic model in speech production. In Peters HFM, Hulstijn W, Starkweather CW (Eds) Speech motor control and stuttering. Amsterdam: Elsevier Science, pp 37–52.

Schmidt RA (1988) Motor Control and Learning: A Behavioral Emphasis. Champaign, IL: Human Kinetics.

Smith A (1997) Dynamic interactions of factors that impact speech motor stability in children and adults. In Hulstyn W, Peters HFM, van Lieshout PHHM (Eds) Speech Production: Motor Control, Brain Research and Fluency Disorders. Amsterdam: Elsevier Science: 143–49.

Stager SV, Ludlow CL (1993) Speech production changes under fluency-evoking conditions in nonstuttering speakers. Journal of Speech and Hearing Research 36: 245–53.

Starkweather CW (1987) Fluency and Stuttering. Englewood Cliffs NJ: Prentice-Hall.

Starkweather CW (1995) A simple theory of stuttering. Journal of Fluency Disorders 20: 91–116.

Van Lieshout PHHM, Peters HFM, Hulstijn W, Starkweather CW (1993) Physiological differences between stutterers and nonstutterers in perceptually fluent speech: EMG amplitude and duration. Journal of Speech and Hearing Research 36: 55–63.

Van Lieshout PHHM, Alfonso PJ, Hulstijn W, Peters HFM (1994) Eloctromagnetic articulography (EMA). In Maarse FJ, Akkerman AE, Brand AN, Mulder LJM, Van der Stelt MJ (Eds) Computers in Psychology 5: Applications, Methods, and Instrumentation. Lisse: Swets, Zeitlinger, pp. 62–76.

Van Lieshout PHHM (1995) Motor planning and articulation in fluent speech of stutterers and nonstutterers. Nijmegen Institute for Cognition and Information, University Press Nijmegen, The Netherlands.

Van Lieshout PHHM, Hulstijn W, Peters HFM (1996a) Speech production in people who stutter: Testing the motor plan assembly hypothesis. Journal of Speech and Hearing Research 39: 76–92.

Van Lieshout PHHM, Hulstijn W, Peters HFM (1996b) From planning to articulation: what differentiates a person who stutters from a person who does not stutter? Journal of Speech and Hearing Research 39: 546–64.

Van Lieshout PHHM, Hulstijn W Alfonso PJ, Peters HFM (1997) Higher and lower order influences on the stability of the dynamic coupling between articulators. In Hulstijn W, Peters HFM, Van Lieshout PHHM (Eds) Speech Production: Motor Control Brain Research and Fluency Disorders. Amsterdam: Elsevier Science, pp. 161–70.

Van Riper C (1982) The Nature of Stuttering (2nd edn). Englewood Cliffs NJ: Prentice-Hall.

Zelaznik HN, Smith A, Franz EA, Ho M (in press) Differences in bimanual co-ordination associated with stuttering. Acta Psychologica.

Zimmermann G (1980) Stuttering: a disorder of movement. Journal of Speech and Hearing Research 23: 122–36.

Chapter 43
Control of Speech Rate and Rhythm in Patients With Left Hemisphere Lesions

KARIN DEGER AND WOLFRAM ZIEGLER

Introduction

Phonetic research on timing control in the speech of brain-damaged patients has shown that left-hemisphere lesions produce timing deficits not only at the segment level but also over larger-sized linguistic units (e.g. Gandour, Dechongkit, Ponglorpisit, Khunadorn and Boongird, 1993; Gandour, Dechongkit, Ponglorpisit and Khunadorn, 1994). The underlying problem of the aberrant timing patterns at the word and sentence level (e.g. 'excess and equal stress') in patients with non-fluent aphasia or apraxia of speech remains still unclear. The deviant metrical structures can be a consequence of articulatory or phonological problems at the segment level. Another possible explanation could be a general timing deficit.

Speech is a rhythmically organized behaviour like almost every skilled complex motor activity, e.g. handwriting or typing. The fundamental unit of the rhythmicity of speech appears to be the syllable (Kent, Mitchell and Sancier, 1991). An influential theory concerning the timing control of rhythmically organized motor sequences is the 'proportionate timing' model (see Viviani and Terzuolo, 1980; Viviani and Laissard, 1991). It predicts that ratios between successive time intervals remain approximately constant, irrespective of the speed at which the movement as a whole is executed. This invariance is also a basic assumption of the 'Generalized Motor Program' (GMP) (e.g. Wulf, 1992). The hypothesis is that the relative durations of the movement sequences are stored in a GMP, while a single rate parameter specifies the absolute durations. For speaking this would mean that the relative durations of successive syllables, the speech rhythm, is prestored in a GMP, whereas a single-rate parameter specifies the speech rate.

Search for evidence of proportional timing through a wide range of movement types led to conflicting opinions of this concept, and it is still unclear whether this model applies to speech (Löfqvist, 1991).

Methods

Procedures

To resolve the underlying problem of suprasegmental speech timing, the ratios of relative syllable durations were investigated in two different experiments. The subjects had to imitate or generate rhythmically structured speech and non-speech utterances at different rates. Two perceptual control experiments were also part of the whole examination procedure.

Experiment 1: syllable reiteration

The first experiment was a syllable reiteration task with minimal articulatory demands. First of all the subjects heard a rhythmically structured stimulus of four clicks. In the first stage of the experiment they had to imitate the rhythm, repeating the syllable 'da'; then they were asked to produce the same rhythm 'twice as fast' and 'still faster'. At the next stage the subjects heard the target rhythm again, but after the imitation they were required to speak the rhythm 'half as fast' and 'still slower'. The whole procedure was repeated twice. Figure 43.1 illustrates the investigation and analysis technique. Using the sound pressure level of the spoken syllables, the inter-syllable intervals were calculated from the onset of the ongoing syllable to the onset of the following syllable. The three acquired values (t1, t2, t3) were matched with the corresponding inter-syllable intervals of the target signal.

Syllable reiteration

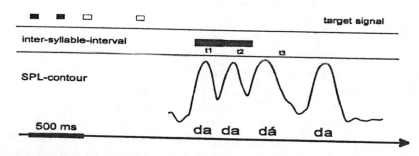

Figure 43.1. Determination of the inter-syllable intervals in the syllable reiteration task.

Experiment 2: word production

In the second experiment the demands from the artificial non-speech syllable reiteration task were stepped up to the level of word production. Two aspects were of interest:

(1) Does the variation of speech rate affect the relative durations of speech rhythm under the more natural, automatized condition of word production?
(2) Do increasing articulatory demands affect the speech rhythm?

The instruction was to speak the German word /apoteke/ ('pharmacy') at different rates. The word accent corresponds to the target stimulus of the syllable reiteration task of Experiment 1.

Experiment 3: perception tasks

Results in the literature hypothesize an 'internal clock' or a common timekeeping mechanism that is not modality-specific but is responsible for the timing in both production and perception (Keele, Pocorny, Corcos and Ivry, 1985; Keele and Ivry, 1990; Ivry and Hazeltine, 1995). If the underlying cause for deviant speech rhythm is a general timing deficit, the perception of time should also be impaired.

We wanted to investigate the perception of time by an interval discrimination task similar to the studies of Keele and co-workers (1985, 1990). Two time intervals were presented, separated by a pause of 1000 ms. The task was to decide whether the duration of the intervals was 'same' or 'different'. Interval-durations varied from 300 ms to 500 ms and were the same in half of the cases. In the remaining half the tones differed by a minimum of 80 ms and a maximum of 200 ms.

A pitch-perception task was designed as a control task for the perception of time. The subjects had to judge whether the pitches of two tones, separated by a pause of 200 ms, were 'same' or 'different'. Pure tones with a duration of 200 ms were chosen. The frequency varied between 487 Hz and 513 Hz. Here again, in half of the cases the tones were the same. In the remaining half the minimum difference was 10Hz, the maximum difference was 26Hz.

Sample

Thirty normal controls and 17 patients with lesions of the left hemisphere participated in the investigation. Eight patients were diagnosed as having apraxia of speech and aphasia, nine patients were diagnosed as having aphasia but no apraxia. In addition, 10 professional musicians were examined to see whether special rhythmic or timing skills affect the abilities investigated in the experiments described above.

Results

Figure 43.2 illustrates the performance of a professional musician whose timing is very likely to be perfect. Each bar represents one utterance. The long syllable (syllable 3) should, in the best case, be twice as long as the short syllables (syllables 1 and 2). The vertical lines show the rhythm of the target signal. As expected, the musician can handle the task very well. He achieves almost perfect imitation, and he precisely follows the instruction to speak 'twice as fast' and 'still faster' or to speak 'half as fast' and 'still slower'.

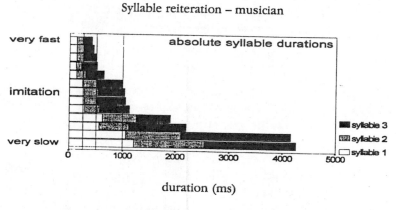

Syllable reiteration – musician

Figure 43.2. Absolute durations of the inter-syllable intervals for a professional musician in the syllable reiteration task.

The pattern found in the whole group of skilled musicians was also found in a group of normal controls, containing even explicitly unmusical subjects (Figure 43.3). The healthy controls can keep the absolute durations (Figure 43.3a), as well as the relative durations (Figure 43.3b) when they are asked to imitate the target signal. The variability increases when they are asked to modify the speech tempo. The diagram of the relative syllable durations shows that the deviation from the target rhythm (symbolized by the vertical lines) is increasing, with a tendency of scaling the syllables equally, under the extreme conditions of speaking very fast or very slowly.

Equally-scaled syllables are a frequent symptom of disordered speech. Figure 43.4a gives an illustrative example of this feature, generally called 'scanning speech'. It clearly shows a decomposition of the target rhythm (symbolized by the vertical lines) into three equally-scaled syllables, irrespective of the speech rate. This particular realization by an apraxic patient is not representative of the whole group of the investigated patients but these equally-scaled performances can be well identified among others in the presentation of the whole patient group (Figure 43.4b). In general, the performances of the whole group of patients with left brain lesions show a great variability over all conditions.

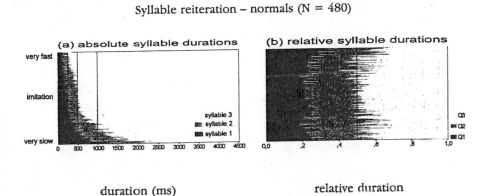

Figure 43.3. Absolute syllable durations (a) and relative syllable durations (b) of the normal controls.

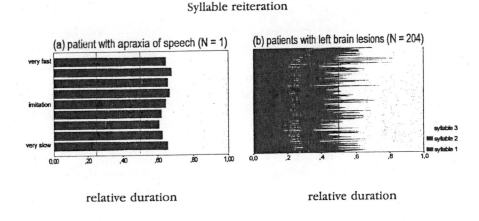

Figure 43.4. Example for equally-scaled syllables of (a) one apraxic patient and (b) performance of all patients with left brain lesions.

To find out the reason for the variability of the patients' performance it was necessary to separate patients with apraxia of speech from patients without apraxia of speech. Furthermore the Euclidean distance was calculated to have one single measure that represents the overall deviation of a subject from the target rhythm. The deviation from target rhythm for all groups and each condition is shown in Figure 43.5. The normals were able to hold the target rhythm very well when they spoke at a normal rate, but the deviation increased when they had to vary the speech rate. The patients with aphasia but no apraxia of speech produced a similar pattern, although at a worse level. They showed the smallest deviations at normal rate and increasing deviations when they had to vary the speech rate. In contrast, the patients with apraxia of speech maintained the rhythm best at slow to normal speaking rates, but the deviation increased abruptly when they spoke the rhythm at a faster rate. This might point to the fact that not the production of relative durations — i.e. the rhythm *per se* — is difficult for the apraxic patients investigated, but that the absolute durations, the speech rate, was their major problem. This explanation would not support a general timing deficit.

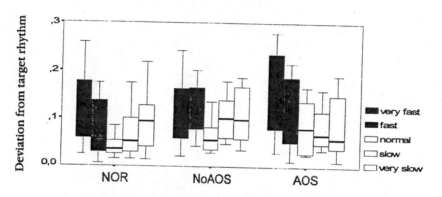

Syllable reiteration

Figure 43.5. Deviation from target rhythm for all groups and each condition in the syllable reiteration task. NOR = normals, NoAOS = patients with aphasia but no apraxia of speech, AOS = patients with apraxia of speech.

In the artificial syllable reiteration task none of the groups provided strong evidence for proportionate timing. Even for the healthy controls it was difficult to maintain the target rhythm under this non-automatized condition when they were asked to speak at faster or slower rates.

Provided that proportionate timing is a feature of skilled automatized movements, the relative syllable durations were investigated under more natural circumstances.

Figure 43.6 shows the deviation from normal rhythm, when speaking the word *Apotheke* ('pharmacy') at different rates. In contrast to the more artificial syllable reiteration task, the fast speaking rate did not affect proportionate timing in the normals. To speak at a faster rate seems to be a natural condition where automatized speaking can take place, but when the normals had to speak at a reduced rate the speech rhythm broke down and changed into controlled, non-automatized speech with a tendency to scale the syllables equally. It appeared difficult, even for the healthy controls, to preserve a normal word accent when speaking at a reduced rate.

The patients with aphasia but no apraxia of speech were able to maintain a normal word accent when they spoke at a normal rate. Probably they were no longer able to produce the word /apoteke/ as automatized speech as soon as they were asked to change the speech rate in any direction

In contrast to the phonologically easier syllable reiteration task, the apraxic patients showed no benefit in this task when they slowed down their speech rate. They showed large deviations from normal speech rhythm, irrespective of the speech rate. In this task they could choose their own speech rate and had no target rate to reach, so they adapted their speaking rate to their articulatory and phonological capabilities and spoke at a reduced rate in all conditions. This might be the reason why they failed to adopt a normal speech rhythm.

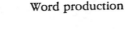

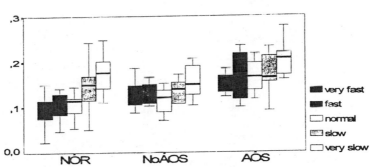

Figure 43.6. Deviation from normal speech rhythm when speaking the word /apoteke/ at different rates. NOR = normals, NoAOS = patients with aphasia but no apraxia of speech, AOS = patients with apraxia of speech.

These observations point to the fact that proportionate timing occurs only within a very narrow velocity range, when speech movement can proceed in an automatized way. Furthermore there are no grounds for the assumption that the underlying problem of aberrant metrical structures in the investigated patients is a general timing deficit.

Before rejecting the hypothesis of a general timing deficit as a possible explanation for deviant metrical structures the perception of time was investigated. As already mentioned, timing is assumed not to be modality specific. If the underlying problem of deviant metrical structures is a general timing deficit, the perception of time should also be problematic.

Figure 43.7 represents the percentage of errors of the three groups in discriminating time intervals (gray boxes) and pitch (white boxes). In each group the control task 'pitch perception' leads to a higher percentage of errors than interval discrimination but the results give no indication for a specific time perception deficit in the patient groups. The generally worse performance of the apraxic and non-apraxic patients could be interpreted as an unspecific result of an overall impairment, like reduced attention or memory deficits.

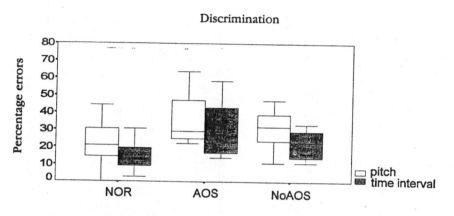

Figure 43.7. Percentage errors in the discrimination of pitch (white boxes) and time intervals (grey boxes). NOR = normals, NoAOS = patients with aphasia but no apraxia of speech, AOS = patients with apraxia of speech.

Preliminary conclusions

The invariance of relative durations, called 'proportionate timing', occurs only in skilled, automatized speech movements, and not under artificial conditions. With decreasing speech rate, the movement comes under 'closed-loop' control (Adams, 1971) and is not longer automatized. It is difficult, even for the healthy controls, to preserve speech rhythm when speaking at a slow rate. This might be the reason for the deviant metrical structures of patients with apraxia of speech. Increasing speech control prevents automatized speech and produces a breakdown of the speech rhythm.

These observations do not support the hypothesis that deficient time structures 'on the surface', i.e. a deviant speech rhythm, result from a general timing deficit in the sense of a defective 'internal clock'.

References

Adams JA (1971) A closed-loop theory of motor learning. Journal of Motor Behavior 3: 111–49.

Gandour J, Dechongkit S, Ponglorpisit S, Khunadorn F, Boongird P (1993) Intraword timing relations in Thai after unilateral brain damage. Brain and Language 45: 160–79.

Gandour J, Dechongkit S, Ponglorpisit S, Khunadorn F (1994) speech timing at the sentence level in Thai after unilateral brain damage. Brain and Language 46: 419–38.

Ivry RB, Hazeltine E (1995) Perception and production of temporal intervals across a range of durations: evidence for a common timing mechanism. Journal of Experimental Psychology: Human Perception and Performance 21: 3–18.

Keele SW, Pocorny R, Corcos D, Ivry RB (1985) Do perception and motor production share common timing mechanisms: a correlational analysis. Acta Psychologia 60: 173–91.

Keele SW, Ivry R (1990) Does the cerebellum provide a common computation for diverse tasks? A timing hypothesis. Annuals of the New York Academy of Sciences 608: 179–211.

Kent RD, Mitchell PR, Sancier M (1991) Evidence and role of rhythmic organization in early vocal development in human infants. In Fagard J, Wolff PH (Eds) The Development of Timing Control and Temporal Organization in Coordinated Action. Amsterdam, Elsevier Science Publishers, pp. 135–49.

Löfqvist A (1991) Proportional timing in speech motor control. Journal of Phonetics 19: 343–50.

Viviani P, Laissard, G (1991) Timing control in motor sequences. In Fagard J, Wolff PH (Eds) The Development of Timing Control Temporal Organisation in Coordinated Action. Amsterdam, Elsevier Science Publishers, pp 1–36.

Viviani P, Terzuolo C (1980) Space time invariance in learned motor skills. In Stelmach GE, Requin J (Eds) Tutorials in Motor Behavior. Amsterdam: North Holland Publishing Company, pp 525–33.

Wulf G (1992) The learning of generalized motor programs a motor schemata: Effects of KR relative frequency and contextual interference. Journal of Human Movement Studies 23: 53–76.

Chapter 44
Speech Encoding and Apraxia of Speech: Evidence from Xhosa

PATRICIA MAVIMBELA, GRZEGORZ DOGIL AND JÖRG MAYER

Introduction

Most of the explanatory approaches in recent research refer to some higher level of motor control to describe the underlying pathomechanisms in apraxia of speech (Darley, 1969; Rosenbek, Kent, LaPointe, 1984; Ziegler and von Cramon, 1989; Lebrun, 1990). What all these approaches have in common is firstly that the crucial distortion that causes apraxia of speech (AOS) lies outside the cognitive language system and, secondly, that all these models emphasize the term *apraxia* rather than the term *speech*. However, since pure AOS affects only oral performance and since patients suffering from AOS produce not only phonetic errors (eg. distortions) but also phonemic errors (eg. substitutions, additions, metatheses, deletions) it is reasonable to consider a linguistically based interpretation of this disturbance. In a number of recent publications we have argued that it is not the precision of the motor control but rather the mapping from the phonological to the phonetic representation that underlies the symptomatic disabilities of patients suffering from AOS (Vollmer, 1993; Mayer, 1995; Dogil, Mayer, Vollmer, 1996). In particular, we have argued that overspecified phonetic representations are responsible for the loss of ability to produce highly encoded speech. We have illustrated this hypothesis by investigating the degree of coarticulation across various phonetic (lip rounding coarticulation at a long distance) and phonological (stress and morphonological boundary) contexts. The sound material that we have used in this research consisted of maximally underspecified sounds, i.e. laryngeals. Laryngeals are underspecified, coarticulatorily transparent and are always strongly encoded within larger linguistic units (Keating, 1988; Stemberger, 1993). This, according to our hypothesis, makes them difficult for patients suffering from AOS. The fact that the patients do show difficulties with laryngeals (cf. Mayer, 1995) presents a challenge to explanatory theories of apraxia based on motor control because the degree of motor complexity required in the production of laryngeals (e.g. the sound [h]) is minimal compared to the motor complexity required for the production of other sounds.

In the present contribution we evaluate the overspecification hypothesis on apraxia of speech with sound material covering the other extreme of speech encoding. We report findings of experiments regarding the performance of a native speaker of Xhosa suffering from AOS. The consonantal system of Xhosa makes use of 3 clicks and 5 different voice qualities, resulting in 15 phonologically distinct click sounds. Clicks, as opposed to laryngeals, require an extreme degree of motor precision and are phonologically highly specified and unencoded. One would expect a large number of errors in click production due to motor complexity according to motor control models of speech apraxia. On the other hand, our overspecification hypothesis predicts fewer problems with clicks because maximally specified and unencoded sounds are supposed to be the 'normal' condition in apraxic speech production.

Gestural properties of velaric initiation

Precise timing and gestural implementation of the individual components of velic suction (oralic initiation) are essential in the production of any click. A lot of research has been devoted to the articulatory description of clicks in various languages and the picture that emerges from this research is relatively clear.[1] The fully-fledged production of any click consists of three distinct phases: (a) the closure phase, which in itself consists of two closures, the initiatory closure, which is velar for all clicks and the articulatory closure, which is coronal for all oral clicks and labial for the labial click; (b) the suction phase, during which the air in the cavity between the two closures is rarefied by the downward movement of the tongue, and (c) the release phase, which again consists of two releases, the articulatory release, which has been called influx in traditional descriptions and which is considered to determine the click type (Ladefoged and Traill, 1994) and the initiatory release, always velar or uvular, called efflux by Beach (1938) and referred to as the click accompaniment in Ladefoged and Traill (1994). All these phases are timed in such a way that an acoustically crisp (cf. Johnson, 1993) and perceptually salient sound is produced (cf. Traill, 1994). The salience is concentrated within the period of the noiseburst (the release phase) itself (cf. Traill, 1994; Dogil, Roux and Mayer, 1996), because clicks do not appear to coarticulate with their phonetic context (cf. Sands, 1992; Dogil et al. 1996).

In summary, we are dealing with sounds that are articulated extremely precisely and that aquire their clear perceptual structure from this complex articulation. Phonetically, these sounds are not encoded in the speech string because the noiseburst properties are unique to them and are not shared with the rest of the speech signal.

Phonological opacity of clicks

Click consonants prove to be resistant to phonological processes induced by their environment. Out of approximately 36 click-using languages on record there is not a single one in which clicks are synchronically substituted by different sounds. This is true both of the indigenous click languages of the Khoisan group and of the Bantu languages. Synchronically, clicks do not undergo phonological changes, neither in a phonetic, phonological or lexical context nor context-independently as a whole class (cf. Dogil and Luschtzky, 1990).

The resistance to context influence and the inability to influence the immediate context is also a feature of clicks in diachronic phonology. Traill and Vossen (1996) provide a complete list of diachronic changes of clicks in Khoisan languages and there appears to be not a single one among them that is phonetically or phonologically conditioned: 'The changes we have been examining are context-free in the sense that they affect a whole class of sounds no matter what the phonological or phonetic context' (Traill and Vossen, 1996: 30).

This context-free behaviour is to be expected of unencoded sounds. In terms of representation, sounds that do not interact with the context should be maximally specified. Indeed, all attempts at representing clicks in terms of feature geometry have assigned very complex structures to them.

A case of apraxia of speech in Xhosa[2]

Subject

The patient MQ, a 23-year-old female, monolingually raised speaker of Xhosa from the Western Cape province, suffered from a cerebro-vascular accident in March 1993. The CVA destroyed large parts of the left perisylvian cortex. Neurologically, the patient suffered a mild paralysis in the right side of her body and a substantial language problem. No other cognitive impairment could be diagnosed. The motor control over the right extremities has been steadily getting better whereas the language impairment turned out to be more severe and lasting. After a phase of initial spontaneous improvement that particularly involved language comprehension as well as the skills of reading and writing, the patient reached a stage at which no further improvement of her language ability could be observed. Due to her normal cognitive capacity MQ was admitted to school again in 1995. Her speech production, however, was so defective that she was referred to the Department of Logopedics of the Groote Schuur Hospital in Cape Town for ambulant speech therapy. It was then that she was diagnosed for apraxia of speech. She had been receiving speech therapy in blocks of weekly sessions ever since.

Her problems were exclusively restricted to speech production. She showed strong articulatory search movements, which are typical for AOS. Her production problems were not caused by any significant deficit of the speech musculature either. The pattern of mistakes, which showed that phonological substitutions and uncertainties at the beginnings of words clearly outnumbered other error types (i.e. phonological insertions and deletions as well as phonetic distortions), suggested a case of AOS. As is the case for most patients suffering from AOS, the patient was aware of her problem and was frustrated by it.

Method

Formal testing of the phonological and phonetic structure of MQ's speech was based on the data collected between March and July 1996. The data consisted of the recordings of a repetition test that had been devised in order to test the pattern and variability of the patient's speech production and of numerous audio and video recordings of spontaneous speech. The repetition test consisted of a list of words that had been selected by the second author from a commercially available dictionary of the most useful (i.e. frequent) Xhosa words and phrases. Words with an unmarked segmental and prosodic structure (e.g. *dada* 'swim'; *lila* 'cry') were placed next to words with several clicks (e.g. *cocisisa* [|ɔ|isisa] 'clean'; nqonqoza [ŋ̊ŋ̊za] 'knock'). The samples of spontaneous speech consisted of audio and video recordings of MQ's speech. The results presented below are based on an analysis of a transcription of a video recording of approximately 15 minutes. Only categorical (i.e. phonological) errors were counted.

Results

Regarding the repetition test, MQ did indeed make variable mistakes. There were, however, very few of them (altogether 17 errors in three test sessions) and they all involved vowels and coronal obstruents [d] and [s]. MQ showed no problems or hesitations in the production of any of the 15 phonemic clicks. Words with ejective affricates were also mastered without difficulty. In general, MQ had rather minor problems in this test situation. This was in sharp contrast to her productions in spontaneous speech.

Let us start reviewing the error patterns in spontaneous speech by analysing the production of vowels. Xhosa has five phonemic vowels [i e a o u] that are highly underspecified and in normal speech coarticulated with the sounds in their context (except for the clicks, cf. Dogil et al. 1996). Of the five vowels in the system, the peripheral ones [i a u] are considered to be less marked — i.e. less specified — than the other two vowels. The overspecification hypothesis predicts a large number of errors for vowels and a quantitative difference in a number of substitutions among the less specified [i a u] and the more specified [e o]. This prediction is supported by the data on vowel errors given in Table 44.1.

Table 44.1. Pattern of errors in Xhosa vowels

	vowels				
Orthography	i	e	a	o	u
IPA	i	e	a	o	u
Errors/Item	30	9	24	6	27
Errors/Class					96

The criteria of underspecification and markedness also appear to be the driving force behind the errors made in the production of approximants and nasals. Among these sounds, most errors are made among the least marked sounds [l m n] (cf. Avery and Rice, 1989; Paradis and Prunet, 1989). Consider the data in table 44.2.

Table 44.2. Pattern of errors in Xhosa approximants and nasals

	approximants				nasals - plain and breathy voiced						
Orth.	r	l	w	j	m	n	ny	n'	mh	nh	nyh
IPA	r	l	w	j	m	n	ɲ	ŋ	m̥	n̥	ɲ̥
Err/Itm	0	15	3	6	21	15	0	0	0	2	0
Err/Class			24								38

A similar vulnerability to errors can be observed in Xhosa pulmonic stops (consider Table 44.3). Across all categories of pulmonic stops (voiceless aspirated, voiced, murmured voiced) the coronal ones show the highest degree of error.

Table 44.3. Pattern of errors in Xhosa pulmonic stops

	aspirated stops				voiced stops			murmured stops				
Orth.	ph	th	tyh	kh	mb	nd	ndy	ng	bh	d	dy	g
IPA	pʰ	tʰ	cʰ	kʰ	b	d	ɉ	g	b̤	d̤	ɉ	g̈
Err/Itm	3	10	0	9	2	36	3	9	0	6	3	1
Err/Class			22					50				10

In the case of pulmonic fricatives presented in Table 44.4. The biggest challenge for the patient seems to be the voiceless coronal [s]. The much more marked lateral fricatives are never substituted (they are frequent in Xhosa, and they are often encountered in a vulnerable, initial position).

Table 44.4. Pattern of errors in Xhosa pulmonic fricatives

	central voiceless					central voiced				lateral	
Orth.	f	s	sh	rh	h	v	z	gr	h	hl	dl
IPA	f	s	ʃ	x	h	v	z	ɣ	ɦ	ɬ	ɮ
Err/Itm	2	30	0	0	0	0	8	0	0	0	0
Err/Class			32				8				0

As far as pulmonic obstruents are concerned, the rendition of affricates is error-free in those parts of MQ's spontaneous speech that we have examined. Note that the degree of motor control (particularly timing control) required for the production of these sounds is probably not smaller than in the articulation of clicks. Still, our AOS patient appears to have no problems with motor control in the timing domain, if this domain is phonologically fully specified.

Table 44.5 lists the phonological errors that MQ made in the production of glottalic obstruents. Xhosa has one implosive stop, four ejective stops and five ejective affricates. Ejective affricates, which are gesturally more complex than the other sounds of this class, apparently provided no problems for our patient. However, these sounds are quite rare in Xhosa (cf. Roux, 1992) and might be underrepresented in our database. The implosive <ɓ> appeared to be very vulnerable, as did the velar and the coronal ejectives. As far as the quality of the errors is concerned, the implosives and ejectives alternated with pulmonic stops.

Table 44.5. Pattern of errors in Xhosa glottalic obstruents

	impl. stop	ejective stops				ejective affricates				
Orth.	b	p	t	ty	k	mf	ts	tsh	kr	ntl
IPA	ɓ	p'	t'	c'	k'	p͡f'	t͡s'	t͡ʃ'	k͡x'	t͡ɬ'
Err./Item	15	0	5	0	30	0	0	0	0	0
Err./Class	15			35						0

Velaric obstruents (clicks) provided no problems for MQ. The data given in table 44.6 illustrate this clearly. In the whole database we found only two cases in which a dental, nasal click <ǀ̃> was replaced. The critical word was *incwadi* [ǀ̃ | vadi] 'book' and the click was replaced with the nasal [m] on one occasion and the nasal [n] on another. None of the remaining 14 phonemic clicks presented any serious challenge to the appraxic patient.[3] It can therefore be stated that the speaker suffering from AOS had perfect control over the timing structure of the influx ([!] is an abrupt click, [|] and [|||] are noisy), the type of a stricture ([|||] is a lateral click, [||] and [!] are central), and the intricacies of the accompaniment (nasality, aspiration, voicing, breathiness).

Table 44.6. Pattern of errors in Xhosa velaric obstruents (clicks)

	voiceless			aspirated			voiced-breathy		
Orth.	c	q	x	ch	qh	xh	gc	gq	gx
IPA	ǀ	ǃ	ǁ	ǀʰ	ǃʰ	ǁʰ	ᶢǀ	ᶢǃ	ᶢǁ
L & T	kǀ	kǃ	kǁ	kǀʰ	kǃʰ	kǁʰ	ɡǀ	ɡǃ	ɡǁ
Err./Item									

		nasal			nasal breathy	
Orth.	nc	nq	nx	ngc	ngq	ngx
IPA	ᵑǀ	ᵑǃ	ᵑǁ	ᵑǀ	ᵑǃ	ᵑǁ
L & T	ŋǀ	ŋǃ	ŋǁ	ŋ̈ǀ	ŋ̈ǃ	ŋ̈ǁ
Err./Item	2					

Discussion

In summary, the pattern of errors produced by MQ supports our phonological hypothesis rather than the classical motor control hypothesis. Notice that practically no errors were found in clicks and affricates, which, within all accounts of speech science, are gesturally complex. On the other hand, most errors were found in vowels and coronal consonants, which in many phonological models have been described as being underspecified. Especially in a relatively simple five-vowel system like the one found in Xhosa, vowels are considered to be highly underspecified and phonetically encoded, i.e. transparent to the influence of the consonantal context. The loss of underspecification and phonetic transparency, which we consider to be the underlying distortion in AOS, is the crucial factor explaining the large number of errors in this group of sounds. Similarly, it has been argued by Avery and Rice (1989), Paradis and Prunet (1989) and others that coronals are the least specified and most transparent of obstruent sounds. The claim is that, from a merely technical point of view, coronals either do not have to be specified for the place features or lack the place node altogether. This makes them as transparent as the laryngeals and therefore, assuming our phonological explanation of the selective impairment found in AOS, particularly vulnerable.

Conclusion

In this paper we have suggested that there exists a selective impairment of the phonology-phonetics interface and that it is illustrated by the syndrome of pure apraxia of speech. We showed in the analysis of clicks and other complex sounds in Xhosa that apraxia of speech can hardly be accounted for by theories of gestural complexity and motor control. We have shown that the theories of motor control make predictions that are not supported by the AOS data. The linguistic overspecification hypothesis that we have advocated predicts that phonologically under-specified and phonetically transparent units of speech are the most difficult to master by AOS patients. The analysis of laryngeals and clicks, which form the two opposite poles of the underspecification/encoding spectrum, points to the validity of our linguistic hypothesis.

References

Avery P, Rice K (1989) Segment structure and coronal underspecification. Phonology 6: 179–200.

Beach DM (1938) The Phonetics of the Hottentot Language. Cambridge: W. Heffer & Sons Ltd.

Darley FL (1969) The classification of output disturbance in neurologic com-munication disorders. Paper presented at the American Speech and Hearing Association Convention, Chicago.

Dogil G, Luschtzky HC (1990) Notes on sonority and segmental strength. Rivista di Linguistica 2: 3–54.

Dogil G, Mayer J, Vollmer K (1996) A representational account for apraxia of speech. In Powell TW (Ed) Pathologies of Speech and Language: Contributions of Clinical Phonetics and Linguistics. New Orleans, LA: ICPLA, pp. 95–9.

Dogil G, Roux J, Mayer J (1996) Unencoded Speech: Clicks and their Accompaniments in Xhosa. Paper presented at Phonologica 1996, Vienna.

Johnson K (1993) Acoustic and auditory analysis of Xhosa clicks and pulmonics. UCLA Working Papers in Phonetics 83: 33–45.

Keating PA (1988) Underspecification in phonetics. Phonology 5: 275–92.

Ladefoged P, Traill A (1994) Clicks and their accompaniements. Journal of Phonetics 22: 33–64.

Lebrun Y (1990) Apraxia of speech: A critical review. Journal of Neurolinguistics 5: 379–406.

Mayer J (1995) Phonologisch-phonetische Überspezifizierung bei Sprechapraxie. Phonetik-AIMS 2(3): 35–155 (Working Papers of the Chair of Experimental Phonetics, University of Stuttgart).

Paradis C, Prunet JF (1989) On coronal transparency. Phonology 6: 317–48.

Rosenbek JC, Kent RD, LaPointe L (1984) Apraxia of Speech: An Overview and Some Perspectives. In Rosenbek JC, McNeil M, Aronson A (Eds) Apraxia of Speech: Physiology, Acoustics, Linguistic Management. San Diego: College Hill Press.

Roux JC (1992) On Ingressive Glottalic and Velaric Articulations in Xhosa. Proceedings of the XIIth ICPhS Aix-en-Provence, pp 158–61.

Roux JC (1993) An Electro-Palatographic Study of Xhosa clicks. Paper presented to the 7th ALASA Conference, Johannesburg.

Sands B (1992) An Acoustic Study of Xhosa Clicks. Proceedings of the XIIth ICPhS Aix-en-Provence, pp 130–33.

Scharf G, Hertrich I, Dogil G, Roux J (1995) An Articulatory Description of Clicks by Means of Electromagnetic Articulography. Proceedings of the XIIIth ICPhS Stockholm, pp 378–79.

Stemberger JP (1993) Glottal transparency. Phonology 10: 107–38.

Traill A (1994) The perception of clicks in !X. Journal of African Languages and Linguistics 15: 161–74.

Traill A, Vossen R (1996) Sound Change in the Khoisan Languages: New Data on Click Loss and Click Replacement. Unpublished manuscript, University of the Witwatersrand, Johannesburg.

Vollmer K (1993) Untersuchung der Koartikulation bei gestörter Sprache: Experimentalstudie. MA thesis: University of Bielefeld.

Ziegler W, Von Cramon D (1989) Die Sprechapraxie - eine apraktische Störung? Fortschritte Neurologischer Psychiatrie 57: 198–204.

Notes

1   Most of this research is summarized in a seminal study by Ladefoged and Traill (1994). For EPG data see Roux (1993); for EMA data see Scharf, Hertrich, Dogil and Roux (1995).

2   This study was made possible by a grant for the second author by the Research Unit for Experimental Phonology of the University of Stellenbosch.

3   Clicks in Xhosa usually occupy the word initial position, i.e. the position in which most phonological substitution errors are expected in AOS. In Khoisan languages clicks are restricted to the word initial position.

Chapter 45
Timing Deficits in Dysarthric Patients: Acoustic and Articulatory Correlates of Vowel Type and Vowel Quantity in Patients with Parkinson's Disease and Cerebellar Ataxia

GABRIELE SCHARF, INGO HERTRICH AND
HERMANN ACKERMANN

Introduction

It is well known that the basal ganglia and the cerebellum play a central role in movement execution (Kandel, Schwartz and Jessell, 1991). However, the contribution of these two subcortical structures to the control of timing is an issue that is subject to ongoing research. Speech production requires the exact temporal adjustment of a variety of acoustic and articulatory events. The investigation of speech production in patients with basal ganglia or cerebellar dysfunction may therefore illuminate the role of these two systems in the control of timing. In the present study a specific linguistic timing task, the production of vowel quantity contrast, was investigated on the basis of acoustic and articulatory data.

Several arguments in favour of the hypothesis that the cerebellum functions as an internal timing device ('internal clock') were discussed in the last decades. Braitenberg (1967, 1996) pointed out the regular anatomical structure of the cerebellum, which might predispose it to compute sequential, temporal information. Furthermore, in patients with cerebellar syndromes, dysmetria and dysdiadochokinesia can be interpreted as mistiming of agonistic and antagonistic muscular activity. Results of EMG recordings corroborate this interpretation (Ivry and Keele, 1989). The failure of cerebellar patients in classical eyeblink conditioning tasks has similarly been interpreted as disturbed impulse-reaction timing (McCormick and Thompson, 1984). The hypothesis of the timing function of the cerebellum was considerably supported by the results of Ivry and Keele (1989); Keele and Ivry (1991) who showed that cerebellar patients present with specific deficits (greater variability) in the perception of duration and velocity. However, the perception of linguistically relevant length parameters such as VOT and phonemic consonant duration could not be shown to be disturbed (Ivry and Gopal, 1992; Ivry, 1993). This led Ivry (1993) to speculate that the cerebellum is not involved in the computation of linguistically relevant durations. This view is questioned by recent findings by Gräber, Ackermann, Hertrich and Daum (1997) and Ackermann, Gräber, Hertrich and Daum (1997) showing a deficit in the perception of consonantal occlusion duration in cerebellar patients. So the question of whether the cerebellum plays an essential role in the timing of speech units has still not been definitely answered.

In the case of the basal ganglia an explicit timing hypothesis has been formulated by Artieda, Pastor, Lacruz and Obeso (1992) and Pastor, Artieda, Jahanshahi and Obeso (1992) who observed abnormal processing of temporal parameters in Parkinson's disease (PD). In time-estimation tasks duration was underestimated and in time-reproduction tasks time intervals were overproduced by PD patients, leading to the assumption that 'the internal clock runs slowly' in these patients. The clinical picture is ambiguous in this regard. On the one hand, PD is characterized by slowing of movements and longer reaction times in the initiation of movement and the change between two different motor patterns. These symptoms are summarized by the term *bradykinesia* (Hallett and Khoshbin, 1980). On the other hand, hastening phenomena are reported in a subgroup of PD patients while walking or speaking: the patients are unable to control movement velocity or to stop the movement at the right moment (Ackermann, Konczak and Hertrich, 1997). In its extreme form the acceleration prevents the implementation of separate sequential movements (freezing). These clinical observations would lead to the assumption that the internal clock runs faster in this group of patients (Ackermann, Gröne, Hoch and Schönle, 1993).

The present study tries to evaluate timing functions in the speech production of patients with basal ganglia (PD) and cerebellar damage (CA), respectively. For this purpose the production of the vowel quantity contrast, which is phonemic in German, was investigated in dysarthric and normal speakers. The analysis included the perceptual evaluation of the contrast, calculation of durational and spectral characteristics of the acoustic signal and elementary kinematic measurements of labial articulation.

Methods

Eleven patients with an ataxic syndrome due to pure cerebellar atrophy (aged between 27 and 69 years), 10 patients with idiopathic Parkinsonian syndrome (aged 48 to 78 years) and 15 normal controls who never suffered from any diseases of the brain or the cranial nerves (aged 30 to 79 years) took part in the study.[1] The three groups did not differ significantly with respect to age ($p > 0.05$). After a trigger signal the subjects were asked to produce sentences of the form: *'Ich habe gepVpe gelesen,'* with the target vowel *V* being one of the tense or lax vowels [a, a:, i, i:, u, u:].

Each target item (*'gepape, gepappe'* etc.) was visually presented *(font 70)* eight times in randomized order so that each subject produced 48 sentences. The labial movements were recorded by means of an optoelectronic two-camera system (BTS-ELITE, Milano / Italy) with a sampling rate of 100 Hz. The following three measurement positions were registered: the midsagittal point of upper and lower lips and the nasion as a reference point for the head movements. The acoustic signal was recorded simultaneously on a digital tape (Sony PCM-2000, Japan; microphone: AKG C410/B, Austria) with a mouth–microphone distance of about 5 cm. The acoustic signal was transferred to a Silicon Graphics Indigo Workstation with a sampling rate of 16 kHz and analysed by means of the signal analysis software ESPS/Waves. Thirteen labels were set manually at the oscillographic signal of each utterance at the following positions: onset of the six vowels in the sequence *'habe gepVpe ge,'* as well as vowel offsets and bursts of the three syllable initial plosives of the target word *gepVpe* each (Figure 45.1). If the localization of a burst event was uncertain, the label was eliminated.

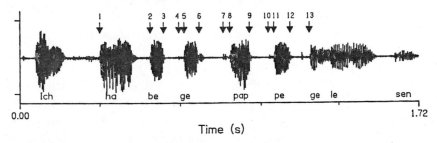

Figure 45.1. Oscillographic signal of the sentence utterance *'Ich habe gepappe gelesen'* produced by a normal speaker with 13 time marks at the relevant vowel onsets, vowel offsets and bursts.

In order to investigate the effect of vowel quantity on the different linguistic units in the three groups, the duration of the following time intervals was calculated from the acoustic time marks: vowel duration (vowel onset to vowel offset), voice onset time (burst to vowel onset), closure duration (vowel offset to vowel onset) and syllable duration (vowel offset to vowel offset except first syllable: vowel onset to vowel offset) of the three syllables of the target word, duration of the target word (vowel onset of first syllable to vowel offset of third syllable), utterance length (vowel onset of /a/ in *babe* to vowel offset of *ge* in *gelesen*) and inter-word pauses. The time interval from one vowel onset to the next one was calculated for all five vowels. This measure is called the 'beat' because it might be relevant for the control of speech rate and rhythm. In order to characterize the durational vowel contrast, three different parameters were calculated: the mean difference between short and long vowels (DIF), the mean difference related to the variability of long and short vowel duration (CON=DIF/ (STDDEVlong+STDDEVshort vowel)) and the quotient of short and long vowel duration (REL=DURATIONshort vowel / DURATIONlong vowel). In addition to the durational measurements, formants of the target vowels were measured at the spectrogram in order to examine the production of the vowel quality contrast between tense and lax vowels. For that purpose the values of F1, F2 and F3 were calculated in the mid position of a relatively stable phase of the formant structure or in the middle of the peak or valley structure of the spectrogram of the target vowel (window width +/– 25 ms, Burg algorithm, Hamming window function, 20 coefficients; cf. Kay, 1988).

Two kinematic signals were calculated: the distance between upper and lower lip marker over time (three-point filtered) and the velocity of the changes of the lip distance in terms of the unfiltered first derivative of this signal. For the target sequence *pap* the maximum and minimum points of lip distance and velocity were automatically detected. Figure 45.2 shows the synchronized lip distance signal (upper panel), the velocity of lip distance (mid panel) and the acoustic signal (lower panel) of the target word *gepappe* with the relevant extreme points marked.

The following kinematic parameters were calculated: amplitude, maximum velocity and movement duration of the opening and closing gesture for the sequence *pap*. The opening and closing amplitude was defined as the difference between minimum and maximum labial distance in the opening (D2 – D1) and closing gesture (D3 – D2) each. The maximum velocity of opening and closing gesture was given by G1 and G2, respectively. Movement duration was defined as the time interval between maximum closing and maximum opening (opening duration) and between maximum opening and maximum closing (closing duration). The position of the vowel onset in the opening gesture was determined by the following quotient: (Vo-DΛ)/(D2-DΛ), time difference (ONS) between prevocalic maximum closure (D1=start of opening gesture) and vowel onset (Vo) divided by the opening duration (D2-D1). This is a relational measure that achieves 100% if ONS has the same duration as the opening duration, i.e., if maximum labial opening and vowel onset are synchronous.

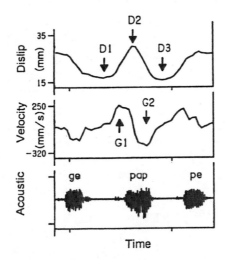

Figure 45.2. Distance between upper and lower lip marker (upper panel), velocity of lip distance (mid panel) and acoustic signal (lower panel) of the target word '*gepappe*' produced by a normal speaker. Extreme points: D1 = minimal labial distance in pre-target closure, D2 = maximum labial distance in target vowel /a/, D3 = minimal labial distance in post-target closure, G1 = maximum opening velocity towards the target vowel, G2 = maximum closing velocity after the target vowel.

The means of the acoustic and kinematic parameters were calculated for each speaker and condition. Analyses of variance were carried out with the six different conditions (vowel quantity x vowel type) as six repeated measurements, with the three independent factors 'group' (PARK, CERE, NORM), 'vowel quantity' (short, long vowel) and 'vowel type' (a, i, u).

Perceptual evaluation was carried out by two young female speech-language pathologists without any hearing disorders who were not involved in the study. They were instructed to listen to the sentence utterances and to transcribe the target word orthographically in such a way that vowel quantity and vowel quality were identified. Any deviation of the perceived word from the stimulus was registered as an error. Errors in vowel quantity were separated from segmental errors (errors in vowel type or consonants). Because of the high inter-rater reliability (the ratings of both listeners agreed in 95.6% of the normal utterances and in 86.1% of all cases) the means of the two raters were used for further analysis. The frequency of quantity errors was calculated for each speaker and condition as well as the respective group means and standard deviations.

Results

Figure 45.3 shows the frequency of quantity errors at perceptual evaluation. In the case of the normal speakers, quantity errors were very rare with respect to all three vowel types. The utterances of the dysarthric groups, however, yielded more quantity errors with large variability between the speakers. Most of these errors were shortening errors of long vowels in the case of vowels /a/ and /u/ and lengthening errors of short vowels in the case of vowel /i/, respectively. That is, the feature *vowel quantity* was perceptually less stable in both patient groups than in the normal speakers.

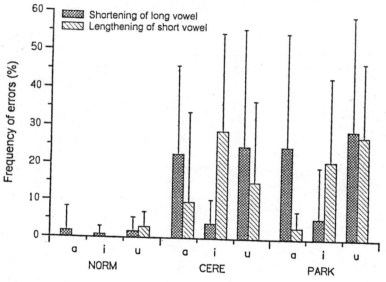

Figure 45.3. Frequency of perceived quantity errors. Group means across both raters and standard deviation for the various vowel types.

The vowel duration for the short and long vowel /a/ as measured in the acoustic signal is shown in Figure 45.4.[2] The normal speakers produced a clear quantity contrast with a distinctive vowel length for short and long vowels. The older control speakers presented with longer tense vowels than the younger ones so that an even greater quantity contrast was found in this subgroup.[3]

The cerebellar patients produced longer vowel durations with a clearly large intra- and inter-speaker variability than the normal controls. The mean difference between short and long vowels (DIF) in the cerebellar group was greater than in the control group ($p < 0.0001$), but related to the increased standard deviation of both short and long vowel duration ($p < 0.05$), the contrast (CON=DIF/STDDEV) was significantly reduced in comparison to the

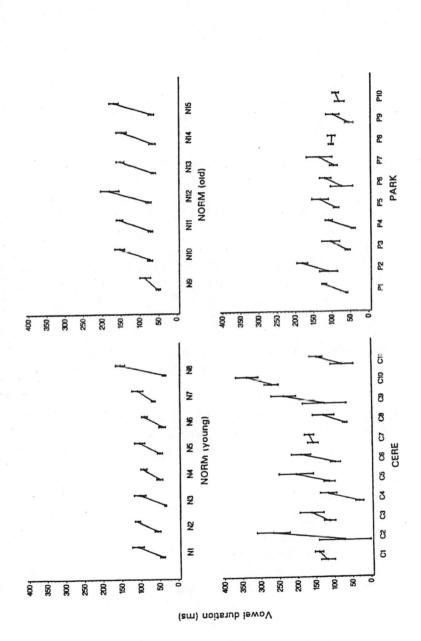

Figure 45.4. Vowel duration for short and long vowel /a/ in normal speakers (young: aged from 30 to 45 years; old: from 59 to 79 years) and patient groups. Means per speaker for short (left) and long vowels (right) are linked, plus/minus one standard deviation.

controls. Two of the cerebellar speakers (C2, C7) presented with overlapping length for short and long vowels instead of distinctive durations. The PD patients showed vowel duration at a normal level but with the tendency to approximate the duration of short and long vowels leading to overlap in subjects P6, P7, P8 and P10. The relational contrast of short and long vowel (REL=DURATIONshort vowel/DURATIONlong vowel) was reduced in PD patients as compared to the controls. The durational vowel quantity contrast is therefore reduced, or at least less stable, in both patient groups as compared to the controls.

Vowel quantity influenced the timing of the sentence utterance at different linguistic levels in the group of normal speakers in the following way. Going from smaller to larger units, quantity affected the duration of the target vowel and the preceding voice onset time, the target syllable, the duration of the beat that contains the target vowel, the word and the utterance. That is, all these units had longer duration in the case of the target being a long vowel (p<0.05). This was the case for the PD patients as well, with the exception of the target vowel, which was less affected by vowel quantity. The group of CA patients showed a different pattern. In addition to the units mentioned, the voice onset time of the first syllable *ge* of the target word, the first syllable as a whole and the two beats preceding the target word (corresponding to *abe g*) were lengthened in the case of the long target vowel. That is, in contrast to the normal speakers, the cerebellar patients seemed to anticipate the feature of vowel quantity prior to the production of the target syllable and even the target word. Furthermore, the cerebellar patients showed a general lengthening of all linguistic units in comparison to the normal group (p<0.01) except the voice onset time before and after the target vowel, which was slightly shorter than in the control group.

No significant difference between the groups could be found with respect to the spectral structure of the target vowel (p>0.05, Figure 45.5). Like the control group, both patient groups showed only very small differences in F1, F2 and F3 between the tense and lax counterparts of vowel /a/ and vowel /u/. A greater contrast related to vowel quality could be seen in F3 of vowel /i/. This was the case for all three groups equally.

Kinematic analysis yielded the following results. In all three groups, movement amplitude and movement duration of the labial opening and closing gesture were larger for the long target vowel than for the short cognate (p<0.0001). The cerebellar patients tended to produce larger closing amplitudes than the control speakers (p<0.05); the PD patients produced normal amplitudes. Figure 45.6 shows the peak velocity in relation to the movement amplitude of the labial closing ges-

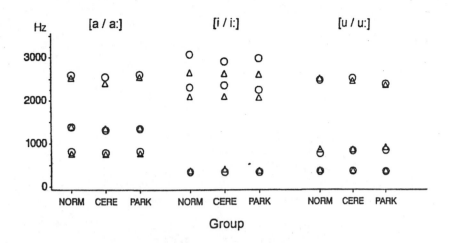

Figure 45.5. Formants 1, 2, and 3 of the target vowel. Triangles: short vowels, circles: long vowels. Group means for the three vowel types.

ture of the short vowel /a/. The normal controls (circles) showed an increase in peak velocity with increasing movement amplitude. The cerebellar patients (dots) presented with clearly smaller peak velocities as related to their movement amplitudes. This result has to be interpreted as a slowing of the labial closing movement in the cerebellar patients. The PD patients (squares) behaved like the normal controls with respect to the relation of amplitude and velocity; they did not show a slowing of labial movement. The slowness of movement in the cerebellar patients was also reflected by the general increase of movement duration of the opening and closing gesture (p<0.0001).

Whereas the PD patients did not differ from the control group in the basic motor parameters like amplitude, velocity and duration of labial movement, they did show a deviant pattern with respect to the position of the vowel onset in the labial opening gesture (Figure 45.7).

The normal speakers exhibited a clear contrast between short (left) and long vowels (right) in this measure. For the short vowel /a/ they tended to synchronize vowel onset and maximum lip opening (position parameter = 100%). For the long vowel /a/ the value is smaller, that is, the vowel starts earlier in the (longer) opening gesture. This contrast, which is realized consistently by every normal speaker, was reduced in the PD patients as can be seen in Figure 45.7. Three patients (as indicated by the dots) levelled this contrast or even showed the reverse pattern.

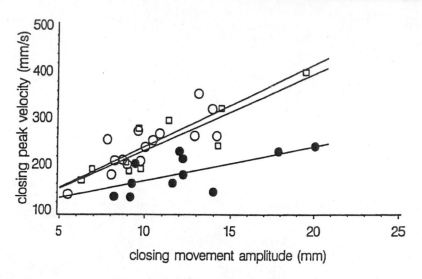

Figure 45.6. Peak velocity and amplitude of closing gesture in the target sequence *papp* with short target vowel. Mean per speaker. Circles: NORM, squares: PARK, dots: CERE.

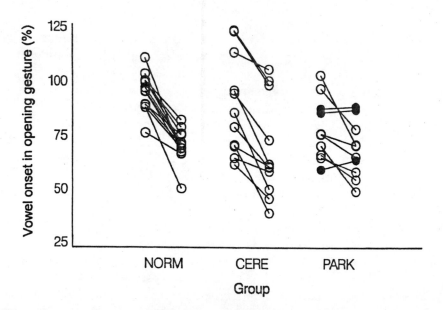

Figure 45.7. Position of vowel onset in lip opening gesture (quotient of time interval from start of opening gesture to vowel onset (ONS) and opening duration) for short (left) and long vowel /a/ (to the right). Mean per speaker.

Summary and discussion

Both groups of dysarthric patients showed a reduced, or at least less reliable, vowel quantity contrast with increased variability and overlap of the duration of short and long vowels. The higher frequency of perceived quantity errors in both patient groups compared to the controls confirms this result. Reduced peak velocity in relation to movement amplitude was found in the labial closing gesture of the target vowel in the cerebellar patients. This finding, concomitant with the overall lengthening of all linguistic units (except the voice onset time) has to be interpreted in terms of a general slowing down of labial and speech movements in CA patients. In addition, an anticipatory effect of the quantity feature was found in cerebellar patients, which might suggest a different overall strategy in these patients in the sense of an augmentation of temporal contrasts in order to reach a higher degree of intelligibility.

In the case of the PD patients, no indication of a slowing down of articulatory movements (bradykinesia) emerged. Instead of this a disorder of the temporal coordination of vowel onset and labial movement (positioning of the vowel onset in the labial opening gesture) could be found. This result might be explained in two different ways: On the one hand, this lack of coordination might be caused by a phonatory disorder, which often accompanies Parkinson's disease. In the present data, however, the PD patients showed an early vowel onset in short and long vowels (cf. Figure 45.7) which would not be expected in cases of phonatory disorders like a breathy or creaky voice, which are typical in PD patients. An alternative approach would be to assume a reduced adaptation of the articulatory coordination to the different timing requirements of long and short vowels in these patients. The realization of the durational vowel contrast, including the positioning of the vowel onset in the lip cycle, requires acceleration and deceleration of the labial movements at different times and to a different degree. It is exactly this 'fine tuning' of articulatory movements according to the specific timing task that seems to be affected in the Parkinsonian patients. The clinical observation of PD patients being unable to start or to stop a movement at the right moment might reflect the same underlying deficit.

Conclusion

Two different patterns of altered vowel quantity contrast emerged in PD and cerebellar patients. Whereas in the case of cerebellar patients the slowing down of labial movements preserves the exact realization of a durational vowel contrast, incorrect timing between lip articulation and phonation might be responsible for the reduced quantity contrast in PD patients.

References

Ackermann H, Gröne BF, Hoch G, Schönle PW (1993) Speech freezing in Parkinson's disease: a kinematic analysis of orofacial movements by means of electromagnetic articulography. Folia Phoniatrica 45: 84–9.

Ackermann H, Hertrich I, Daum I, Scharf G, Spieker S (1997) Kinematic analysis of articulatory movements in central motor disorders. Movement Disorders (in press).

Ackermann H, Gräber S, Hertrich I, Daum I (1997) Categorical perception in cerebellar disorders. Brain and Language (in press).

Ackermann H, Konczak J, Hertrich I (1997) The temporal control of repetitive articulatory movements in Parkinson's disease. Brain and Language (in press).

Artieda, J, Pastor MA, Lacruz F, Obeso JA (1992) Temporal discrimination is abnormal in Parkinson's disease. Brain 115: 199–210.

Braitenberg V (1967) Is the cerebellar cortex a biological clock in the millisecond range? Progress in Brain Research 25: 334–46.

Braitenberg V (1996) Flutwellen in den Parallelfasern des Kleinhirns. Talk presented at Wissenschaftliches Kolloquium, Neurological Department, University of Tübingen, October 1996.

Gräber S, Ackermann H, Hertrich I, Daum I (1997) Speech perception and production in cerebellar disorder: the contribution of timing. In Ziegler W, Deger K (Eds) Clinical Phonetics and Linguistics. Proceedings of the Fifth Annual Conference of the International Clinical Phonetics and Linguistics Association. London: Whurr. pp 439–43.

Hallett M, Khoshbin L (1980) A physiological mechanism of bradykinesia. Brain 103: 301–14.

Ivry R (1993) Cerebellar involvement in the explicit representation of temporal information. Annals of the New York Academy of Sciences 682: 214–30.

Ivry RB., Gopal HS (1992) Speech production and perception in patients with cerebellar lesions. Meyer DE, Kornblum S (Eds) Attention and Performance. Vol XIV: Synergies in Experimental Psychology, Artificial Intelligence and Cognitive Neuroscience. MIT Press: Cambridge MA, pp 771–802.

Ivry RB, SW Keele (1989) Timing functions of the Cerebellum. Journal of Cognitive Neuroscience 1: 136–52.

Kandal E, Schwartz J, Jessell T (1991) Principles of Neural Science. Amsterdam: Elsevier.

Kay SM (1988) Modern Spectral Estimation: Theory and Application. Englewood Cliffs, NJ: Prentice-Hall.

Keele SW, Ivry RB (1991) Does the cerebellum provide a common computation for diverse tasks? A timing hypothesis. Annals of the New York Academy of Sciences 608: 179–211.

McCormick D, Thompson R (1984) Cerebellum: essential involvement in the classically conditioned eyelid response. Science 223: 296–99.

Pastor MA, Artieda J, Jahanshahi M, Obeso JA (1992) Time estimation and reproduction is abnormal in Parkinson's disease. Brain 115: 211–25.

Notes

1   A further description of the subjects can be found in Ackermann, Gräber, Hertrich, Daum (1997).

2   Vowel /a/ is shown as the clearest example of the three vowel types. The deviations of the dysarthric speakers in general show the same pattern in the cases of vowel /i/ and /u/. The durational quantity contrast in these two vowel types, however, is slightly less stable in the younger control speakers (there is some overlap between short and long vowels).

3   The older normal speakers are shown in a separate panel because of the difference in vowel quantity contrast. Young and old normal speakers together constitute a single control group for the statistical analysis.

Chapter 46
Speech Perception and Production in Cerebellar Disorders: The Contribution of Timing Deficits[1]

SUSANNE GRÄBER, HERMANN ACKERMANN,
INGO HERTRICH AND IRENE DAUM

Introduction

Based on neuroanatomical findings, Braitenberg was the first to postulate that the cerebellar cortex plays an important role as a 'timing device'. (Braitenberg and Atwood, 1958). This theory found further support in later electrophysiological (Heck, 1995) and clinical investigations (Jueptner, Rijntjes, Weiller, Faiss, Timmann, Mueller and Diener, 1995). The studies conducted by Keele and Ivry (1991) stressed the contribution of the cerebellum to timing functions within the motor domain and revealed cerebellar involvement in the discrimination of time intervals. For example, patients with cerebellar lesions showed a marked deficit in estimating time intervals extending from 400 to 550 ms. Keele and Ivry (1991) therefore conceived of the cerebellum as a supramodal timing device. In a later experiment Ivry and Gopal (1992) used verbal stimuli to test the performance of cerebellar patients on durations smaller than 100 ms and surprisingly failed to show any deficits. These results are all the more noteworthy since Braitenberg's anatomical model predicted a cerebellar involvement at that time scale (1958).

With regard to speech production, cerebellar patients show deficits in tasks requiring high-speed repetition of syllables. The impairments are characterized by syllable prolongations and greater variability at the acoustic speech signal (e.g. Keller, 1990).

From these findings we would expect specific deficits of speech perception and production in cerebellar patients if processing of durational

parameters is required. Since it is unclear so far whether the postulated impairments exclusively reflect cerebellar dysfunctions, or
whether they are more general in nature and thus could be expected
with lesions of other subcortical structures, we included patients with
Parkinson's disease as clinical controls.

Methods

Subjects

Eight subjects with an exclusively cerebellar disorder were tested. All
of these patients suffered from a diffuse atrophy of the cerebellum
(for details see Ackermann, Gräber, Hertrich and Daum, 1997). These
subjects were compared with ten normal controls and a group of
seven patients with Parkinson's disease. The three groups were
matched according to age and education. All subjects were native
German speakers and there was no evidence of auditory deficits or
dementia.

Speech perception

In this task we manipulated three German minimal pairs by varying the
duration of several parameters, using the paradigm of categorical perception. The dimensions used were voice onset time (VOT; 'Tick'–
'dick'; 'tic' and 'fat'), vowel length (VL; 'Gram' – 'Gramm'; 'grief' and
'gram') and duration of stop consonant closure (DCL; 'Boten' –
'Boden'; 'messenger' and 'ground'). The utterances of each word
pair member were produced by a professional actress and then
manipulated on the CSL (Computerized Speech Lab) from Kay
Elemetrics (Pine Brook, NJ). A continuum of 10 stimuli was derived
for each word pair by subdividing the respective temporal and spectral parameters into nine equally spaced intervals. These stimuli were
recorded on a DAT recorder and applied in a random order in a
sound-attenuated room. The subjects had to listen to individual stimuli and to indicate which member of the respective word pair they
heard.

The probability of each of the 10 stimuli pertaining to each word
pair being rated as the end-point stimulus with the longest duration
was calculated (for details see Ackermann et al., 1997).

Speech production

In the speech production task the subjects were asked to produce a list
of word pairs embedded into a carrier phrase differing either in the

parameter VOT (e.g. 'Tank' – 'Dank'; 'tank' and 'thanks') or VL of the vowel 'a' (e.g. 'Rate'– 'Ratte'; 'rate' and 'rat'). The utterances of each subject were recorded on a DAT recorder and the acoustic analysis was undertaken using the CSL. The length of the parameters VOT and VL were measured in order to quantify speech variability at the oscillograms using the CSL.

Results

In the perception task there was no significant difference between the subjects with cerebellar disorders and the normal control group for the parameters VOT and VL. The CERE patients, however, exhibited a highly significant impairment with respect to the duration of closure (DCL) relative to the normal control subjects. Contrary to that, the PD group showed a comparable normal performance in all of the three parameters (Figure 46.1).

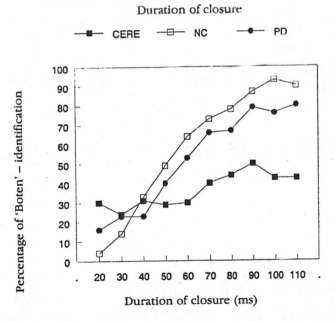

Duration of closure

Figure 46.1. Percentage of identifications of the word 'Boten': Group means for cerebellar (CERE), Parkinsonian (PD) and healthy control subjects (NC).

It is crucial for the interpretation of the data to note that both variables VOT and VL provide duration as well as acoustic energy as discriminating features, while words manipulated in the DCL paradigm distinguish themselves solely by the closure length. This strongly suggests that the deficits seen in cerebellar patients are due to the miscalculation of the time intervals at the speech signal.

A similar pattern emerged for the patients' performance in the production tasks. Specifically, the CERE group had abnormalities in speech production whereas the PD groups did not show any significant impairment. The means of absolute durations of the VOT and the VL were comparable for all groups. However, the CERE patients showed a significantly higher variability in producing the VOT (Figure 46.2). For the variance of VL the differences did not reach significance.

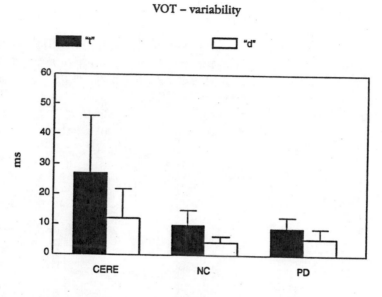

Figure 46.2. Group means of within-subject variance of VOT in cerebellar (CERE), Parkinsonian (PD) and healthy control subjects (NC).

Conclusions

The results of the present study indicate that the cerebellum is critically involved in the processing of linguistically relevant time intervals shorter than 100 ms both in speech perception as well as speech production. The cerebellum can thus be interpreted as a supramodal timing device.

References

Ackermann H, Gräber S, Hertrich I, Daum I (1997) Categorical speech perception in cerebellar disorders. Brain and Language (in press).

Braitenberg V, Atwood RP (1958) Morphological observations on the cerebellar cortex. Journal of Comparative Neurology. 109: 1–34.

Heck D (1995) Sequential input to guinea pig cerebellar cortex in vitro strongly affects Purkinje cells via parallel fibers. Naturwissenschaften 82: 201–3.

Ivry RB, Gopal HS (1992) Speech production and perception in patients with cerebellar lesion. In Mayer DE, Kornblum S (Eds) Attention and Performance. Vol. XIV. Hillsdale/NJ: Erlbaum, pp 771-801.

Jueptner M, Rijntjes M, Weiller C, Faiss JH, Timmann D, Mueller SP, Diener HC (1995) Localization of a cerebellar timing process using PET. Neurology 45: 1540-5.

Keele SW, Ivry R (1991) Does the cerebellum provide a common computation for diverse tasks? A timing hypothesis. Annals of the New York Academy of Sciences. 608: 179–211.

Keller E (1990) Speech motor timing. In Hardcastle WJ, Marchal A (Eds) Speech Production and Speech Modelling. Dordrecht: Kluwer, pp. 343–64.

Note

1   This research was supported by the Deutsche Forschungsgemeinschaft (SFB 307, B10).

Chapter 47
Orofacial and Forefinger Force Control in Parkinson's disease

MICHELE GENTIL, SABINE PERRIN, PIERRE POLLAK AND ALIM LOUIS BENABID

Force control tasks may provide quantitative information about motor control and may elucidate the functional role of different motor structures and systems (Mai, Bolsinger, Avarello, Dieber and Dichgans, 1988). Parkinson's disease (PD) is a neurodegenerative disease with prominent neuropathology of the basal ganglia (Marsden, 1984). It is characterized clinically by four major symptoms: inability to initiate movements (akinesia), slowness of voluntary movements (bradykinesia), muscular rigidity, and tremor (Wichmann and DeLong 1993). Some previous works have studied force production in patients with PD. Stelmach and Worringham (1988) and Stelmach, Teasdale, Philips and Worringham (1989) observed isometric forces generated by elbow flexors. Sheridan, Flowers and Huller (1987) were interested in isometric forces of the upper limbs. These authors noted force production impairments in PD. With regard to orofacial force control, several studies are relative to neurologically impaired subjects (Barlow and Abbs, 1986; Barlow and Burton, 1990; Dworkin, Aronson and Mulder, 1980) but very few investigations concern patients with PD (Abbs et al. 1987). We have extended previous work by studying force control in lips, tongue and forefingers. Our study aimed at answering two questions : (a) Do the disorders of orofacial and forefinger force control resemble each other in PD, and (b) what is the fine force control of the orofacial structure in PD?

Methods

Subjects

Fourteen patients (seven males and seven females) diagnosed with idiopathic PD (duration of the symptoms 9 ± 3 years), and exhibiting an akinetic-rigid type of PD were examined. Their mean age was 58 ± 7 years. Moreover, 14 age- and sex-matched healthy, control subjects participated in this study. All subjects had functionally normal occlusion. Patients were treated with levodopa, and were tested after a medication-free interval of at least 10 hours, before their first morning dose of levodopa. Immediately before the force study, overall motor disability of patients was assessed using the unified Parkinson's disease rating scale motor examination (Fahn et al., 1987), and a timed hand-tapping test. The patients were classified 'moderately impaired' with regard to perceived speech intelligibility.

Instrumentation

A load-sensitive cantilever (Neuro Logic Incorporated, Bloomington/ Indiana, USA) adjustable in the inferior-superior and anterior-posterior dimensions was used to sample, at midline, compression forces generated by the upper and lower lips. The cantilever slid along a jaw yoke that was encapsulated in a moldable dental impression block and placed between the molars. The upper lip transducer is shown in Figure 47.1. The load sensitive cantilever was inverted for sampling lower-lip force. A tongue force transducer with a simple dimensional strain gauge was used for sampling anterior tongue force toward the alveolar ridge. For testing the forefingers, the lip transducer was installed on the right and on the left of a tabletop, which was fixed to a dental arm-chair. The subject rested his arm on the tabletop with his forefinger extended on the strain gauge device and his other fingers loosely curled up. Control subjects began on their dominant side, and PD patients began on their less affected side. A two-channel oscilloscope provided visual feedback. Data were acquired on-line.

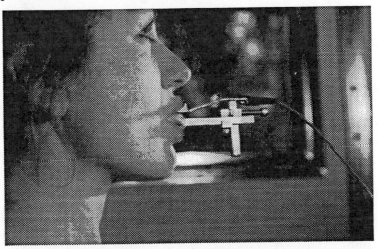

Figure 47.1. Upper lip force transducer *in situ* to sample upper lip depression.

Experimental tasks

Subjects were seated in a dental armchair. Target feedback signals were delivered by the computer and presented to the subject in the booth. The target force levels used in the present study included 0.25, 0.5, 1 and 2 newtons (N) corresponding to fine forces presumably involved in speech production. Subjects were given the instruction to generate forces from baseline 'as rapidly and as accurately as possible' in response to the target signal that appeared on the screen. A 'ready' signal preceded the target. The rapid phase of force increase to reach the target was followed by a stabilization for the duration of the hold phase. Ten consecutive contractions were obtained at each of the four target force levels. Moreover, two maximal contractions were sampled for articulatory organs.

Measures

Maximal voluntary forces of lips and tongue were evaluated. The following measures were completed on each record of force for each structure:

- Reaction time, defined as the interval from the time the target signal appeared on the screen until the force has reached 10%.
- Peak force during the force ramp. That is the highest force level occuring in the first one-second period following 0.1 N above the base line.
- Peak rate of force change taken from the maxima of the first derivative of force.
- Mean and standard deviation of force ouput during the first 1.5 second period of the hold phase.
- The data were submitted to sequential one-way ANOVAs and Tukey tests, alpha level chosen was $p = 0.05$ to characterize the significance of the main effects : sex, group, force level.

Results

Maximal voluntary forces

Concerning maximal voluntary forces (MVF) of the lips and tongue, a one-way analysis of variance revealed no significant differences between males and females for each articulatory organ in both groups, control subjects and patients. A significant difference was, however, found between both groups of subjects for the upper and lower lips. Figure 47.2 shows the MVF across sex for upper lip, lower lip and tongue. In both groups significant differences were observed between lower lip and upper lip on the one hand, and lower lip and tongue on the other hand, lower lip having a greater MVF in comparison with the other articulatory organs. Thus, our results confirm that lower lip compressional forces were greater than the maximum closing forces generated by the upper lip (Barlow and Rath, 1985; Amerman, 1993). Moreover, it was clear from our results that the Parkinson's group yielded a significantly reduced level of lip force production compared to the controls. Wood, Hughes, Hayes and Wolfe (1992) had shown lower lip weakness in PD patients.

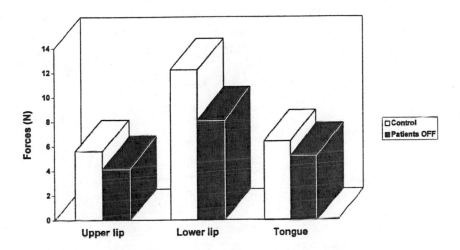

Figure 47.2. Maximal voluntary forces of the upper lip, lower lip and tongue for control subjects and Parkinsonian patients off of medication. Values are in newtons.

Average reaction times

For each structure, average reaction times were always significantly greater for the patients than for the control subjects. Moreover, Parkinsonian patients exhibited a larger variability as indicated by greater standard deviations. Some authors have observed that PD patients were slower in initiating a limb-force production (Stelmach et al. 1989). Our results support these previous observations, though we should point out that reaction time was differently defined in our study.

Peak force

In order to estimate the precision of the peak force in relation to the target and to compare this estimation between both groups of subjects, we calculated the difference between the amplitude of the actual peak force and that of the target force for each trial, that is 0.25 N and 2 N respectively (extreme levels) and we tested whether these differences were significant with a two-tail t-test. No significant difference in the articulatory organs was observed at the 0.25N target level between both groups of subjects, and we noted an overshoot of the target at this level. On the contrary, at the 2 N target level a significant difference was examined between both groups. The group of control subjects overshot the target and the group of patients undershot the target. Concerning the forefingers, similar results were obtained, i.e. no difference at the 0.25 N target level, but a significant difference at the 2 N target level with a large undershoot of the target for the patients. This is probably a matter of strategy rather than of hypokinesia. However, Stelmach *et al.* (1989) found a smaller peak force for PD patients.

In patients, we noted in particular at 2 N target level that the peak force of the upper lip was further from the target than that of the lower lip or tongue. On muscular grounds, the upper lip is not well suited for reaching relatively high target levels. This weakness was most remarkable in Parkinsonian patients.

Peak rate of force change

Maximal values for the first derivative of force, regarded as the peak rate of force change, increased with the target level in both groups of subjects. For the patients, this increase went from a mean of 2.83 N/s at 0.25 N target level to 11.71 N/s at 2 N target level. We observed significant differences in peak rate of force change between both groups of subjects as estimated by a one-way analysis of variance across structures. At any target level, the peak rate of force change for the control subjects was always greater than that of the patients. Stelmach (1989) also found a slower rate of force development in PD. Moreover, the peak rate of force change for the articulatory organs was significantly different from that of the forefingers, the higher values being associated with the articulatory organs in both groups. Figure 47.3 shows this effect of structure at 2 N target level.

Hold phase

The hold phase was studied with regard to static force control. The average amplitude of the force during the hold phase was significantly different between control subjects and patients except for the 0.25 N target level. Patients held the force further from the target, and the variability of the averages indicated by the standard deviations was greater, indicating that PD patients had more difficulty in maintaining a given contraction. Abbs, Hartman and Vishwanat (1987) noted that PD patients manifested greater instability in articulators than normal subjects.

In order to estimate the precision of the hold phase in relation to the target and to compare this precision between the articulatory organs and

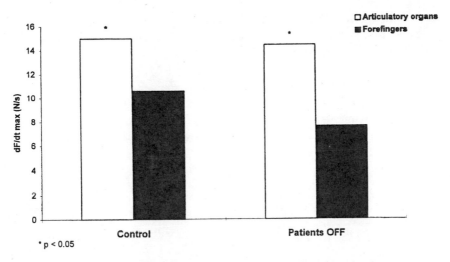

Figure 47.3. Peak rate of force change at 2 N target level for the articulatory organs and forefingers in the control and PD groups. * = significant difference between articulatory organs and forefingers. Values are in newtons/second.

forefingers across sex at each target level, we calculated, for each trial, the difference between the mean amplitude of the actual force and that of the target force, and we tested whether the differences relative to the articulatory organs were equal to those of the forefingers with a two-tail t-test. At each target level the hold phase of the articulatory organs was significantly different from that of the forefingers. Concerning the articulatory organs, patients as well as control subjects held the force below the target at each target level, but the undershoot observed for patients was four to 12 times greater than the undershoot noted for control subjects. Behaviour of the forefingers was different from that of the articulatory organs. Subjects in a general way hold the force above the target, except for patients at 2 N target level, and the forefingers were more precise than the articulatory organs.

With regard to the hold phase, differences between the articulatory organs were observed in the patients. At 2 N target level, for example, lower lip was closer to the target than tongue and upper lip, and a significant difference existed between lower lip and upper lip means, as indicated by a one-way analysis of variance. For the control subjects, on the other hand, no significant difference was noted between the three articulatory organs (Figure 47.4).

Conclusion

This study examining the production of isometric forces in PD patients and healthy control subjects shows force production impairments in PD – that is: longer reaction time, slower rate of development, difficulty in maintaining a given contraction, and increased variability. The disorders of orofacial and forefinger force control present differences in PD. These divergences could be explained by the specific anatomical and physiological characteristics of the orofacial system. At last, the force production impairments of the various articulatory organs are not identical. It seems likely that combined measures of fine force control and interstructure speech force dynamics in patients with PD provide useful insights in the speech motor disorders in PD.

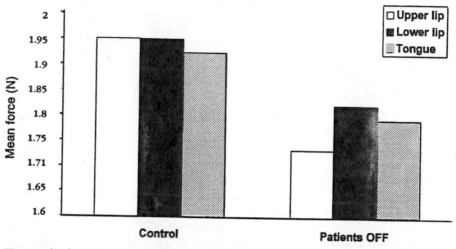

Figure 47.4. Difference between the articulatory organs at 2 N target level during the hold phase in the control and PD groups. Values are in newtons.

References

Abbs JH, Hartman DE, Vishwanat B (1987) Orofacial motor control impairment in Parkinson's disease. Neurology 37: 394–8.

Amerman JD (1993) A maximum force dependent protocol for assessing labial, force control. Journal of Speech and Hearing Research 36: 460–5.

Barlow SM, Abbs JH (1986) Fine force and position control of selected orofacial structures in the upper motor neuron syndrom. Experimental Neurology 94: 699–713.

Barlow SM, Burton MK (1990) Ramp-and-hold force control in the upper and lower lips: developing new neuromotor assessment applications in traumatically brain injured adults. Journal of Speech and Hearing Research 33: 660–75.

Barlow SM, Rath E (1985). Maximum voluntary closing forces in the upper and lower lips of humans. Journal of Speech and Hearing Research 28: 373–6.

Dworkin JP, Aronson AE, Mulder DW (1980) Tongue force in normals and in dysarthric patients with amyotrophic lateral sclerosis. Journal of Speech and Hearing Research 23: 828–37.

Fahn S, Elton RL and members of the UPDRS development committee (1987) Unified Parkinson's disease rating scale. In Fahn S, Marsden CD, Calnem DB, Goldstein M (Eds) Recent developments in Parkinson's disease. New Jersey: Macmillan Healthcare information, pp 153–64.

Mai N, Bolsinger P, Avarello M, Dieber HC, Dichgans J (1988) Control of isometric finger force in patients with cerebellar disease. Brain 111: 973–98.

Marsden CD (1984) Which motor disorder in Parkinson's disease indicates the true motor function of the basal ganglia? In Evered D, O'Connor M (Eds) Functions of the basal ganglia. Ciba Foundation Symposium N°107. London: Pitman, pp. 225–37.

Sheridan MR, Flowers KA, Huller J (1987) Programming and execution of movement in Parkinson's disease. Brain 110: 1247–71.

Stelmach GE, Teasdale N, Phillips J, Worringham CJ (1989) Force production characteristics in Parkinson's disease. Experimental Brain Research 76: 165–72.

Stelmach GE, Worringham CJ (1988) The preparation and production of isometric force in Parkinson's disease. Neuropsychologia 26: 93–103.

Wichmann T, DeLong MR (1993) Pathophysiology of parkinsonian motor abnormalities In Narabayashi H, Nagatsu T, Yanagisawa N, Mizuno Y (Eds) Advances in Neurology 60. New York: Raven Press.

Wood LM, Hughes J, Hayes KC, Wolfe DL (1992) Reliability of labial closure force measurements in normal subjects and patients with CNS disorders. Journal of Speech and Hearing Research 35: 252–8.

Chapter 48
Gender-specific Phonatory Dysfunctions in Disorders of the Basal Ganglia and the Cerebellum: Acoustic and Perceptual Characteristics

INGO HERTRICH, SYBILLE SPIEKER AND HERMANN ACKERMANN

Introduction

Normal speakers show gender-specific mechanisms of laryngeal control (Nittrouer, McGowan, Milenkovic and Beehler, 1990). Sexual dimorphism of neurogenic dysphonias must therefore be expected. In accordance with this suggestion, Parkinson's disease gives rise to gender-specific phonatory deficits (Hertrich and Ackermann, 1995). The present study addresses the question of whether other neurogenic dysphonias are also characterized by sexual dimorphism in voice abnormalities. Both acoustic parameters and perceptual ratings were considered for analysis. Besides the description of gender-specific voice disorders, the investigation thus provides the opportunity to compare these two measures and to examine the acoustic correlates of perceived voice dimensions.

Method

As a part of an extensive investigation of the speech and voice abnormalities in central motor disorders, sustained phonations of the vowel /a/ (6 repetitions) were obtained from patients with Huntington's chorea (HD; eight males, five females; age 30–64 years), Parkinson's disease (PD; 12 males, four females; age 47–76 years), Friedreich's ataxia

(FA; five males, six females; age 21–35 years), or cerebellar atrophy (CA; nine males, five females; age 32–76 years) as well as from a healthy control group (seven males, five females; age 26–66 years). Some patients failed to sustain the vowels for a duration of at least 800 ms (four male HD patients and a single subject from the male PD, the female PD, the female FA and the female CA groups each). These subjects were excluded from further analysis (for further details see Hertrich, Ackermann, Braun and Spieker, 1996).

The following acoustic parameters were computed using the 'Multidimensional Voice Program' (MDVP; Kay Elemetrics, USA):

(1)	FO	=	average fundamental frequency (F0)
(2)	JITT	=	period-to-period jitter in percent
(3)	RAP	=	deviation from the 3-point smoothed F0 contour
(4)	PPQ	=	deviation from the 5-point smoothed F0 contour
(5)	SPPQ	=	deviation from the 55-point smoothed F0 contour
(6)	VFO	=	variation coefficient of F0
(7)	SHIM	=	period-to-period shimmer in percent
(8)	APQ	=	deviation from the 11-point smoothed amplitude contour
(9)	SAPQ	=	deviation from the 55-point smoothed amplitude contour
(10)	VAM	=	variation coefficient of F0-period amplitudes
(11)	SPI	=	'soft phonation index' (harmonic energy 70–1600 Hz divided by harmonic energy 1600–4500 Hz)
(12)	VTI	=	'voice turbulence index' (unharmonic energy 2800–5000 Hz divided by harmonic energy 70–4500 Hz)
(13)	NHR	=	'noise-to-harmonic ratio' (unharmonic energy 1500–4500 Hz divided by harmonic energy 70–4500 Hz).

In order to eliminate outliers due to erroneous pitch extraction, individual medians of the acoustic parameters across repetitions were computed.

Five certified speech pathologists rated all vowel productions with respect to the dimensions 'breathy', 'harsh', 'strained', 'creaky', 'quiver', 'pitch fluctuations', and 'loudness fluctuations' (0 = unremarkable, 1 = slight, 2 = moderate, 3 = severe). 'Overall performance' was assessed on a scale extending from 1 (= good) to 6 (= severely impaired). The scores obtained at perceptual evaluation were averaged across the five listeners.

Results

Multivariate analysis of group differences

Several acoustic parameters (RAP, PPQ, SPPQ, APQ, SAPQ) showed high correlations with JITT and SHIM and, thus, do not provide additional information. These measures were therefore excluded from multivariate analysis.

The first five principal components derived from the acoustic parameters accounted for 93% of variance and the first five components obtained from the perceptual ratings for 92% of variance of the respective data corpus. MANOVAs were performed with each of these two sets of five principal components as dependent variables and with 'group' and 'sex' as independent factors. The acoustic measures yielded significant main effects for 'group' (F[20,146] = 2.59; p< 0.001) and 'sex' (F[5,44] = 9.99; p< 0.001) as well as a significant 'group' x 'sex' interaction (F[20,146] = 2.97; p< 0.001). In contrast, the perceptual scores showed a significant group effect only (F[20,146] = 3.28; p< 0.001).

Post hoc pairwise comparisons (Kruskall Wallis test; alpha = 0.05) were performed for each principal component separately with the male and female subgroups. Apart from a few exceptions (acoustic data: NC / HD; perceptual data: CA / PD, CA / HD), significant differences for at least one of the five components emerged within the male subgroups, both with respect to the acoustic as well as the perceptual data. As regards the female subjects, most comparisons in the acoustic domain did not yield significant effects (exceptions: NC/HD and HD/PD). All female patient groups differed from the controls in the obtained perceptual ratings. In addition, the comparison of HD and FA patients achieved significance.

Descriptive characterization of the patient groups

The group means of the perceptual and acoustic parameters are listed in Tables 48.1 and 48.2. It is noteworthy that the perceptual data showed significantly (p< 0.05) increased values for at least one dimension in all patient groups as compared to the respective controls. By contrast, the acoustic measures failed to reach significance for the male HD as well as the female PD groups. Perceptual analysis thus seems to be more sensitive to the overall voice impairment than acoustic analysis. Considering the relatively small sample sizes and the large number of possible tests, 'alpha' as well as 'beta' errors cannot be ruled out.

Specific profiles of acoustic and perceptual features emerged within the various patient groups to some degree. In accordance with a previous study, the PD subjects showed a largely gender-specific dysphonia. Increased values of 'breathiness', jitter, and F0 were obtained in the male patients. Furthermore, a loss of harmonic energy in the high frequency range was observed as indicated by a high 'soft phonation index'. By contrast, the females presented with strained voice quality and long-term instabilities in terms of 'loudness fluctuations' and 'quivering'.

The vowel productions both of male and female HD subjects were characterized by increased harshness and quivering as well as by loudness fluctuations. Breathy voice quality concomitant with high jitter values was observed in the female subgroup only. As concerns breathiness and jitter, the gender-specific profiles of the HD subgroups showed a pattern that was the reverse of the one obtained in PD patients.

Both gender groups with Friedreich's ataxia had a reduced ability to keep the sound pressure at a constant level, as indicated by a large amplitude variability (VAM) as well as high ratings on the dimensions 'loudness fluctuations' and 'quiver'. Furthermore, all other perceptual scales showed moderately increased values.

Males with CA seemed to be less impaired than females. The latter group had increased values on almost all parameters, and even six of the acoustic dimensions reached significance. The long-term instability scores ('pitch' and 'loudness fluctuations', 'quiver', VF0, and VAM) were particularly high, whereas the soft phonation index was remarkably low.

Correlation analysis

All correlations among the perceptual dimensions were positive and most of them achieved significance at the 1% level. In particular, those between 'overall performance' and the specific perceptual dimensions were all above 0.60 (Table 48.3). As concerns the acoustic parameters, high positive correlations emerged among all pitch (JITT, RAP, PPQ, SPPQ) and amplitude (SHIM, APQ, SAPQ) perturbation measures respectively. Furthermore, a high correlation between the two measures of the harmonics-to-noise ratio, i.e. NHR and VTI, was observed (Table 48.4).

Perceptual and acoustic data were compared by means of canonical correlation analysis. Three canonical functions were significant, accounting for 55%, 21%, and 12% of common variance, respectively. These dimensions can be interpreted as (a) overall performance (positively linked to all perceptual and acoustic parameters, with a particularly high loading on 'breathiness' and jitter), (b) the distinction between long-term versus short-term perturbation (highest positive loading on 'loudness fluctuations'), and (c) spectral distribution of harmonic energy (particularly high negative loading by the soft phonation index and 'breathiness').

Conclusions

Perceptual ratings were superior to acoustic analysis with respect to the differentiation of patients and controls, but failed to discriminate between the various patient groups. A gender-specific dysphonia profile emerged in three patient groups (HD, PD, CA). Canonical correlation analysis relating the acoustic data to the perceptual scores revealed three interpretable common factors.

Table 48.1. Group means (standard deviations) of the perceptual parameters obtained from sustained vowel productions

| | Male subgroups | | | | | Female subgroups | | | | |
	NC	HD	PD	FA	CA	NC	HD	PD	FA	CA
breathy	0.69 (0.38)	0.65 (0.50)	1.91* (0.68)	1.36 (0.59)	1.44 (0.81)	0.96 (0.50)	1.84* (0.57)	1.27 (0.70)	1.84* (0.57)	1.80* (0.52)
harsh	0.46 (0.25)	1.05* (0.38)	1.58* (0.69)	1.04* (0.46)	1.18* (0.70)	0.40 (0.24)	1.24* (0.74)	1.00* (0.40)	1.12 (0.70)	1.35* (0.55)
strained	1.06 (0.56)	1.65 (0.34)	1.56 (0.79)	1.32 (0.69)	1.37 (0.60)	0.48 (0.39)	1.84* (0.78)	1.73* (0.23)	1.41* (0.66)	2.20* (0.82)
creaky	0.57 (0.37)	0.95 (0.50)	1.09 (0.74)	1.40 (0.97)	0.84 (0.79)	0.36 (0.43)	0.92 (0.70)	1.00 (0.53)	1.12 (0.81)	1.15 (0.97)
quiver	0.43 (0.14)	1.10* (0.53)	1.24* (0.61)	1.40 (0.76)	0.84 (0.64)	0.24 (0.26)	1.84* (1.01)	1.33* (0.50)	1.33* (0.82)	1.65* (0.87)
pitch fl.	1.00 (0.48)	1.70 (0.93)	0.93 (0.61)	1.60 (0.47)	1.04 (0.53)	0.52 (0.52)	1.36 (0.77)	1.00 (0.20)	1.32 (0.82)	1.40* (0.52)
loudn. fl.	0.31 (0.20)	0.70* (0.26)	0.51 (0.29)	1.12* (0.63)	0.42 (0.25)	0.20 (0.14)	0.68* (0.23)	0.73* (0.23)	0.92* (0.46)	1.15* (0.60)
perform.	2.66 (0.52)	3.40* (0.37)	3.78* (1.03)	3.88* (0.88)	3.27 (0.99)	2.08 (0.66)	4.16* (0.55)	3.53* (0.42)	3.68 (1.33)	4.40* (0.82)

pitch fl. = pitch fluctuations, loudn. fl. = loudness fluctuations, perform. = overall performance; NC = controls, HD = Huntington's chorea, PD = Parkinson's disease, FA = Friedreich's ataxia, CA = cerebellar atrophy. * = significantly above the control group (Kruskall–Wallis test; p<0.05).

Table 48.2. Group means (standard deviations) of the acoustic parameters

	Male subgroups					Female subgroups				
	NC	HD	PD	FA	CA	NC	HD	PD	FA	CA
FO	140.45	135.43	170.84*	121.96	128.62	198.71	210.27	186.03	200.37	215.30
	(53.20)	(29.67)	(44.45)	(23.77)	(22.54)	(23.61)	(27.36)	(25.58)	(30.86)	(44.55)
JITT	0.75	0.72	2.65*	1.01	1.00	1.45	2.84	1.04	2.18	2.41
	(0.46)	(0.33)	(2.35)	(0.60)	(0.51)	(1.09)	(1.42)	(0.13)	(1.26)	(2.02)
RAP	0.43	0.40	1.54*	0.56	0.57	0.88	1.67	0.60	1.31	1.37
	(0.28)	(0.22)	(1.36)	(0.33)	(0.30)	(0.67)	(0.83)	(0.12)	(0.73)	(1.18)
PPQ	0.44	0.40	1.60*	0.59	0.58	0.85	1.77	0.56	1.32	1.54
	(0.27)	(0.20)	(1.42)	(0.37)	(0.30)	(0.64)	(0.93)	(0.11)	(0.80)	(1.40)
SPPQ	0.79	1.13	2.12*	1.19	0.94	0.87	2.54*	1.17	1.72	3.44*
	(0.23)	(0.53)	(1.56)	(0.37)	(0.34)	(0.41)	(1.34)	(0.41)	(1.03)	(2.51)
VFO	1.76	2.19	3.25	3.25*	1.79	1.98	4.44	2.05	3.63	10.75*
	(0.86)	(0.59)	(2.16)	(1.41)	(0.66)	(1.25)	(1.57)	(0.58)	(1.97)	(12.88)
SHIM	4.29	4.45	6.15	5.19	4.44	5.11	6.98	3.17	5.74	8.53
	(1.47)	(1.95)	(3.14)	(3.17)	(3.22)	(1.36)	(2.42)	(0.39)	(2.65)	(4.27)
APQ	3.68	3.88	4.96	4.95	3.48	3.75	5.24	2.69	4.20	6.44
	(1.22)	(2.25)	(2.31)	(4.02)	(2.44)	(0.84)	(1.88)	(0.58)	(2.18)	(3.53)
SAPQ	6.52	7.28	7.58	8.40*	6.30	6.30	11.06	6.72	7.41	13.81*
	(1.18)	(2.55)	(2.75)	(1.67)	(3.37)	(0.58)	(1.46)	(1.09)	(4.20)	(9.42)
VAM	12.38	19.01	18.58*	41.18*	24.70*	16.60	35.74*	26.32	30.54*	44.13*
	(2.74)	(6.92)	(6.45)	(10.99)	(12.89)	(2.42)	(4.11)	(4.64)	(11.67)	(17.31)
SPI	14.07	12.46	23.98*	16.49	18.82	15.33	22.19	13.11	15.38	7.25
	(11.89)	(7.06)	(11.80)	(2.37)	(13.91)	(6.43)	(15.35)	(9.11)	(4.52)	(1.76)
VTI	0.044	0.052	0.044	0.044	0.053	0.034	0.049	0.041	0.047	0.084*
	(0.012)	(0.005)	(0.030)	(0.008)	(0.026)	(0.006)	(0.016)	(0.004)	(0.013)	(0.048)
NHR	0.140	0.160	0.151	0.153	0.142	0.142	0.166	0.159	0.163	0.274*
	(0.017)	(0.016)	(0.042)	(0.025)	(0.023)	(0.018)	(0.035)	(0.029)	(0.047)	(0.149)

* = significantly above the control group (Kruskall–Wallis test; $p < 0.05$); see Table 1 for abbreviations.

Table 48.3. Correlation analysis with the perceptual parameters

	harsh	strained	creaky	quiver	fluctuations of pitch	fluctuations of loudness	overall performance
breathy	0.71*	0.29	0.32	0.60*	0.21	0.34*	0.62*
harsh		0.60*	0.71*	0.62*	0.33	0.30	0.76*
strained			0.65*	0.55*	0.40*	0.51*	0.74*
creaky				0.55*	0.45*	0.39*	0.67*
fluctuations of pitch					0.65*	0.65*	0.83*
fluctuations of loudness						0.69*	0.64*
overall performance							0.64*

* = significant (p<0.01).

Table 48.4. Correlation analysis with the acoustic parameters

	JITT	RAP	PPQ	SPPQ	VFO	SHIM	APQ	SAPQ	VAM	SPI	VTI	NHR
FO	0.30	0.32	0.31	0.28	0.24	0.05	-0.11	0.17	0.15	-0.15	0.03	0.04
JITT		0.99*	0.99*	0.88*	0.61*	0.60*	0.49*	0.31	0.08	0.39*	0.14	0.46*
RAP			0.99*	0.87*	0.60*	0.60*	0.48*	0.31	0.07	0.40*	0.13	0.44*
PPQ				0.89*	0.64*	0.62*	0.50*	0.33	0.09	0.38*	0.17	0.48*
SPPQ					0.78*	0.63*	0.54*	0.48*	0.25	0.27	0.33	0.70*
VFO						0.51*	0.39*	0.32	0.18	-0.01	0.22	0.66*
SHIM							0.95*	0.67*	0.33	-0.02	0.57*	0.71*
APQ								0.66*	0.35*	-0.02	0.58*	0.66*
SAPQ									0.58*	-0.09	0.55*	0.52*
VAM										-0.12	0.42*	0.38*
SPI											-0.43*	-0.17
VTI												0.67*

* = significant (p<0.01).

Table 48.5. Cross-correlations: perceptual versus acoustic parameters

	breathy	harsh	strained	creaky	quiver	fluctuations of		overall performance
						pitch	loudness	
FO	0.29	0.02	0.16	−0.11	0.14	−0.09	0.20	0.12
JITT	0.64*	0.52*	0.24	0.31	0.47*	0.17	0.19	0.46*
RAP	0.65*	0.52*	0.24	0.30	0.46*	0.17	0.19	0.45*
PPQ	0.65*	0.52*	0.24	0.29	0.46*	0.17	0.19	0.47*
SPPQ	0.56*	0.48*	0.31	0.31	0.52*	0.27	0.27	0.53*
VFO	0.32	0.22	0.19	0.10	0.24	0.14	0.30	0.30
SHIM	0.55*	0.69*	0.38*	0.49*	0.49*	0.24	0.24	0.59*
APQ	0.48*	0.66*	0.34*	0.52*	0.46*	0.26	0.22	0.58*
SAPQ	0.44*	0.46*	0.40*	0.40*	0.60*	0.35*	0.44*	0.56*
VAM	0.33	0.35*	0.46*	0.44*	0.53*	0.37*	0.61*	0.55*
SPI	0.37*	0.18	−0.19	0.06	0.12	0.08	−0.13	0.05
VTI	0.22	0.46*	0.56*	0.38*	0.31	0.17	0.22	0.52*
NHR	0.20	0.44*	0.45*	0.42*	0.33	0.24	0.23	0.45*

* = significant (p<0.01)

References

Hertrich I, Ackermann H (1995) Gender-specific vocal dysfunctions in Parkinson's disease: electroglottographic and acoustic analyses. Annals of Otology, Rhinology and Laryngology 104: 197–202.

Hertrich I, Ackermann H, Braun S, Spieker S (1996) Geschlechtsdimorphismus pathologischer Stimmerkmale bei zentralnervösen Dysphonien: eine vergleichend auditiv-akustische Studie. Sprache-Stimme-Gehör 20: 169–74.

Nittrouer S, McGowan RS, Milenkovic PH, Beehler D (1990) Acoustic measurements of men's and women's voices: a study of context effects and covariation. Journal of Speech and Hearing Research 33: 761–75.

Chapter 49
A Case of Spasmodic Dysphonia Restricted to Propositional Language Tasks

ERNST G. DE LANGEN

Introduction

Spasmodic dysphonia has long been considered a psychogenic voice disorder resulting from a conversion reaction. At present there is some consensus that it is – in most cases – a neurogenic voice disorder. Spasmodic (also called spastic) dysphonia or laryngeal dystonia is an action-induced laryngeal movement disorder. Voice quality can be effortful, squeezed, grunting, choked, stuttering-like, jerky, strained-strangled or pinched. Sometimes periodic breaks in phonation can be discerned. Voice quality is usually normal during laughter, singing, shouting, or anger. Aronson (1980) distinguishes between adductor spastic dysphonia, abductor spastic dysphonia, and mixed adductor-abductor spastic dysphonia.

Patients with spasmodic dysphonia are forced to phonate during involuntary effortful closure of the larynx in cases of the adductor type. Abductor spasmodic dysphonia leads to a breathy, effortful, voice quality with abrupt termination of voicing resulting in aphonic whispered segments of speech. Spasmodic dysphonia is resistant to voice therapy. The onset of the disorder is slow with progressive deterioration stabilizing after three to five years. The onset is usually in middle age with a greater incidence in females. The site of the neurological disorder is uncertain so far, but the condition seems to originate in the extrapyramidal system. Since spasmodic dysphonia is a focal dystonia it can be restricted to the vocal cords but in most cases it combines with other focal symptoms like blepharospasm, oromandibular dystonia, torticollis, or writer's cramp. In some cases the distribution is segmental (cranial, axial or crural), multifocal, or generalized (Brin, Fahn, Blitzer, Olson, Stewart., 1992). Dystonia can be primary, with or without a hereditary pattern, or secondary, i.e. associated with other neurological disorders, most of them known as basal ganglia disorders.

In a study of 45 subjects with spasmodic dysphonia Pool et al. (1991) found the majority (71.1%) had abnormal neurological characteristics. They found a considerable heterogeneity among these patients with respect to neurological signs and brain imaging results. They concluded that spasmodic dysphonia is a manifestation of disordered motor control involving systems of neurons rather than single anatomical sites. They suggested that the pallidothalamic – supplementary motor area (SMA) – system could be responsible for the pathogenesis of spasmodic dysphonia. Thalamocortical projections to the SMA are mainly from the pars oralis of the ventrolateral nucleus of the thalamus (Vlo). The input to the Vlo is primarily from the globus pallidus in the basal ganglia. Involvement of the globus pallidus, projections from the globus pallidus itself to the Vlo, the Vlo itself, projections from the Vlo to the SMA, or the SMA itself might produce spasmodic dysphonia. The co-occurence of basal ganglia signs, however, supports the hypothesis that spasmodic dysphonia arises from a disorder in a system that is located in the basal ganglia or directly functionally connected with them.

Case report

A 42-year-old woman, EL, with a diagnosis of psychogenic dysphonia lasting for more than five years, was assessed because she was totally unresponsive to speech therapy and psychotherapy. She reported that before onset of her voice problems she had twitching of her eyelids for several months which, in a video demonstration of movement disorders, she identified as blepharospasm. She had a feeling of tension in her face during speaking and eating and sometimes a retroflexion of the head. She indicated that during emotionally loaded situations like anger and quarrels, and also immediatly after sleeping and during singing, she experienced her voice as rather normal. One year ago she had to deliver an address at a dinner on the occasion of her husband's birthday. She learned the text by heart and delivered it in a normal voice quality in the presence of 50 people, as demonstrated by a video tape. Immediately afterwards her voice deteriorated again. An extensive interview revealed some evidence of psychosocial problems.

Since the onset of her voice problems there was a slowly progressing alteration of her voice, in the beginning with intermittent remissions. For more than one year her voice problems were persistent without considerable changes.

Neuroradiological examination with CT (non-contrast and contrast) and MRI (T1 and T2) did not produce any evidence of structural changes.

An intensive clinical phonetic examination included the following aspects:

- spontaneous speech
- diadochokinesis
- vowel prolongation
- assessment of articulation
- voicing onset and voice quality
- fundamental frequency-intensity profile
- contrastive and sentence stress
- speech respiration
- posture of head and trunk
- motility of jaw, lips and tongue in chewing and swallowing.

Additional assessment included the examination of automatized speech like counting to 20, reciting the alphabet, the days of the week, the names of the seasons and of European countries, and the completion of word pairs, antonyms, proverbs, songs and sentences.

There was an independent 'second-opinion' examination by an experienced speech-language pathologist, two experts in phoniatrics, and two experts in neurologic movement disorders. An acoustic analysis of speech samples was made by spectograms.

Results

During spontaneous speech a mild facial dyskinesia and sometimes episodes of visible dystonic contractions of the neck were observed and also a discrete focal myoclonus of a part of the upper lip. During spontaneous (propositional) speech the voice was abnormal with a relatively low fundamental frequency. The voice quality was strained and effortful with intermittent episodes of breathiness and hypernasality, especially at the end of an expiration phase. During non-propositional speech-like sentence repetition, reading, automatized speech, vowel prolongation, singing and diadochokinesis the voice was completely normal as judged by the patient, her husband and the phonetician. Laryngoscopy showed almost normal movements of the vocal cords. A fundamental frequency-intensity profile registered some slight reduction and tension in phonation. Articulation, prosody, motility of jaw, lips and tongue as well as chewing and swallowing were normal.

Spectrographic analysis (narrow band and broad band) of propositional speech revealed a fundamental frequency of 140 Hz. The formant structure included only F1 and the harmonic structure contained only up to three partial tones. The analysis of samples of non-propositional speech showed a fundamental frequency of 180–200 Hz and a formant structure with F1 and F2, and in parts also F3. The harmonic structure contained up to 15 partial tones.

The clinical and phonetic investigation resulted in the unanimous diagnosis of a spasmodic dysphonia (adductor – abductor type) restricted to propositional language caused by focal dystonia. At present EL is treated with botulinum toxin and respiration training by a speech-language therapist. This treatment is successful and the voice quality is also nearly normal in propositional language tasks.

Discussion

Does phonation in propositional language and in non-propositional language rely on different neural mechanisms? Are distinct processes involved, mediated by disparate brain regions or systems, and is the dimension of these processes specific to language or can some analogy to this also be found in other domains of human behaviour?

Two types of facial expressions may be distinguished (Moscovitch and Olds, 1982; Borod, 1993): posed expressions and spontaneous expressions. Posed facial expressions are, by definition, intentional and volitional, whereas spontaneous expressions are involuntary reactions to emotionally stimulating situations. Neurological evidence suggests that posed facial expressions involve the cortical pyramidal system, whereas spontaneous expressions involve the subcortical extrapyramidal system.

In a study of akinesia, Heilman and Watson (1989) distinguish between movements that are generated primarily in response to an external stimulus (exo-evoked movements) and movements that are generated based upon motivations internal to an organism (endo-evoked movements). In a review of the structure of the supplementary motor area Goldberg (1985) defines similar phenomena using different terminology. Goldberg discusses two motor-programming systems with a 'projectional system', in which action is derived from an internal model that permits prediction of a future state of affairs, and a 'responsive system', in which action is based upon an explicit external input. The first system involves the supplementary motor area, the basal ganglia, and the portion of the ventral lateral nucleus of the thalamus receiving pallidal input whereas the latter system is associated with the lateral premotor cortex, the cerebellum and the portion of the ventral lateral nucleus receiving cerebellar input. In the thalamus the 'pars oralis' of the ventral lateral nucleus is receiving direct input from the medial globus pallidus and indirect input from the lateral globus pallidus. The caudal part and the pars extrema of the ventral lateral nucleus receive input from the cerebellar dentate nucleus.

In a study of 15 dystonic patients with positron emission tomography (PET) and (18F)-2-fluoro-2-deoxy-D-glucose (FDG) Karbe, Holthoff, Rudolf, Herholz and Heiss (1992) confirmed the concept that dystonia is caused by impaired connections between the basal ganglia, the thalamus, and frontal association areas. In these patients the reduction of rCMR(Glu) in frontal areas known to receive major input from different thalamic nuclei, which in turn receive input from pallidothalamic projections, shows that dystonia can be caused by metabolic abnormality without any changes in basal ganglia morphology. These findings agree with Marsden, Obeso, Zarranz and Lang's (1985) concept of dystonia, which assumes that functional lesions of the thalamus, as well as of the caudate and lentiform nuclei, have the common ability to disrupt the thalamic input to the frontal cortex, and ultimately to the motor area. The pathways described in idiopathic dystonia seems to be the same loop that is involved in the projectional system of Goldberg (1985) and which is similar to the concept of endo-evoked movements of Heilman and Watson (1989).

Ceballos-Baumann *et al.* (1995), on the basis of a study with H2 15O and positron emission tomography, state that a decrease in inhibitory output from the internal globus pallidus secondary to striatal overactivity should produce dystonia. In a review about focal dystonia Csala and Deuschl (1994) postulate an idiopathic dysfunction of the putamen and the globus pallidus, which results in an increase of activity of the direct inhibitory pathway to the globus pallidus. Albin, Young and Penney (1989) conclude that dystonia represents a clinical equivalent of a generalized insufficiency of all basal ganglia pathways, which leads to a decrease of pallidothalamic inhibition. Both interpretations implicate an overactivity of thalamocortical afferents.

Since a reproductional and responsive task like repetition is absent in Van Lancker's (1987) propositional/non-propositional dimension, it is necessary to consider whether this task, as well as reading aloud and automatized speech, belong to the non-propositional part of the continuum. Repetition is not overlearned and it does not necessarily contain fixed forms and conventional meaning. To some degree, however, it seems to be reflexive and therefore not endo-evoked.

It is interesting that repetition is spared or only minimally impaired in most cases of thalamic aphasia (Papagno and Guidolti, 1983; Crosson, 1985; Kirk and Kertesz, 1994). Thus, lesions to thalamic nuclei in most cases do not hinder aphasic patients in producing a response to an external stimulus although there is an overall paucity of spontaneous speech.

It is not intended to equalize concepts of motor and linguistic behaviour. In the production of propositional language, however, it should be considered that phonation and articulation are planned and programmed continuously during language formulation. According to the concept of incremental sentence production (Kempen and Hoenkamp, 1987; Levelt, 1989) there is a close relationship between the stages of conceptualization, formulation and articulation, provided that an utterance is newly created and expresses a unique predicate or statement, itself the product of a voluntary, intentional cognitive act. In communicative acts, language is propositional in the sense that it is made up of novel sentences to express particular thoughts. This always requires a unique and novel cooperation between linguistic and motor behaviour.

Non-propositional language utterances are familiar, conventionalized and more-or-less holistic, with stimulus-bound, overlearned or high frequency cohesive sentences. They involve little conceptual or semantic contribution on the part of the speaker. So, coordination of linguistic and motor processing is prepared or learned in some way and does not require neuronal systems normally used in unprepared tasks.

Thus, if symptoms of dystonia become apparent only in the course of spontaneous propositional speech production, this means that these newly created, original and novel utterances must involve the cortico-striato-pallido-thalamo-cortical loop, whereas non-propositional speech production seems to rely mainly on other projections which result in normal phonatory control.

This interpretation does not exclude a right-hemisphere contribution to the production of non-propositional speech. In the present case, however, the preservation of phonatory control is not primarily demonstrated on the basis of unitary and cohesive forms of non-propositional expressions like stereotyped utterances, social formulae and serial speech, which seem to be intact in some aphasic patients, but rather on tasks like repetition, reading aloud and sentence completion, which are usually impaired in aphasia and are considered to involve mainly left-hemisphere structures.

In experimental studies with squirrel monkeys, Jürgens and Zwirner (1996) demonstrated the existence of two separate vocal fold control pathways at mid-brain level: one limbic, responsible for non-verbal emotional vocal utterances, and one neocortical, responsible for the production of learned vocal patterns. These two forms of vocalization are clearly different from human patterns of phonation. The existence of separate pathways of neural control of phonation in squirrel monkeys however shows that there is some phylogenetic evidence for the development of distinct neuronal pathways dependent on the underlying intention of communication behaviour and subsequent phonatory motor control. Similar proposals were also made by Myers (1968) and by Botez and Barbeau (1971).

We are still far from understanding how it may work in humans. The differentiation of motor behaviour with respect to exo-evoked and endo-evoked movements in relationship with the underlying linguistically defined communicative intention may throw some light on the question of why spasmodic dysphonia may be restricted to propositional language tasks, at least in some cases. A further conclusion from this case study is that examination of these patients should always include different tasks of linguistic behaviour in order to detect potentially distinct performance in phonatory control.

References

Albin RL, Young AB, Penney JB (1989) The functional anatomy of basal ganglia disorders. Trends in Neuroscience 12: 366–75.

Aronson AE (1980) Clinical Voice Disorders. New York: Thieme-Stratton, pp. 157–69.

Borod JC (1993) Cerebral mechanisms underlying facial, prosodic, and lexical emotional expression: A review of neuropsychological studies and methodological issues. Neuropsychology 7: 445–63.

Botez MI, Barbeau A (1971) Role of subcortical structures and particularly of the thalamus in the mechanisms of speech and language. International Journal of Neurology 8: 300–20.

Brin MF, Fahn FS, Blitzer A, Olson Ramig L, Stewart C (1992) Movement disorders of the larynx. In Blitzer A, Brin MF, Sasaki CT, Fahn S, Harris KS (Eds) Neurological Disorders of the Larynx. New York: Thieme, pp 248–78.

Ceballos-Baumann, Passingham RE, Warner T, Playford ED, Marsden CD, Brooks DJ (1995) Overactive prefrontal and underactive motor control areas in idiopathic dystonia. Annals of Neurology 37: 363–72.

Crosson B (1985) Subcortical functions in language: a working model. Brain and Language 25: 257–92.

Csala B, Deuschl G (1994) Kraniozervikale Dystonien. Nervenarzt 65: 75–94.

Goldberg G (1985) Supplementary motor area structure and function: review and hypotheses. Behavioral and Brain Sciences 8: 567–615.

Heilman KM, Watson RT (1989) Intentional-activation disorders. Paper presented at the 15th Annual Course in Behavioral Neurology and Neuropsychology of the Florida Society of Neurology and the Center for Neuropsychological Studies, Tampa, FL.

Jürgens U, Zwirner P (1996) The role of the periaquaductal grey in limbic and neocortical vocal fold control. Neuroreport 7: 2921–3.

Karbe H, Holthoff VA, Rudolf J, Herholz K, Heiss WD (1992) Positron emission tomography demonstrates frontal cortex and basal ganglia hypometabolism in dystonia. Neurology 42: 1540–4.

Kempen G, Hoenkamp E (1987) An incremental procedural grammar for sentence formulation. Cognitive Science 11: 201–58.

Kirk A, Kertesz A (1994) Cortical and subcortical aphasias compared. Aphasiology 8: 65–82.

Levelt WJM (1989) Speaking: From Intention to Articulation. Cambridge, MA: The MIT Press, pp 236–246.

Marsden CD, Obeso JA, Zarranz JJ, Lang AE (1985) The anatomical basis of symptomatic hemidystonia. Brain 108: 463–83.

Moscovitch M, Olds J (1982) Asymmetries in spontaneous facial expressions and their possible relation to hemispheric specialization. Neuropsychologia 20: 71–81.

Myers RE (1968) Neurology of social communication in primates. Proceedings of the 2nd International Congress of Primatology, Atlanta 3: 1–9

Papagno C, Guidolti M (1983) A case of aphasia following left thalamic hemorrhage. European Neurology 22: 93–5.

Pool KD, Freeman FJ, Finitzo T, Hayashi MM, Chapman SB, Devous MD, Close LG, Kondraske GV, Mendelsohn D, Schaefer SD, Watson BC (1991) Heterogeneity in spasmodic dysphonia. Archives of Neurology 48: 305–9.

Van Lancker D (1987) Nonpropositional speech: Neurolinguistic studies. In Ellis AW (Ed) Progress in the Psychology of Language, Vol 3. London: Lawrence Erlbaum, pp 49–118.

Chapter 50
Velar Function in Normal and Dysarthric Speakers

CHRISTIAN LEDL, SUSANNE HOLZLEITER AND
GERHARD HOCH

Introduction

Velopharyngeal valving mechanisms have received considerable attention in phonetic research. It is assumed that during the production of
oral sounds the velum moves backward and upward in order to
achieve a velopharyngeal closure, whereas for nasals it is lowered and
the airflow passes through the nasal cavity. According to this description, Thompson and Hixon (1979) reported that nasal airflow was zero
for isolated productions of /i/, /s/ and /z/ as well as for oral CV combinations with C= /t,d,s,z/ and V=/i/ and postulated that velar function in
isolated sound production could be described as a simple binary
mechanism. An important shortcoming of this study, however, results
from the selection of the speech material because the high vowel /i/
and the fricatives /s, z/ are known to be highly invariant in an articulatory, acoustic and aerodynamic way (Shadle and Scully, 1995; Hoole
and Tillmann, 1991).

Analyses of broader speech samples rejected the binary hypothesis.
Moll (1962) in an x-ray study, revealed that low vowels exhibited less
velopharyngeal closure than high vowels, and vowel height has been
shown to have an effect on velopharyngeal port opening and velum
height (Moll, 1962; Lubker, 1968; Fritzell, 1969). Additionally, Lubker
and Moll (1965) measured small nasal airflow during the production
of /p/. Their data seemed to be consistent with findings from Emanuel
and Counihan (1970) which also indicated the occurrence of nasal
airflow in totally oral plosive-vowel sequences and changes in oral
and nasal airflow rates depending on the consonantal and the vocalic
category.

Nasalization of vowels in nasal consonant-vowel syllables has been
confirmed by all investigators. Anticipatory coarticulation, i.e. the low-

ering of the velum in the vocalic segment that precedes a nasal consonant, has been found by Moll for speakers of American English.
Benguerel (1977) in an EMG-study of the levator veli palatini and the
palatoglossus muscles observed predominant anticipatory coarticulation for French speakers and nearly no carryover processes. Contrary to
these results, both carryover and anticipatory coarticulation of velar
movement have been described in German (Künzel 1979) and have
been interpreted as active preplanning (anticipatory) and mechanical
inertia of the velum (carryover).

Up to now, most normative data for assessing resonance have been
collected with English-speaking individuals and clinical studies were
mainly concerned with acoustic or kinematic deviations in children
with cleft palates. On the clinical side, Thompson and Murdoch (1995)
investigated neurological patients by means of a nasal accelerometer.
They included 19 English-speaking subjects who suffered from a cerebrovascular accident (CVA) and who had been judged by perceptual ratings
as being hypo- or hypernasal. Unfortunately, the instrumental findings
could not confirm the clear perceptual ratings. In some of the hypernasal patients a significant increase in nasality indices was found in
the oral, but not in the nasal, speech tasks. It is therefore unclear
whether the latter findings reflect a general mechanism in dysarthric
speech production or, rather, whether they result from an inadequate
measurement principle.

By using the Rothenberg instrumentation for measuring oral and
nasal airflow in the present study, we aim to describe differences
between normal and dysarthric speech in German and to compare the
results with the existing clinical data. Furthermore, we want to investigate
whether German speakers demonstrate patterns of velo-pharyngeal closure similar to speakers of English and French.

Method

Subjects

We investigated three male and two female dysarthric speakers who
were rated by three trained speech therapists as being hypernasal.
Two of the subjects (P1 and P4) suffered from two-sided velar dysfunction, and three subjects (P2, P3, P5) from one-sided velar dysfunction caused by closed head injury (CHI) or cerebro-vascular accident (CVA). The patients' mean age was 46;4 and time since onset
ranged from three months to 100 months. The control group (N1 to
N5) for this study included three female and two male speakers ranging in age from 29 to 47 years (mean 38;0) with no history of speech
disorders.

Table 50.1. Demographic and clinical data of (a) normal controls and (b) patients

(a)

Subject no.	sex	age at assessment (years)
N1	f	29
N2	m	43
N3	m	31
N4	f	47
N5	f	37

(b)

Subject no.	sex	age at assessment (years)	time post-onset (months)	aetiology	velar incompetence
P1	m	26	100	CHI	two-sided
P2	f	62	9	CVA	one-sided
P3	m	58	3	CVA	one-sided
P4	m	37	10	CHI	two-sided
P5	f	49	10	CVA	one-sided

CHI = closed head injury CVA = cerebro-vascular accident

Speech material

The speech material used in this study consisted of a series of sustained phonemes (Corpus 1) and CV reiterations (Corpus 2). Corpus 1 included the vowels /a:/, /i:/, /u:/, the nasals /m:/, /n:/ and the fricatives /f:/, /s:/. Each phoneme had to be sustained for approximately five seconds during a single breath and was repeated 10 times in a randomized order. Corpus 2 consisted of the following CV combinations: nasal consonant-vowel with C=/m, n/ and V= /a, i, u/ as well as oral consonant-vowel combinations with C=/p, t, k/ and V=/a, i, u/. CV-reiterations were produced at a moderate speech rate in time with a metronome (80 beats/minute) and were repeated 10 times.

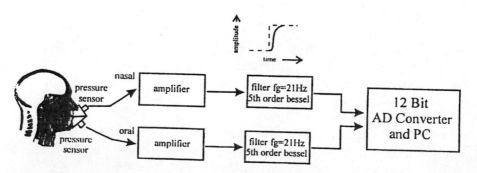

Figure 50.1. Experimental design.

Instrumentation

Measurements were made by means of a Rothenberg Mask. Details of the measurement principle are given elsewhere (Rothenberg, 1973; Rothenberg, 1977). In the present study, the two separated chambers of the mask were used for simultaneous measurements of oral and nasal airflow. The analog signals were amplified, low-pass and filtered with a fifth-order Bessel filter at a cut-off frequency of 21 Hz, and AD converted (12 bit).

Data analysis

Sustained phonemes

To quantify the absolute airflow during the production of sustained phonemes, the integrals of nasal and oral airflow were computed for a period of three seconds starting from the first maximum of the oral airfow signal. These segmentations were adopted for the oral and the nasal channel. Relative oral airflow (ROA) was computed by dividing the values of the absolute oral airflow by the sum of the absolute oral and nasal airflow.

CV-reiterations

In the first stage of analysis, the beginning (minimum 1) and ending (minimum 2) of airflow for each target phoneme were marked. Segmentations were made in the oral channel for oral sounds and in the nasal channel for nasal sounds. These boundaries were used to compute integrals of both the absolute nasal and the absolute oral airflow using a 10% onset and offset criterion. Values of relative oral airflow (ROA) were calculated as indicated above.

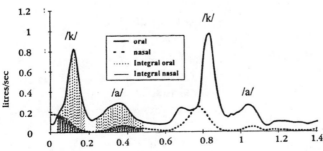

Figure 50.2. Example of airflow signals during a Rothenberg mask recording of /ka/ (dotted line = nasal airflow, solid line = oral airflow), illustrating the method of segmentation and the calculation of integrals (integrals of oral and nasal airflow for each phoneme).

Furthermore, we wanted to determine the amount of vocalic nasalization – the coarticulatory influence of nasals on vowels. We therefore calculated the amount of overlap of oral and nasal airflow at the phoneme boundaries (Int1 and Int2) and hypothesized that we would observe a carryover type of coarticulation if the overlap at the beginning of the vowel (Int1) were higher than the overlap at its ending (Int2) and an anticipatory type in the opposite case.

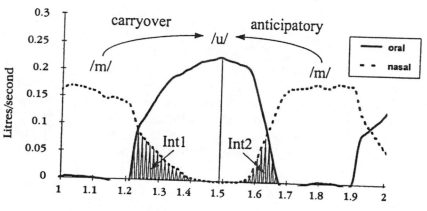

Figure 50.3. Example of oral and nasal airflow during a /mu/-reiteration with sections of nasal and oral airflow curves (Int1, Int2). Arrows indicate carryover and anticipatory coarticulation.

Results

Sustained phonemes

Relative oral airflow during the production of the sustained vowels /aː/, /iː/ and /uː/ is shown in Figure 50.4 for the normal speakers (N1 to N5) and for the dysarthric speakers (P1 to P5). The patients' productions are clearly hypernasal and they therefore exhibit less relative oral airflow when compared to the normal realizations. In the latter, the contribution of oral airflow to the sound production never falls below the 75% level (minimum 75.7% for /a/; 79.1% for /i/; 83,6% for /u/). Generally, the relative oral airflow is least for /aː/, indicating the highest degree of nasality for this vowel. Except in the case of speakers P1 and P2, high vowels show less nasality than the low vowel with /uː/ being even less nasal than /iː/.

Single sound
Vowels: relative oral airflow

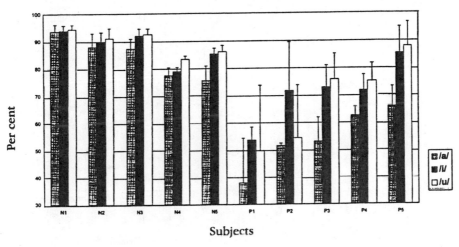

Figure 50.4. Sustained vowels: values of relative oral airflow (ROA) for /a:/, /i:/, /u:/ produced by normal (N1–N5) and dysarthric speakers (P1–P5).

Fricatives are more resistant to nasalization than vowels. Relative oral airflow always exceeds the 87% level (87.5% for /s/; 90.2% for /f/) in the productions of the normal and of the dysarthic speakers who suffer from a one-sided velar dysfunction. Only speakers P1 and P4, who suffer from a two-sided velar dysfunction, show a clear increase in nasal airflow and are much more variable in their productions. Furthermore, all subjects except P1 demonstrate higher relative oral airflow values for /f:/ than for /s:/.

CV-reiterations

Consonants

Analyses of the CV-reiterations were divided into the consonantal and the vocalic segments. Firstly, we looked at the consonantal segment and wanted to quantify changes in relative and absolute airflow. The relative airflow measurements revealed few structural differences between the two speaker groups but displayed generally lower values of relative oral airflow for nasals and plosives uttered by the patients.

Their various vowels did not have any effects on plosives in normal production (see Figure 50.6a). Percentages of ROA were stable across all vowels and ranged from 98% for /a/ and /i/ to 99% for /u/. Besides somewhat lower values of ROA, the dysarthric productions showed a slight decrease of nasality according to the vocalic environment (/a/: ROA=86%; /i/: ROA=90%; /u/: ROA=93%) (see Figure 50.6b).

Single sounds
Fricatives: relative oral airflow

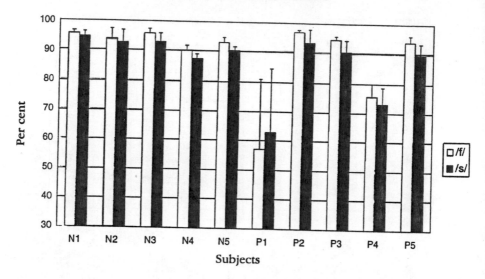

Figure 50.5. Sustained fricatives: values of relative oral airflow (ROA) for /f:/, /s:/ produced by normal speakers (N1–N5) and dysarthric speakers (P1–P5).

Consonant: relative oral airflow normal speakers

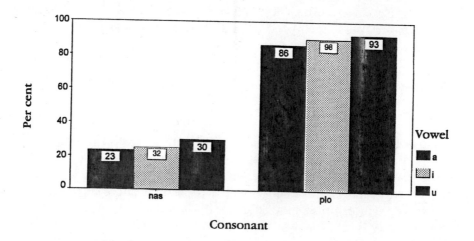

Figure 50.6a. CV-reiterations: values of relative oral airflow (ROA) for nasals and plosives (consonantal segment) depending on the vowels /a/, /i/, /u/ produced by normal speakers.

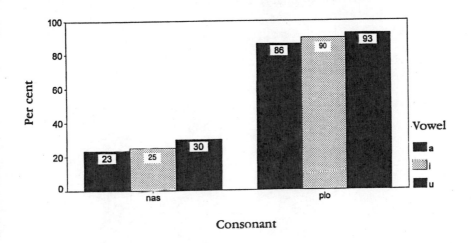

Figure 50.6b. CV-reiterations: values of relative oral airflow (ROA) for nasals and plosives (consonantal segment) depending on the vowels /a/, /i/, /u/ produced by dysarthric speakers.

In both groups the nasal consonants /m/ and /n/ were coarticulated with the following vowel so that the vowel /a/ causes more nasalization than /i/ or /u/.

Analyses of absolute oral and nasal airflow, however, revealed clear differences between the two speaker groups. We measured a considerable increase in both airflow channels during the dysarthric productions (see Figure 50.7). The values of absolute nasal airflow for the plosives /p, t, k/ grew from 1.1 ml per phoneme in the normal utterances to 13.6 ml (difference = 12.5 ml) in the dysarthric realizations; the values of the absolute oral airflow were from 67.8 ml to 96.3 ml (difference = 28.5 ml). For the nasal consonants /m/ and /n/ there was a significant increase of nasal (difference = 45.4 ml) and only a slight increase (difference = 8.0 ml) of oral airflow for speakers P1 to P5.

Vowels

In the vocalic segment we also observed a coarticulatory effect induced by the consonant environment. As could be expected, there was a significant nasalization of all vowels by the nasal consonant for both speaker groups. Compared to the sustained productions mean values of ROA (normal speakers) were decreased for /a/ from 84.5% in isolation to 58% in the nasal consonant-vowel sequence, for /i/ from 88.0%

to 74% and from 89.6% to 82% for /u/ (see Figures 50.4 and 50.8a). The values of the dysarthic speakers are decreased from 54.3% to 46% for /a/, from 71.3% to 53% for /i/ and from 68.8% to 53% for /u/ (see Figures 50.4 and 50.8b). Our control speakers maintained vowel intrinsic differences in ROA (these have already been observed in isolated productions) whereas dysarthric speakers tended to obliterate the pattern and were much more hypernasal, especially in the production of high vowels.

Cv-reiterations
Consonantal airflow by speaker – and consonantal category

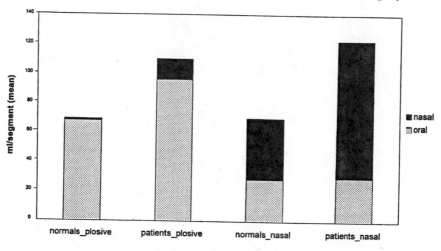

Figure 50.7. CV-reiterations: values of absolute oral and nasal airflow for plosives and nasals (consonantal segment) produced by normals and patients.

In the plosive-vowel sequences there was no vowel-intrinsic difference of ROA but there was rather an 'oralization' of the vowel. This phenomenon is especially evident for the dysarthic utterances in which values of ROA varied from 54.3% in the sustained productions of /a/ to 76% in the CV-sequences, from 71.3% to 82% (/i/) and from 68,8% to 81% (/u/).

Regarding the absolute values of oral and nasal airflow, differences between the two speaker groups mainly result from an increase of nasal airflow in the dysarthric utterances (see Figure 50.9). There was a simultaneous increase in oral airflow in the plosive vowel sequences which, however, seems to play a minor role when compared to the considerable changes in the consonantal segment. The difference in oral airflow between normals and patients in CV-reiterations with C = plosive amounted to 13 ml and in nasal airflow to 12.3 ml, with C = nasal to 0.9ml (oral airflow) and to 46 ml (nasal airflow).

Vowel: relative oral airflow normal speakers

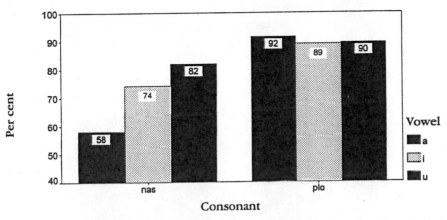

Figure 50.8a. CV-reiterations: values of relative oral airflow (ROA) for /a/, /i/, /u/ (vocalic segment) depending on the preceeding consonant (nasal, plosive). Productions by normal speakers.

Vowel: relative oral airflow patients

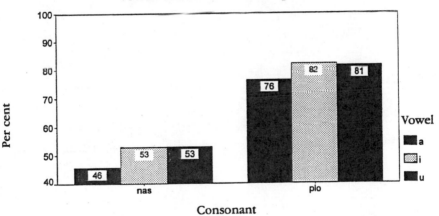

Figure 50.8b. CV-reiterations: values of relative oral airflow (ROA) for /a/, /i/, /u/ (vocalic segment) depending on the preceeding consonant (nasal, plosive). Productions by dysarthric speakers.

Coarticulation: anticipatory versus carryover

As described above, vocalic nasalization is assumed to be induced mainly by anticipatory processes. Analyses of Int1 and Int2, however, show influences of both the preceding and the following nasal in CV-sequences. The blending of the nasal and the vocalic segment was enlarged for the dysarthric speakers except P5, whose patterns did not differ from normal. Moreover, all speakers except N5 and P2 demonstrated higher values for Int1 and therefore exhibited a predominance of carryover processes. Speaker P2 clearly inverted the pattern, whereas N5 showed only a slight predominance of anticipatory coarticulation.

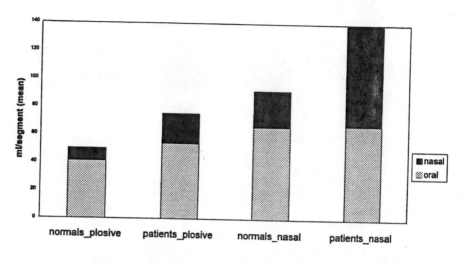

Figure 50.9. CV-reiteratons: values of absolute oral and nasal airflow for plosives and nasals (vocalic segment) produced by normals and patients.

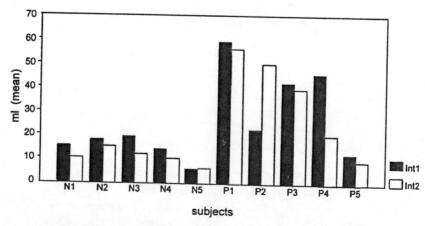

Figure 50.10. Nasal-vowel reiterations: patterns of carryover (Int1) and anticipatory (Int2) coarticulation for normal (N1-N5) and dysarthric (P1-P5) speakers.

Summary and discussion

German speakers' patterns of velopharyngeal closure during sustained phoneme production are largely comparable to those reported for other languages. Vowel height has a clear effect on velum height and nasality is highest for the low vowel /a/ and lower for the high vowels, with /u/ being less nasal than /i/. This ordering is preserved in nasal-vowel reiterations, but not in plosive-vowel sequences. The greater velo-pharyngeal closure for /u/ compared to /i/ is certainly surprising. However, it might be hypothesized that the high back position of the tongue for /u/ supports elevation of the velum. Analyses also revealed a lesser degree of nasality for the labio-dental fricative in comparison to the alveoalar fricative /s/. In CV-sequences, plosives are not influenced by neighbouring vowels, whereas vowels are influenced by plosives and show an increase in oral airflow. In consequence, coarticulation of plosive-vowel sequences has to be described as being unidirectional in nature, coarticulation of nasal-vowel sequences is bi-directional with vowels and nasals being influenced by each other. We therefore observe three phenomena:

(a) vowels and fricatives show an intrinsic ordering of nasality;
(b) nasal consonants nasalize the vowel and intensify vowel-intrinsic differences;
(c) plosives 'oralize' the vowel and extinguish vowel-intrinsic differences.

Differences in the degree of nasality are therefore not only phoneme-intrinsic, as suggested by the notion of coarticulatory resistance (Bladon and Al Bamerni, 1976), but they have to be described as a function of vocalic and consonantal variation.

In contrast with English and French speakers, who exhibited little or no carryover coarticulation, German speakers showed both carryover and anticipatory nasalizations with a slight predominance of the first type. Similar results for German have been reported by Künzel (1979). In view of these cross-linguistic differences it is doubtful whether carry-over processes should be explained by mechanical factors. It rather seems that they should be explained by postulating language-specific timing patterns of velar gestures leading to variations in the temporal extent of vowel nasalization across languages (Cohn, 1990).

Comparing dysarthric to normal productions, dysarthric speakers maintain the structural properties of nasalization in German. This is expressed by largely comparable patterns of relative oral airflow for isolated and reiterated productions. Differences between the two speaker groups can be explained by an increase in nasal and oral airflow that can be especially observed in totally oral sequences. This phenomenon might be interpreted as a compensatory strategy to increase intraoral pressure by reinforcing expiration in speech. Therapists might use the fact that dysarthric speakers perform best during the production of fricatives, plosive-vowel combinations and isolated high vowels but they should control pathological changes or increase of airflow pressure.

Acknowledgement

We gratefully acknowledge the assistance of Erich Hartmann for program delivery and data analysis.

References

Benguerel A-P, Hirose H, Sawashima M, Ushijima T (1977) Velar coarticulation in French: an electromyographic study. Journal of Phonetics 5: 149–58.

Bladon RAW, Al Bamerni A (1976). Coarticulation resistance of English /l/. Journal of Phonetics 4: 135–50.

Cohn AC (1990) Phonetic and phonological rules of nasalization. UCLA Working Papers in Phonetics 76.

Emanuel FW, Counihan D T (1970) Some characteristics of oral and nasal air flow during plosive consonant production. Cleft Palate Journal 7: 249–60.

Fritzell B (1969) The velopharyngeal muscles in speech: an electromyographic and cineradiographic study. Acta Otolaryngologica, Suppl. 250.

Hoole P, Tillmann HG (1991) An articulatory investigation of front rounded and unrounded vowels. Proceedings XIIth International Congress of Phonetic Sciences, 2: 362–5.

Künzel HJ (1979) Videofluoroscopic evaluation of a photo-electric device for the registration of velar elevation in speech. Folia Phoniatrica 31: 153.

Moll KL (1962) Velopharyngeal closure for vowels. Journal of Speech and Hearing Research 5: 30–77.

Lubker JF (1968) An electromyographic-cineradiographic investigation of velar function during normal speech production. Cleft Palate Journal 5:1–18.

Lubker J, Moll K (1965) Simultaneous oral-nasal air flow measurements and cinefluorographic observations during speech production. Cleft Palate Journal 2: 257–72.

Rothenberg M (1973) A new inverse-filtering technique for deriving the glottal airflow waveform during voicing. Journal of the Acoustical Society of America 53: 1632–45.

Rothenberg M (1977) Airflow in speech. Journal of Speech and Hearing Research 20: 155–76.

Shadle CH, Scully C (1995) An articulatory-acoustic-aerodynamic analysis of [s] in VCV sequences. Journal of Phonetics 23: 53–66.

Thompson AE, Hixon TJ (1979) Nasal airflow during normal speech production. Cleft Palate Journal 16: 412–20.

Thompson EC, Murdoch BE (1995) Disorders of nasality in subjects with upper motor neuron type dysarthria following cerebrovascular accident. Journal of Communication Disorders 28: 261–76.

PERIPHERAL PROCESSES

Chapter 51
Surgical Mapping and Phonetic Analysis in Intra-Oral Cancer

JANET MACKENZIE BECK, ALAN WRENCH, MARY JACKSON, DAVID SOUTAR, A.GERRY ROBERTSON AND JOHN LAVER

Introduction

It is well documented that surgery for oral cancer may result in a range of articulatory deficits and hence reduced intelligibility (Fletcher, 1988). Many patients compensate surprisingly well for the loss or structural change of the articulators (Greven, Meijer and Tiwari ,1994) but we are not able to predict with any accuracy what the phonetic consequences of any particular type of surgical intervention are likely to be. If any conclusion can be drawn from the literature, or from clinical observations, it is that individuals vary enormously in their ability to compensate for oral surgery; some people have speech that sounds nearly normal following an almost complete glossectomy, whereas others may suffer much more severe speech distortion following more limited surgery. At present we cannot really judge to what extent these variations in compensatory ability are due to differing strategies used by the patient and to what extent they depend on precisely which parts of the speech production mechanism are damaged.

The study reported here was motivated initially by oral surgeons, who were anxious to be able to predict the speech outcome for patients undergoing surgery for oral cancer and to minimize the extent of surgically induced speech impairment. Concern for long-term survival of oral cancer patients dictates that additional tissue may be removed from the area surrounding a tumour in order to minimize the risk of spread. The dilemma faced by surgeons is that, because they do not know which muscles and nerves are most critical for intelligible speech, they have difficulty in judging how much tissue can be removed without catastrophic consequences for speech production. The issues involved in solving this dilemma and in predicting speech impairment are complex, involving knowledge of the relationships between oro-motor function and speech output, and between speech patterns and intelligibility.

Initial discussion with the surgeons highlighted an immediate difficulty in trying to correlate speech output with surgical pattern, which is that it is not common practice for surgeons to map with any accuracy the site and extent of tissue damaged or excised. A typical report might be, for example, 'tumour excised from dorsum of tongue, right side'. It was not always clear from medical notes whether or not excisions crossed the midline, or what volume of tissue had been excised. Development of an improved system for recording surgical patterns was obviously a priority.

This study was therefore a collaborative effort involving oral surgeons, speech and language therapists, phoneticians and a speech scientist. Funding was provided by the Cancer Research Campaign ('Objective Speech Quality Assessment in Patients with Intra-oral Cancers': University of Edinburgh and Canniesburn Hospital, Glasgow). The aims of this study were:

(a) to develop a method for mapping surgery that would be quick and easy to complete and to interpret, which would show the site and extent of tissue removal and damage, and which would allow predictions about speech impairment;
(b) to test the mapping and prediction technique by the analysis of actual speech output of patients undergoing surgical removal of intra-oral tumours.

A third aim of the overall project, which is not addressed in this paper, was to develop a computer-based work station for automatic analysis of voiceless fricatives, which were thought to be good indicators of articulatory quality. This work station, which can be used for assessment and for visual feedback during therapy, has been described elsewhere (Wrench, Beck, Jackson, Jack, Laver, Soutar and Robertson, 1993).

Development of a protocol for surgical mapping

A simple graphic protocol was developed, which allows mapping of surgery in three dimensions. This protocol is based on a variety of sources, including xeroradiographic tracings and tomographic images as well as standard anatomical descriptions. For each case, the site of surgery is mapped on to 6 diagrams of the oral structures. Figure 51.1 shows the mapping protocol, illustrating the way in which it might be

Intra-oral surgery mapping protocol

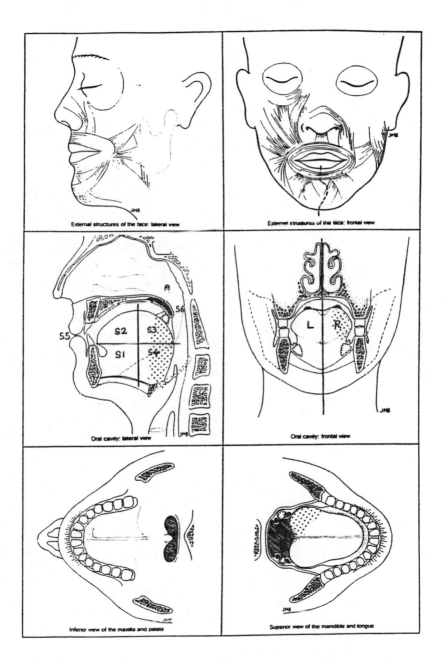

Figure 51.1. The surgical mapping protocol, showing a surgical map for a patient undergoing surgical excision of a tumour from the posterior surface of the tongue.

completed following surgical removal of a tumour affecting the posterior of the tongue. The upper two external views of the face are used to indicate the route of surgical entry, where relevant, and the intra-oral views are used to indicate areas of tissue excised or damaged within the oral and pharyngeal cavities. Trials involving over 100 patients show that the protocol provides much more detailed information about the site and extent of surgery than was previously available, and the protocol is now in routine use.

This approach to mapping could be criticized on the grounds that it is somewhat simplistic and lacking in detail, but this can be justified by two observations. Firstly, there is so much inter-individual variation in orofacial anatomy that the addition of too much detail could be misleading. Secondly, the surgeons report that during the operating procedure structures are often so distorted that they do not feel that they can be accurate enough in their drawing to justify any more detail.

An initial classification of each case can be made in terms of the sector(s) affected (see lateral view), and whether the site of surgery crosses the midline (see frontal, superior and inferior views). The main sectors can be described as follows:

Sector 1 = anterior lower quadrant of the tongue and anterior floor of mouth
Sector 2 = anterior upper quadrant of the tongue
Sector 3 = posterior upper quadrant of the tongue (posterior dorsum of tongue)
Sector 4 = posterior lower quadrant of the tongue (root of tongue)
Sector 5 = the labial area
Sector 6 = the soft palate and adjacent structures (i.e. the area involved in velopharyngeal valving).

It can be seen that the case illustrated involves unilateral excision of tissue affecting sectors 3 and 4 on the left side.

Predicting the phonetic consequences of surgery

In formulating predictions about speech output on the basis of surgical mapping, two assumptions need to be made explicit:

(a) Changed morphology of the vocal tract, in particular changes in resonating cavity volumes, will result in changes in the perceived voice quality. For example, excision of a large amount of tissue from the dorsum of the tongue will enlarge the space within the oral cavity. The perceived voice quality will mimic that of a normal speaker who adopts a lowered tongue posture. In other words, the speaker will be judged as having a lowered tongue body setting.

(b) Damage to individual muscles or muscle groups, or to their inner-vation, will be reflected in difficulties with articulatory movements, which normally involve action of those muscles or nerves. For ex-ample, damage to the hyoglossus muscle will inhibit median depres-sion of the tongue and may therefore cause difficulties in production of central lingual fricatives and approximants.

Coloured acetate overlays showing the major muscle groups can be used to help predict the type of speech impairment likely to be associ-ated with each surgical map, and knowledge of the extent of tissue removal can indicate possible changes in volume of the resonating cav-ities. An illustration of the use of muscle overlays to predict speech out-put is shown in Figure 51.2, using a case with bilateral excision, pre-dominantly affecting sector 1 but extending into sector 2. For the sake of clarity, and because colour cannot be used here, only some of the main lingual muscles are shown. The purpose is simply to indicate the general approach to the formulation of predictions.

In this case, it can be seen that the anterior part of the genioglossus muscle is probably affected, and also the geniohyoid. In addition, a con-siderable volume of tissue has been removed, thus significantly en-larging the oral cavity. From this information, we can make some pre-dictions about the speech impairments that are likely to result from this pattern of surgery.

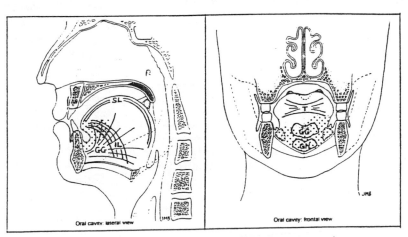

GG = Genioglossus muscle; GH = Geniohyoid muscle; T = Transverse muscle;
IL = Inferior longitudinal muscle; SL = Superior longitudinal muscle

Figure 51.2. An illustration of the use of muscle overlays in the prediction of speech output following surgery affecting the anterior floor of the mouth.

(a) Damage to the anterior part of the genioglossus will cause difficulty in lowering the centre of the tongue, causing distortion of /r/ and front oral fricatives.

(b) Damage to the geniohyoid will cause difficulty in raising the larynx, and also possibly in expanding the lumen of the pharynx. There may also be secondary effects on the control of phonation

(c) Loss of tissue mass will increase the volume of the front of the oral cavity. This may result in an auditory quality which is similar to that produced by a speaker with a normal vocal tract who retracts the tongue, thus increasing the volume ratio between the front oral cavity and the pharynx.

Some preliminary results, using this predictive approach, are reported in the next section.

Evaluating predictions about speech output.

A preliminary study of 10 patients undergoing surgery for intra-oral cancer attempted to relate surgical mapping data to speech output, using the predictive approach described above.

Subjects

The subjects were all aged between 50 years and 70 years, and underwent surgery at Canniesburn Hospital in Glasgow. These subjects would previously have been classified either as floor of mouth cases (N = 5) or dorsum of tongue (N = 5). The subjects are summarized in Tables 51.1 and 51.2, and partial surgical maps are shown in Figures 51.3 and 51.4.

Table 51.1. Summary information about subjects in group A (floor of mouth lesions)

	Gender	Type of excision
A1	Female	Unilateral, minimal loss of tongue tissue
A2	Male	Unilateral, minimal loss of tongue tissue
A3	Female	Unilateral, extensive loss of tissue
A4	Female	Midline, with mandibular involvement
A5	Male	Bilateral and extensive, with mandibular involvement

Predicted speech impairment

General predictions about likely speech impairment were formulated for each subject, using the approach outlined above. These were then compared with actual speech output (see the section on speech data and analysis below).

Table 51.2. Summary information about subjects in group B (dorsum of tongue lesions)

	Gender	Type of excision
B1	Female	Unilateral, dorsum of tongue
B2	Female	Unilateral, extending to sector 2
B3	Male	Unilateral, with buccal involvement
B4	Male	Unilateral, with buccal involvement
B5	Female	Unilateral, extending to sector 4 and epiglottis

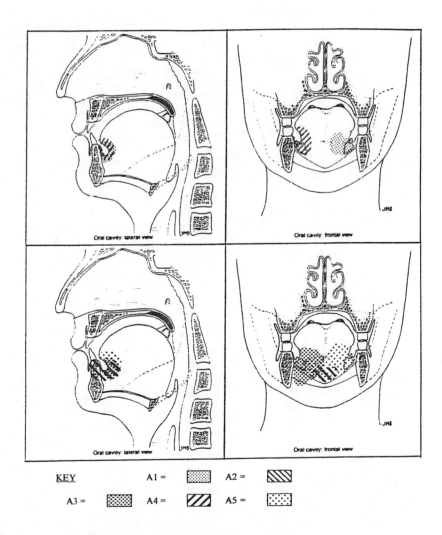

Figure 51.3. Partial surgical maps for subjects in group A.

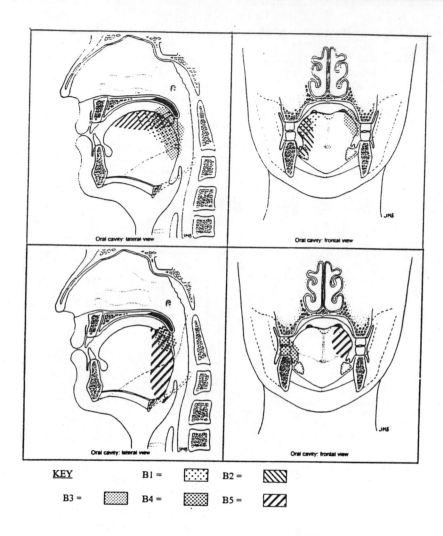

Figure 51.4. Partial surgical maps for subjects in Group B.

Speech data and analysis

Speech data were collected for each speaker, firstly a few days before surgery and then at intervals after surgery. Only the pre-surgery data and data collected 20 weeks after surgery are discussed here. The 20-week stage is chosen because by that stage any radiotherapy was completed, inflammation resulting from surgery and/or radiotherapy had subsided, and dentures had been fitted. Data consisted of digital recordings of six read sentences (taken from a larger sentence set), which included examples of all consonant classes of Scottish English.

Long-term average settings of the vocal tract and laryngeal voice quality were analysed perceptually using the Vocal Profile Analysis

Scheme (Laver, Wirz, Mackenzie and Hiller, 1991; Beck, 1988). Consonant phonemes were transcribed as narrowly as possible. It was found that segmental transcription of post-surgery data using standard IPA and extIPA symbols was extremely difficult for some subjects. This supports the view that the value of fine phonetic transcription is rather suspect in the presence of significant distortion of oral anatomy and physiology. A less detailed analysis was therefore included, which identified phonemes that were realized in any way considered to be atypical for a speaker's habitual accent.

Results

Speech analysis of the pre-surgery cases showed no identifiable speech abnormalities, so only post-surgery analysis results are discussed here.

Group A (floor of mouth)

It is clear from the surgical maps for this group that a two-dimensional representation of surgery can be very misleading; the group appears to be fairly homogeneous when mapped on the lateral view, but the frontal view shows significant variation in both site and extent of surgery. This lack of homogeneity is reflected in differing predictions about likely speech outcome. These are summarized in Table 51.3. Difficulties in production of central fricatives and approximants, as a result of anterior genioglossus involvement, are predicted for all cases, but other predictions vary.

Table 51.3. A summary of predicted speech outcomes for Group A

	Structure affected	Predicted problems
All	genioglossus muscle (anterior segment)	difficulty in lowering central part of tongue → distortion of /r/ + and central lingual fricatives
A1, A2, A3, A5	inferior longitudinal muscle	difficulty in pulling tip down → possible distortion of /j/, /i/
A4, A5	geniohyoid muscle	difficulty in expanding lumen of pharynx → disturbed oral vs. pharyngeal resonance difficulty in raising larynx
A3, A5	extensive loss of tissue in anterior part of mouth	expanded front oral cavity volume → perception of backed and/or lowered tongue body setting

The speech findings, which are summarized in Table 51.4, also vary. Not surprisingly, given that the approach to predictions is still relatively crude, there is not a perfect match between predictions and speech findings, but there are some clear links. For example, A5, where there was expected to be geniohyoid involvement and hence difficulty in raising the larynx, was perceived to have a lower larynx following surgery. A3 and A5 were both predicted to have altered resonance as a result of expanded front oral cavity volume, and both were perceived to have either lowered or backed tongue-body settings following surgery.

Table 51.4. A summary of predicted speech outcomes for Group B

	Structure affected	Predicted problems
B1, B5, (B2)	transverse muscle	difficulty in narrowing and extending tongue → possible distortion of /j/, /i/
B1, B5	superior longitudinal muscle	difficulty in curling tip and sides → distortion of /r/, central fricatives
B3, B4, B5	palatoglossus + ? palatpharyngeus muscles	impaired velopharyngeal control → disturbed nasal resonance
B1, B2, B5	Extensive loss of tissue in posterior part of mouth	expanded back oral cavity and/or pharyngeal cavity volumes → perception of fronted and/or lowered tongue body setting

Group B (dorsum of tongue)

Surgical maps show that all of these cases had surgery affecting sector 3, although in some cases surgery extends to sectors 2 or 4. Table 51.5 shows that, as with group A, the predictions vary in accordance with differing surgical maps. Whereas speech findings broadly follow predictions, there is not a perfect match. For example, the prediction that extensive loss of tissue in B1, B2 and B5 would result in the perception of more fronted and/or lowered tongue body settings fits with the speech findings. B1, however, showed increased nasal resonance and audible nasal escape of air, but this had not been predicted from the surgical map.

Table 51.5. A summary of speech findings for Group A

	Distorted phonemes	VPA changes
A1	/r/ → minor distortion	slightly tenser phonation
A2	/r, l, s/ → minor distortion	tongue body slightly lower, larynx lower, phonation more tense and whispery
A3	/r, l/ and all lingual fricatives	tongue body lower, phonation tenser and creakier
A4	/r/ very distorted. /s, ʃ/	tongue body fronted
A5	/r, l/ and all lingual fricatives	backed tongue body, lower larynx, harsher phonation

Table 51.6. A summary of speech findings for Group B

	Distorted phonemes	VPA changes
B1	/r, j/ and somtimes /l/	increased nasality, ANE*, lower tongue body
B2	/r, s/ + /k/ → frication	slightly increased nasality, occasional ANE* lower, fronted tongue body
B3	/r, l, ʃ/	greatly increased nasality, ANE*, fronted tongue body
B4	/l/	increased nasality, ANE*, tense, harsh, whispery phonation
B5	/l/ (slight distortion was evident pre-operatively	Greatly increased nasality, fronted and raised tongue body, raised larynx, creakier phonation

* ANE = audible nasal escape of air

Conclusions

This paper has attempted to illustrate a possible approach to exploring the relationship between surgical intervention within the oral cavity and speech output. Despite the evident individual differences in compensatory ability, the results do suggest that surgical mapping may help us to make informed predictions about the degree of communication impairment resulting from surgery for intra-oral cancer. The small subject groups, and the lack of homogeneity within each group, make statistical evaluation of the results inappropriate. It must be accepted, too, that predictions, however good, may be confounded by individual variations in compensatory skills.

More data are becoming available, and it is hoped that as this is analysed the predictive power of surgical mapping can be more fully tested. One important comment that arises from observation of the mapping data is that group studies that classify subjects according to the area of surgery may be inappropriate. Quite minor inter-subject differences in either site or extent of surgery may result in major differences in predicted speech outcome if different muscle groups are affected. Further research in this area may therefore need to use methodologies that allow analysis of a series of individual case studies, matching detailed predictions for each subject to extensive speech analysis before and after surgery.

Increasing the sophistication of mapping protocols by utilizing three-dimensional graphic techniques, and linking this to our expanding understanding of the anatomical and physiological bases of speech production, could eventually allow more detailed predictions of the differential effects of oral surgery. These could be relevant to a range of disorders in addition to oral cancer, including cleft lip and palate and traumatic injury. The information gained may, in some cases, allow surgeons to modify surgical intervention in order to minimize speech disturbance. At the very least, it should allow speech and language therapists to make better informed decisions about effective management of these cases.

References

Beck, JM (1988) Organic Variation and Voice Quality. University of Edinburgh: PhD dissertation.

Fletcher, SG (1988) Speech production following partial glossectomy. Journal of Speech and Hearing Disorders 53: 232–38.

Greven A, Meijer MF, Tiwari RM (1994) Articulation after total glossectomy: a clinical study of the speech of six patients. European Journal of Disorders of Communication 29: 85–93.

Laver J, Wirz S, Mackenzie J, Hiller SM (1991) A perceptual profile for the analysis of vocal profiles. In Laver J (Ed) The Gift of Speech. Edinburgh: Edinburgh University Press, pp 265–80.

Wrench AA, Beck J, Jackson M, Jack MA, Laver JS, Soutar DS, Robertson AG (1993) A speech therapy workstation for the assessment of segmental quality: voiceless fricatives. In Proceedings of the Third European Conference on Speech Communication and Technology, Berlin, pp 219–22.

Chapter 52
Which Phonetic Features are Available to Cochlear Implant Patients?

WALTER F. SENDLMEIER AND MICHAEL RIEBANDT

Introduction

Speech transformed by the Nucleus Cochlear Implant (CI) is characterized by rough place-pitch-ranking and reduced dynamic range. Only an approximate understanding of natural speech is attainable. To improve a patient's speech perception ability it can be helpful to focus his or her perception strategies on those phonetic features that his or her CI-system transforms in the best way. The importance of any cue may vary for the individual patient (Sendlmeier, 1989). Some speech signal cues contain more information and are more relevant for the individual patient than others. From the articulation point of view, for consonants, these features are (1) place of articulation, (2) manner of articulation, and (3) voicing. We know from literature that voicing, in particular, may be recognized quite well by patients with cochlear implants (Mülder, Van Olphen, Bosman and Smoorenburg, 1992; Tyler, 1990). The identification of place of articulation, however, seems to be rather difficult (Tyler, Lowder, Parkinson, Woodworth and Gantz, 1995). The aim of our study is to determine which manner of articulation and places of articulation can be discriminated particularly well by CI-patients and which cannot be discriminated.

Method

A consonant recognition test was carried out with four postlingually deaf patients. The duration of deafness varied between six months and 25 years. The patients were at first provided with a 22-channel Nucleus-cochlear implant and a Mini Speech Processor (MSP) using the Multipeak speech-coding strategy. Later they were provided with the

Spectra 22 speech processor, which uses the Speak speech-coding strategy. Between the patients' implantations and the tests with the MSP, two to 17 months passed; the time interval between implantation and test with the Spectra 22 was 15 to 38 months.

The stimuli used for the tests contained 16 German consonants (/p, t, k, b, d, g, m, n, l, r, f, s, ʃ, v, z, x/) in various vowel contexts. They followed a VCV pattern with constant vowel quality in every stimulus. In a psycho-acoustic test we presented the signals to the patients by loudspeaker. They knew the vowel context, and they were asked to repeat the perceived consonant. The loudness and the switch positions of the speech processor were adjusted to the patients' convenience. The tests were carried out with the MSP 19 times and 14 times with the Spectra 22.

The data were calculated by means of a non-metric multi-dimensional scaling procedure (MDS) in order to evaluate the structure underlying the consonant confusions. The frequency of the confusions served as a measure for the similarities. The direction of confusions (e.g., /t/ recognized as /d/ or vice versa) remained unconsidered, although this assumption of symmetry can only be made to a restricted extent with respect to the phoneme perception by cochlear implant patients. For the description of results, two-dimensional MDS solutions (with stress values between 0.19 and 0.28) are considered. Three- and four-dimensional MDS solutions showed a better adaptation with stress values ≤ 0.10, but brought no further information about the perception strategies of the patients.

General results

The average consonant recognition rate of all patients increased from 19% with the Multipeak strategy to 33.9% with the Speak strategy. Voicing showed the highest average recognition rate of all features with 51.1% (Multipeak) and 76.5% (Speak), followed by manner of articulation and place of articulation (Figure 52.1). All phonetic features were identified to a higher degree with the Speak strategy by all patients.

The MDS evaluation underscores the importance of the voicing feature as an essential criterion for the distinction of consonants in almost all cases. With only one exception (patient 4 using MSP), it contributed significantly to one of the two dimensions differentiating the stimuli in both speech coding strategies. Moreover, it divided the first or the second dimension when all patients were pooled. For the Multipeak – and Speak – strategies this confirmed earlier results obtained with the simpler FOF1F2 strategy (Mülder et al. 1992).

Consonant feature recognition MSP – Spectra 22

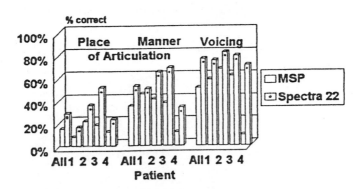

Figure 52.1. Comparison of recognition rates with the Mini Speech Processor (Multipeak coding strategy) and Spectra 22 speech processor (Speak coding strategy).

Manner of articulation was the second essential feature for the recognition of consonants in the patients, with average recognition rates of 35.3% and 52.6% for Multipeak and Speak, respectively. Average recognition rates for place of articulation were 15.3% and 29.0%. The sonorant—obstruent opposition also proved to be important; it explained the distribution along one of the two dimensions for patients 1 and 2 in both strategies. In the groups of phonemes classified as similar by the MDS, differentiation by manner of articulation was far more frequent than by place of articulation. In the patterns obtained for each patient, the voiceless and the voiced plosives were particularly close in at least one dimension for both the Multipeak and the Speak strategy.

The MDS patterns for the individual patients demonstrate a difference between the two coding strategies. With the older speech-coding strategy, Multipeak, confusions between groups of consonants with the same manner of articulation were particularly frequent. With the Speak strategy, however, phonemes with different manners of articulation could be better differentiated, especially by patients 2 and 3.

Results in detail

Multipeak coding

Pooling the four patients' data, Figure 52.2 shows that the voiced consonants were clearly separated from the voiceless consonants along the first dimension. On dimension 2, the plosives scored highest, followed by the fricatives and the sonorants. The sonorant /r/, which was realized as an apical intermittent stop, was placed in the middle between the voiced plosives and the other sonorants.

Consonant similarities All patients

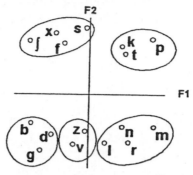

Figure 52.2. Consonant similarities of all patients using Multipeak.

Figure 52.3 presents the results for patient 1. Along the second dimension, the stimuli were divided into voiceless and voiced consonants. Along the first dimension, the voiceless consonants clustered in two groups according to manner of articulation, with plosives on the left and fricatives on the right, whereas the voiced consonants clustered into nasals and the lateral versus plosives and fricatives. The phoneme /r/ could not be integrated into this division according to manner of articulation.

Consonant similarities Patient 1

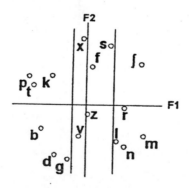

Figure 52.3. Consonant similarities of patient 1 using Multipeak.

For patient 2, a linear combination of F_1 and F_2 clearly divided the stimuli into voiced and voiceless consonants, whereas dimension 2 separated sonorants from obstruents (Figure 52.4).

For patient 3, a subdivision of the phonemes along the first dimension could be interpreted in terms of the voicing feature. Dimension 2 was less conclusive, clustering the nasals with the liquid /r/ and the voiceless fricatives /ʃ/ and /x/ against the remaining obstruents and the lateral. The representation of the similarities in the two dimensions for patient 4 showed fewer possibilities of structuring from a phonetic point of view. Merely in the projection on the first dimension, some consonants could be clustered according to place of articulation. Concerning the features voicing and manner of articulation, neither the first nor the second dimension seemed to order or differentiate the stimuli. Whereas otherwise the three-dimensional solution provided no additional information, a complete division of the plosive and fricative stimuli.

Consonant similarities Patient 2

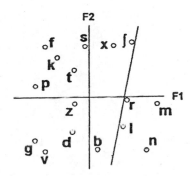

Figure 52.4. Consonant similarities of patient 2 using Multipeak.

Speak coding

Figure 52.5 represents the similarities in the judgements of all four patients together. F_2 very clearly divided the stimuli into voiced and voiceless consonants. Within these two groups they were completely differentiated along the first dimension according to the manner of articulation.

Figure 52.6 represents the similarities of the consonants in the perception of patient 1. The distribution allows a separation along the first dimension according to manner of articulation. The plosives are found in the left part of the diagram, the fricatives in the middle, and the sonorants on the right. The phoneme /ʃ/ was an exception since it lay in the proximity of the other voiceless fricatives, but also near the nasals. The second dimension completely divided the items into voiced and voiceless consonants.

The distribution of the stimuli for patient 2 is shown in Figure 52.7. A linear combination of F_1 and F_2 partitions the items into sonorants and obstruents, while F2 more-or-less represents the voicing dimension. This patient's voiceless fricatives and voiced plosives lay narrowly together along this dimension.

Consonant similarities All patients

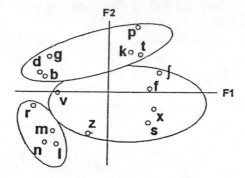

Figure 52.5. Consonant similarities of all patients using Speak.

Consonant similarities Patient 1

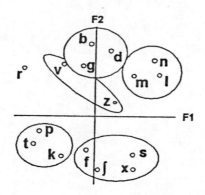

Figure 52.6. Consonant similarities of patient 1 using Speak.

Consonant similarities Patient 2

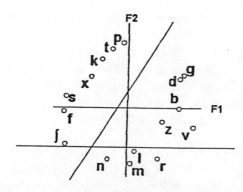

Figure 52.7. Consonant similarities of patient 2 using Speak.

For patient 3, the subdivision of the phonemes along the first dimension could be interpreted with respect to the voicing feature. Along the second dimension, there was a division according to manner of articulation. The voiceless plosives constituted a group in the upper part, directly followed by the voiced plosives. The fricatives, the nasals and the lateral were placed in the lower half. In these stimuli the phoneme /r/ was articulated as an apical trill; it lay consistently in the proximity of the homorganic plosive /d/. For patient 4, again, no phonetically plausible structure could be found along the second dimension of the configuration. A linear combination of F_1 and F_2 divided the configuration according to the voicing feature. Within the voiced group the fricatives were detached.

Summary and discussion

A consonant recognition test was carried out with four patients who first used the MSP (Multipeak strategy) and then the Spectra 22 speech processor (Speak strategy). Consonant recognition rates increased considerably when using the Speak strategy as compared with the Multipeak strategy. Multi-dimensional scaling revealed that consonant voicing showed the highest average recognition rate of all features followed by manner of articulation, place of articulation and the sonorant–obstruent opposition. With the Multipeak speech coding strategy, confusions basically occured between groups of consonants with the same manner of articulation, whereas with the Speak strategy, phonemes articulated in different ways could better be differentiated from each other.

Patient 4 showed a somewhat different pattern of consonant recogniton from the other three patients. This patient was a 32-year-old woman who was born with impaired hearing and who had lost her hearing completely at the age of seven following mumps. In comparison with the other patients, her 'memory' of the hearing experience from early childhood might have been considerably reduced because of her long-term deafness. The division of phonemes into zones of articulation might be interpreted as resulting from the recognition performance of the lip-reading process, which the patient was dependent on during her deafness. The patient obviously also used these structures to recognize speech with cochlear-implant and Multipeak. In contrast to this, the MDS representation of the confusions with the Speak strategy failed to show any considerable division according to place of articulation. At the same time the patient reported an increasing loss of her ability to lip-read. Obviously, the voicing feature now was additionally at her disposal for the distinction of consonants.

The analyses outlined here make it possible to determine hierachies of difficulty in phoneme recognition for individual patients and thereby develop optimally graded training materials. By using a more detailed classification of the speech features according to distinctive phonetic cues we hope to gain further information. Possibly we may find those cues that have a crucial function for the perception of speech in individual patients. This knowledge might be useful both for the development of a training programme for patients with a cochlear implant and for the further development of cochlear implant systems.

References

Mülder HE, Van Olphen AF, Bosman A, Smoorenburg GF (1992) Phoneme recognition by deaf individuals using the Multichannel Nucleus cochlear implant. Acta Otolaryngol (Stockholm): 112: 946–55.

Sendlmeier WF (1989) Speech cue enhancement in intervocalic stops. Clinical Linguistics and Phonetics 3: 151–61.

Sendlmeier WF (1992) Sprachverarbeitung bei pathologischem Gehör. Stuttgart: Thieme Verlag.

Tyler RS (1990) What should be implemented in future cochlear-implants? Acta Otolaryngol (Stockholm) Suppl. 469: 268–75.

Tyler RS, Lowder MW, Parkinson AJ, Woodworth GG, Gantz BJ (1995) Performance of adult Ineraid and Nucleus CI patients after 3.5 years of use. Audiology 34: 135–44.

Chapter 53
The Testing and Evaluation of a New Visual Speech Aid Incorporating Digital Kymography

KENNY R. COVENTRY, JOHN CLIBBENS AND
MARGARET COOPER

Introduction

Speech production is under the control of a variety of distinct and highly autonomous articulators, each of which contributes finely tuned gestures to the flow of speech: the larynx, the tongue, the lips, the velum. Articulate speech results from (a) the proper functioning of each of these articulators and (b) just as important, the proper relative timing of the gestures they initiate. The phonemic difference between /t/ and /d/, for example, is achieved by the relative timing of voice-onset (a laryngeal gesture) and stop-release (an alveolar gesture). It is essential, then, that the articulators are precisely coordinated in order to produce intelligible speech.

In cases where auditory feedback is not available (i.e., with hearing impairment), and where there is some interruption to the articulatory system (e.g., cleft palate), the gestural system is incomplete, and ill-coordinated. The consequences of this are poorly intelligible speech (Markides, 1970). In order to combat this, a number of teaching methods have been developed which attempt to replace the auditory feedback circuit with a visual feedback loop. The use of visual speech aids (VSAs) for speech production training over the last two decades has been relatively widespread (for reviews see Bernstein, Goldstein and Mashie, 1988; Braeges and Houde, 1982; Lippmann, 1982; Povel and Arends, 1991; Strong, 1975). However, it would be premature to suggest that these aids are regarded as successful as therapeutic tools. Coventry, Clibbens, Cooper and Rood (in press) have recently conducted a study of the use of VSAs throughout the UK by eliciting ratings and comments from speech and language therapists. All speech and language therapy managers in the UK were sent questionnaires, tapping information about the VSAs currently used, the client groups with which they are used, the main therapeutic uses for each and the limitations and advantages of each piece of equipment. A total of 193 speech and language therapists completed a questionnaire (58% of all the managers sampled). The conclusion from this study was that VSAs are inaccurate in terms of feedback, and that display appearance has been put before accuracy of feedback. Aside from a mean low rating for accuracy and quality of feedback, the vast majority of written limitations were in the accuracy of feedback category. Additionally, and most importantly, speech and language therapists, the users of the equipment, in the main, have not been consulted in the design of such equipment (such consultation provided one of the main motivations for the study). A follow-up study by Coventry, Clibbens and Cooper (in press) eliciting ratings from specialist speech and language therapists also found that VSA ratings were no better than average ratings and, crucially, individual VSAs did not score differently between specialist types. Given that in this study and the previous study by Coventry, Clibbens, Cooper and Rood (in press) ratings of the 'range of uses' for particular VSAs were especially low, this finding is worrying. Whereas many VSAs may be thought to be more applicable to particular specialist groups, the ratings do not reflect this. At the same time, VSAs are not appropriate for use with a wide range of client groups.

Other reviews of VSAs (reviews by individual researchers, rather than views employing the comprehensive sampling techniques employed by Coventry et al.) have distilled the desirable features of VSAs down to a number of main characteristics (e.g., Ball, 1991). When considering the existence of such features in VSAs, Coventry et al. found that no system scored significantly better than chance on all features combined. There was also a significant interaction between feature type and VSA type. When a particular VSA scored well on one feature, it tended to score below chance on other features. There thus appear to be a large number of trade-offs in the design of VSAs which need to be ironed out.

The development of a new VSA incorporating air flow measures

It appears to be the case that the visual speech aids currently available, the majority of which use acoustic information as the tool for feedback, do not give accurate feedback about speech production. The type of feedback required must give information such that the articulators can be taught to act in concert so that the gestural score can be complete. The instrumental techniques investigated in this paper (the Portable Speech Laboratory (PSL), developed in Edinburgh and Dundee, and the Son of the Nasal Oral Ratiometry System (SNORS) developed at the University of Kent at Canterbury) make this metaphor concrete. The equipment has all the benefits of a product-oriented approach while also giving feedback about the process of speech production/articulation directly. A criticism of process-oriented approaches has been that the articulators cannot be pointed out as readily as the fingers can in the case of piano playing, for example. However, the use of airflow measures in addition to acoustic and laryngographic information (c.f. Fourcin and Abberton, 1971; Fourcin, 1990) does precisely this, as there is a direct correlation between airflow and articulatory activity. The amount of airflow in the nasal trace correlates with the extent of lowering of the velum. The difference between a voiced and a voiceless sound is clearly indicated by the relative onset of the oral and laryngographic traces. The height, length and shape of peaks in the oral trace correlates with the amount of blockage in the oral cavity, hence can distinguish between plosives and fricatives, for example. Furthermore, the relative onsets and offsets of different types of articulatory coordination are readily displayed as a feedback tool in real time. The equipment therefore meets most of the important criteria outlined by Ball (1991).

In the case of the PSL and SNORS, each trace records a distinct articulatory system: the larynx (bottom trace in Figures 53.1, 53.2, 53.3 and 53.4), the oral cavity (next above), and the nasal cavity (above that). The activity of the oral and the nasal articulators is measured by monitoring airflow at 'microscopic' levels. The audio signal is included to show the onset and offset of constrictions in the oral cavity (when the oral cavity is constricted there is low amplitude in the audio signal).

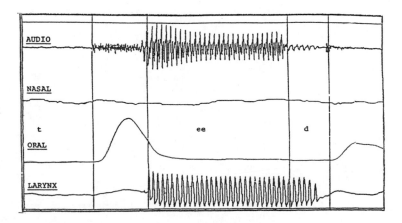

Figure 53.1. Printout of /teed/ from PSL.

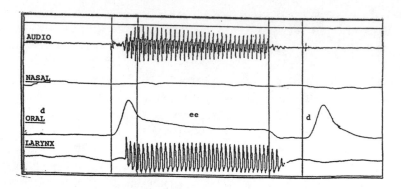

Figure 53.2. Printout of /deed/ from PSL.

Figures 53.1 and 53.2 represent the distinction between a voiced/voice-less minimal pair, between /t/ and /d/, with examples of 'teed' and 'deed' (produced by the PSL). One can focus on the bottom two traces (laryngeal and oral). At the beginning of 'teed' the oral airflow in-creases dramatically, forming a lump or spike as the tongue comes away from the roof of the mouth and air rushes out. Only when the first puff of air is dispelled does the larynx initiate voicing (bottom trace). By contrast, in 'deed' the spike of the stop release is coordinated exactly with the onset of voicing. In both these words there is no activity at all in the nasal trace: the velum – a muscular flap at the back of the roof of the mouth – is raised throughout, sealing off the nasal cavity to airflow. Figures 53.3 and 53.4 illustrate the clear difference between a nasal consonant and an oral consonant in the initial position.

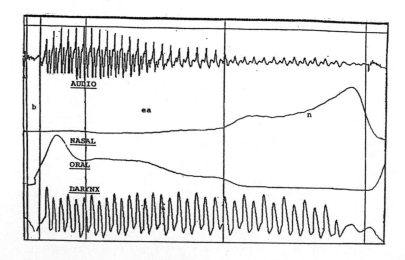

Figure 53.3. Printout of /bean/ from PSL.

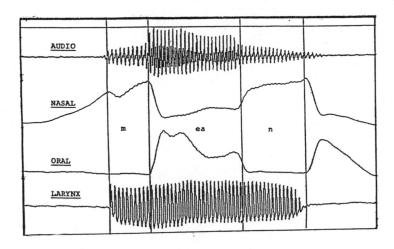

Figure 53.4. Printout of /mean/ from PSL.

It is notable that this technique, displaying articulation change over time, provides clear and unambiguous information about final consonant production, for example, which is regarded as one of the main problems with hearing-impaired speech and which has largely been overlooked in the literature and consequently in the design of VSAs (Abraham, 1989).

Testing and evaluation — validation experiment

Although the outputs from the equipment appear to give clear and unambiguous information related to articulatory processes, the ease with which they can be interpreted remains open to question. Therefore, the first stage in testing this equipment was to evaluate whether naive linguistic subjects (hearing subjects with no linguistic training) could reliably recognise and differentiate between different voiced/voiceless and nasal/oral contrastive pairs.

Method and results

Twenty-six subjects (10 male, 16 female, age range 16–45 years) were given printouts from the portable speech laboratory in a one-sample design experiment. The first set consisted of single sound contrastive pairs (all consonants matched for place of articulation); the second set of simple word pairs with one contrastive change at the start, and the third set of simple words with a contrastive change at some point in the word (other than at the start). For each trial, subjects were given two words/single sounds and two printouts, one for each word/sound. Their task was to match the words/sounds to their corresponding print-outs. Before the experiment, subjects were given a five-minute training session illustrating what each of the four wave traces displayed represented in terms of articulatory activity. Thus, the training session was to establish a link between the visual representations of speech production and the sensory-motor knowledge that subjects possess. Overall subjects correctly identified 91% of the contrastive pairs, which was highly significant (one-sample t-test; $t = 15.35$; $p < 0.01$ (N = 26)). We thus have evidence that the outputs from the portable speech laboratory do map on to speech production in that contrastive pairs, illustrating different combinations of articulatory activity, can be easily and reliably identified and differentiated.

Testing and evaluation — preliminary intervention data

This initial study suggesting that the equipment provides unambiguous information about speech production, gave a clear indication that the feedback may be of the right type to use with those with severe hearing impairment. However, there was no guarantee at this stage that, despite the accurate feedback, the hearing impaired could modify articulation leading to greater intelligibility as a consequence of such feedback. The second study was therefore designed to address this issue. A profoundly deaf client, named here as Emma, was given therapy over a two-week period and a pre- and post-test design was used to evaluate whether the training had been effective.

Participant

Emma (aged 16) was referred to the study by the local speech and language therapy service. She was regarded as being highly motivated to learn and, therefore, as a good participant. Main target areas from referral were (non-visual plosives) – /t/ and /k/ in word final positions – increased frequency and appropriate use of /s/ – increased frequency of /ch/ /dj/ in word final positions.

Method

A pre-test/post-test design was employed. The initial assessment took the form of recordings of the materials from the PACS (Phonological Assessment of Child Speech). Each word (of 100 in total) was read by the client and recorded. After the training sessions, Emma was given the same test. The words were read in the reverse order to control for priming effects from the pre-test. None of the words used in the pre- and post-test were used during intervention. From these initial 100 words, 20 were selected by the therapist to be rated blindly by a group of raters. The words selected were chosen independently as words that reflected the difficulties Emma encountered prior to therapy on referral.

Intervention procedure

Training sessions were split into three phases.

Phase 1 — learning to interpret the waveforms

During this phase Emma was set tasks which allowed her to link the different waveforms to oral and nasal airflow, and to the laryngographic trace. She was required to identify firstly where the word began and ended, and gradually to identify oral/nasal, plosive/fricative and voiced/voiceless contrasts. A progressive programme began with single sound recognition and proceeded to simple CV, VC, CVC, words.

Phase 2 — learning to control the waveforms

This phase offered Emma an opportunity to learn how to gain control of the visual representation and produce waveforms that conformed to a certain expectation.

Phase 3 — self-evaluation and meta-phonological awareness

The final phase of therapy involved tasks that promoted trial-and-error learning, and self-evaluation of speech attempts. For example, Emma was asked to create a list of her best friends' names and to select one of the names for production. She was left alone in the room and encouraged to repeat the word as often as necessary until she had produced a visual representation that conformed to her expectation. The therapist on return was required to identify the name stored on the screen from the list created.

Results

The 20 words recorded pre-test and post-test on DAT were randomized and put together on a new tape. Subjects were played each pair of tokens (one pre- and one post-test) together in a random order. They were instructed to listen carefully to both recordings of the word, and then to give an intelligibility rating for each word (from 0 – 100 where 0 = completely unintelligible and 100 = completely intelligible/normal speech).

A two-way within-subjects ANOVA was performed on the data. A main effect of session was found ($F(1, 6) = 46.13$, $p<0.0005$). The mean level of intelligibility for the pre-test session was 52.64 as compared with a mean rating of 75.43 for the post-test. There was also a main effect for 'word' ($F(19, 114) = 3.17$, $p< 0.0001$): some words were more intelligible overall than others. Finally, there was a significant interaction between session and word ($F(19, 114) = 3.02$, $p< 0.0005$). Some words improved more than others. Most notably, all words improved except for 'clouds'.

Table 53.1. Mean ratings of words pre- and post-test

Word	Pre-test	Post-test
matches	47.6	74.1
spider	66.0	70.4
elephant	59.6	77.3
milk	46.3	90.0
bridge	54.3	90.3
scissors	66.0	69.7
lipstick	56.0	69.3
scribbling	35.3	66.0
kitchen	56.4	76.7
clouds	51.9	50.7
dentist	50.6	72.3
tent	58.1	77.4
sink	58.9	81.0
bus stop	64.3	81.7
that	62.9	86.7
desk	51.3	90.0
torch	33.1	81.9
present	54.3	73.7
stamp	31.0	62.1
hedge	49.1	67.1

General discussion

The results of the pilot intervention study and the initial validation study indicate that the equipment may be a significant therapeutic tool that may be of benefit across a range of client groups. However, these conclusions must remain preliminary until controlled intervention studies can be conducted. Further work evaluating the equipment is presently under way.

References

Abraham S (1989) Using a phonological framework to describe speech errors or orally trained hearing-impaired school-agers. Journal of Speech and Hearing Research 54: 600–9.

Ball V (1991) Computer-based tools for the assessment and remediation of speech. British Journal of Disorders of Communication 26: 95–113.

Bernstein LE, Goldstein M, Mashie J (1988). Speech training aids for profoundly deaf children I; overview and aims. Journal of Rehabilitation Research and Development 25: 53–62.

Braeges JL Houde RA (1982) Use of speech training aids. In Sims D, Walter G, Whitehead R (Eds). Deafness and Communication: Assessment and Training. Baltimore: Williams & Wilkins.

Coventry KR, Clibbens J, Cooper M, Rood B (in press). Visual speech aids: a British survey of use and evaluation by speech and language therapists. European Journal of Disorders of Communication.

Coventry KR, Clibbens J, Cooper M, (in press). Specialist speech and language therapists' use and evaluation of visual speech aids. European Journal of Disorders of Communication.

Fourcin AJ (1990) Prospects for speech pattern element aids. Acta Otolaryngol (Stockholm), Supplement 469: 257–67.

Fourcin AJ and Abberton E (1971) First applications of a new laryngograph. Medical and Biological Illustration 21: 172–82.

Lippmann RP (1982) A review of research on speech training aids for the deaf. In Lass NJ (Ed) Speech and Language: Advances in Basic Research and Practice 7: 105–33.

Markides D (1970) The speech of deaf and partially hearing children with special reference to factors affecting intelligibility. British Journal of Disorders of Communication 5: 126–40.

Povel DJ and Arends N (1991) Visual speech apparatus: theoretical and practical aspects. Speech Communication 10: 59–80.

Strong WJ (1975) Speech aids for the profoundly/severely hearing impaired: requirements, overview and projections. Volta Review, 77: 536–56.

Chapter 54
Application of Spectrographic Feedback for Improvement of Speech Production Skills

REGINE BECKER

Introduction

Computer speech training aids are considered a possible way of improving the speech of deaf children (Bernstein, Goldstein and Mahshie, 1988; Arends, Povel, Van Os, Michielsen, Claasen and Feiter, 1991; Pratt, Heintzelman and Deming, 1993; Ruoß and Schildhammer, 1992). These technical aids are aimed to compensate for the lack of auditory feedback. Most speech training systems are using the acoustic signal from microphone. The visual feedback in real time is based on spectrograms, oscillograms and waveform envelopes. These aids provide external control over different motor functions (e.g. phonation, articulation and prosody), depending on the kind of visual feedback.

Visual feedback systems (e.g. IBM SpeechViewer) are also used as effective tools for the modification of speech attributes and intelligibility in dysarthric subjects (Thomas-Stonell, McClean and Hunt, 1991; Bouglé, Ryalls and LeDorze, 1995). Biofeedback is used to facilitate learning to regulate selected physiological processes (e.g. breathing). (Rubow, 1984). While computer treatment is not necessarily more effective than traditional speech therapy, the computer provides objective measures of treatment efficacy, increases speech motor drill, and supports the planning of new goals.

Most studies deal with the instrumental aspect of computer-based speech training and do not focus on the learning conditions in which visual feedback helps to improve speech production skills. The decoding of speech sounds requires higher-level linguistic knowledge because there is no linear relationship between the acoustic signal and the perceived speech code (Liberman, Cooper, Shankweiler and

Studdert-Kennedy, 1968; Cole, Rudnicky, Zue and Reddy, 1980). These top-down processes must be taken into account through special instruction concerning the interpretation and learning of the visual speech patterns. In particular, a training programme for deaf students must build up phonological knowledge and consider symbolic meaning from signed and written language.

A visible speech device providing spectrographic feedback and a training programme for deaf students were developed. A study by Schildhammer (1996) with 24 deaf students showed significant increase of the intelligibility of rehearsed and non-rehearsed words after training with the visible speech aid. The system has now been tested in five German schools for the deaf over a six-month period. In addition, qualitative data were collected in two single case studies with dysarthric subjects. The following questions were asked:

1. What do teachers of the deaf experience when using the visible speech aid in speech-training deaf students? What level of performance do students reach after training as measured by the number of corrected speech errors? How do the successive stages of the training programme influence the learning achievements?
2. Does the spectrographic feedback support perceptual-motor learning in dysarthric subjects with mild-to-moderate articulatory and phonatory deficits?

Method

Participants

Sixteen teachers from five German schools for the deaf participated in the study of the training of deaf students, together with a total of 75 deaf students of different school grades. The sample was devided into two groups. The distribution of age and grade level is shown in Table 54.1.

Table 54.1. Age and grade level of the deaf students

group 1 (n = 38)	group 2 (n = 37)
preschool, X = 4;06 (n = 5)	5th grade, X = 12;02 (n = 17)
1st grade, X = 7;10 (n = 26)	7th grade, X = 14;00 (n = 8)
2nd grade, X = 8;06 (n = 4)	10th grade, X = 16;08 (n = 12)
3rd grade, X = 9;04 (n = 3)	

For the dysarthria study, a 52-year-old male (JM) and a 54-year-old male (DZ) were chosen as subjects. They had suffered a cerebrovascular accident in the left cerebral hemisphere two months before testing. They had mild to moderate mixed dysarthria as measured by the Frenchay Dysarthria Assessment (Enderby, 1991).

Table 54.2. Speech disorders of the dysarthric subjects

J.M.	D.Z.
- reduced breath support, slightly breathy voice	- harsh voice and low pitch
- hypernasality	- –
- reduced pitch and loudness ranges	- reduced pitch and vocal intensity
- consonant imprecision in single word production, substitutions of stops with nasals	- deviant production of /s/ in single words
- reductions of consonant clusters, deletions of final consonants in conversational speech	- occasional reductions of consonant clusters, deletions of final consonants in conversational speech

Apparatus

The real-time visible speech device developed by Hobohm (1993) was used. It consists of a DOS PC, TIGA graphic card and a signal processing card (AT&T DSP 32c). A Fast-Fourier-Transformation (128 point-FFT, Hamming window, time resolution 8.4 ms) is used for speech analysis. The linear frequency scale runs from 50 to 5800 Hz. The intensity of energy in the speech signal is indicated by colour values. High spectral energy is displayed in dark colours and low spectral energy is indicated by light colours. A split-screen device is used for the display of the target of the teacher/speech therapist and the speech output of the student/patient. The duration of the speech segment display is 2.5 seconds.

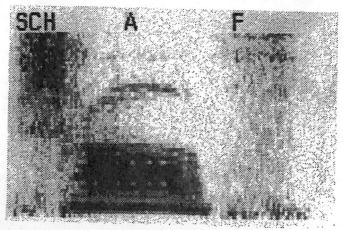

Figure 54.1. Spectrographic display of the german word 'Schaf' /ʃaːf/ (sheep).

Training programme

Our training programme for deaf students (Ruoß and Schildhammer, 1992; Becker, 1993; Schildhammer 1996) included exercises to teach basic skills like breathing control, phonation, nasality, rhythm and phoneme contrasts, and successive training stages in which correct production of different vowels and consonants was taught in the context of words. The sequential order of training stages considered the articulatory difficulty and acoustic characteristics of the speech sounds that were treated. Word meanings were worked out through the presentation of pictures, signed and written words. Further prompts (such as tactile cues, lipreading the sound aloud, and listening to the sound) were given to support speech production if necessary.

Table 54.3. Successive training stages for word production

	phonemes	german words like
stage 1	/p t k/ /a o u/	Opa, Tag
stage 2	/f ʃ s/	Schaf, Fuß
stage 3	/n m h/	Nuß, Oma
stage 4	/h/	Haus, Hof
stage 5	/x/	Fach, Tuch
stage 6	/ç/ /i l e ɛ ø œ y Y aI/	Teich, Fisch
stage 7	/b d g/	Biene, Geige
stage 8	/v z j/	Junge, Wiese
stage 9	/l/	Lippen, Welle

Training sessions with the two dysarthric subjects were conducted using the following visible speech exercises according to the individual deficits of the subjects. Speech training started with the production of single sounds followed by exercises with larger units (syllables and words). It included instruction and exercises for the segmentation, labelling and interpretation of spectrograms. The goal of the trainining programme was to improve the patients' perception of speech deficits, self-regulation and speech naturalness.

Table 54.4. Speech exercises for the dysarthric subjects

JM	DZ
- sustained production /s ʃ f z/	- sustained production /a o u/
- CV-syllables with fricatives (prolonged, different durations)	- diphthongs, vowels
- voice-voiceless contrast /s z/	- sonorant-obstruent contrast
- words with /s/ in initial and medial	- minimal pairs contrasting nasals and stops in initial position
- CV-syllable repetitions	- CV-syllable repetitions

Measurements

An instrument was developed to recording the learning and speech performance of deaf students. For each stage of the training programme, data about the amount and type of training words, speech errors (like substitution, omission and addition of sounds, phonatory deficits and unclassified errors) and corrections were collected. We differentiated between two types of word corrections: short-term corrections occurring within one training session and habitual corrections occurring over two consecutive sessions. The number of corrections in each speech-error category and training stage was counted and quantified in three categories: corrected, partly corrected and non-corrected words.

Procedure

The subjects were required to produce targeted speech units (see training programme) with feedback. Each session provided selected repetitions of previous speech exercises. Depending on individual speech performance, a training stage could include several sessions. Training sessions took place at least twice a week and lasted for 15 minutes for the deaf students and for 30 minutes for the dysarthric subjects. The dysarthric subjects received 10 training sessions with feedback and five sessions without the aid; the deaf students were trained over a six-month period.

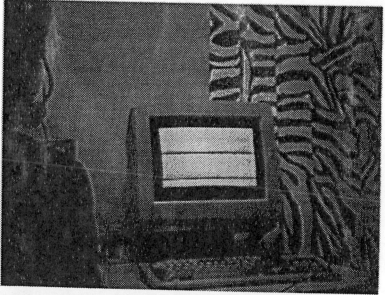

Figure 54.2. Application of the spectrographic feedback.

Results

Teachers' judgements regarding the use of the device were generally very positive concerning the students' acceptance and motivation, the efficacy of speech training and the ease of handling the device. Preferences for further use in speech lessons are given in Table 54.5.

Table 54.5. Preferences for the use of the visible speech aid

two teachers per class	50%
individual training	31%
available in the classroom	38%
improvement of articulation	94%
speech error assessment	31%

Deaf students' learning achievements

The suggested order of phonemes could not be completed with younger children because some sounds were not yet acquired. Only with the older students was it possible to keep the learning conditions constant. A detailed analysis of learning achievements is therefore given only for a subsample of the older students (n = 17) with a mean hearing loss of between 82 and 108 dB. Analysis of error corrections showed a significant effect of the type of speech correction (F (2.32) = 48.33; p<0.01). This means that trained words were more likely to be corrected completely than partly or not at all. Speech correction was very effective in most of the cases and students did not repeat the same mispronunciations in subsequent sessions (F (2.32 = 12.85; p<0.01).

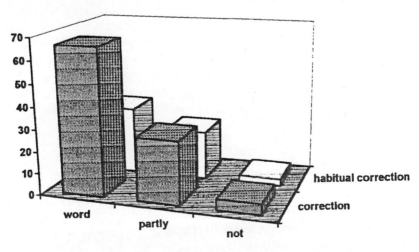

Figure 54.3. Mean of standardized scores (%) of short-term and habitual correction of words over all students and training stages.

We examined speech error corrections depending on training stage. In nine consecutive training stages, students learned words with a successively increasing phoneme repertoire. The visual discrimination and the articulatory difficulty of training words increased step by step (see Table 54.3) as more and more sounds are introduced. The repeated measures factor 'training stage' was aggregated to three levels. This was necessary to make sure that a sufficient number of cases occurred at each level. The relative number of complete word corrections served as the dependent variable. There was a small training effect although the articulatory and visual difficulty of the training words increased with training stage. Articulatory errors occurring on the more difficult words of training stages seven to nine were more often corrected than errors occurring during the first training stages.

Table 54.6. Mean and standard deviation of standardized scores (in percentages) of speech correction in nine subsequent training stages (aggregated into three levels)

training stage	Mean	Standard deviation
L1 – L3	61.9	24.5
L4 – L6	61.5	33.6
L7 – L9	78.9	40.8

Results with dysarthric subjects

The qualitative results indicate that spectrographic display in real time supports perceptual-motor learning. With the help of visual feedback the patients learned to recognize their speech deficits and were able to modify their speech patterns according to the target given by the therapist. The accurate on-line measurement of speech deviations and corrections had a positive effect on the development of self-regulation. The two dysarthrics were able to improve their speech outcome in terms of phonatory, articulatory and prosodic variables and of speech naturalness with the aid of spectrographic feedback. Improvements were reflected in the development of their spontaneous speech. Further systematic investigation is necessary to substantiate these qualitative data.

Conclusion

The visible speech aid can be used as a convenient and effective tool for speech instruction and assessment.

The training programme for deaf students is age-dependent and has to be tailored to individual speech performance. Speech training should be accompanied by the development of phonological knowledge and the presentation of symbolic word meanings with the help of signed and written words. The programme can be easily integrated into the speech lessons of schools for the deaf as a supplementary tool.

Spectrographic feedback provides accurate measurement of speech production skills in real time and can support the perception and self-regulation of motor-disordered speech. The active and more autonomous role of the dysarthric patients may have a positive effect on the speech-remediation process. Higher-level linguistic knowledge of phonetic and phonological decoding strategies should be taken into account by teaching segmentation, labelling and interpretation of the visible speech patterns.

References

Arends N, Povel D-J, Van Os E, Michielsen S, Claasen J, Feiter I (1991) An evaluation of the visual speech apparatus. Speech Communication 10: 404–14.

Becker R (1993) Sprechfertigkeit und Verständlichkeit gehörloser Sprecher: Möglichkeiten der Fehlerdarstellung über eine Lautsprachvisualisierung. Frankfurt/M: Peter Lang.

Bernstein LE, Goldstein MH, Mahshie JJ (1988) Speech training aids for hearing-impaired individuals: I. Overview and aims. J. Rehabilitation Research and Development 25: 53–62.

Bouglé F, Ryalls J, Le Dorze G (1995) Improving fundamental frequency in head trauma patients: a preliminary comparison of speech-language therapy conducted with and without IBM's SpeechViewer. Folia Phoniatr Logop 47: 24–32.

Cole RA, Rudnicky AI, Zue VW, Reddy RD (1980) Speech as patterns on paper. In Cole RA (Ed) Perception and Production of Fluent Speech. Hillsdale, NJ: Lawrence Erlbaum Associates, pp 3–49.

Enderby P (1991) Frenchay Dysarthrie-Untersuchung. Stuttgart: Fischer.

Hobohm K (1993) Verfahren der Spektralanalyse und Mustergenerierung für die Realzeitvisualisierung gesprochener Sprache. Dissertation, TU-Berlin.

Liberman AM, Cooper FS, Shankweiler DP, Studdert-Kennedy M (1968) Why are speech Spectrograms hard to read? Amer. Ann. Deaf 113: 127–33.

Pratt SR, Heintzelman AT, Deming SE (1993) The efficacy of using the IBM SpeechViewer vowel accuracy module to treat young children with hearing impairment. J. Speech Hearing Research 36: 1063–74.

Rubow R (1984) Role of feedback, reinforcement, and . . . In McNeil MR, Rosenbek JC, Aronson AE (Eds) The Dysarthrias. San Diego: College Hill, pp 207–30.

Ruoß M, Schildhammer A (1992) Lautanbildung mit 'visible speech' bei gehörlosen Sprechanfängern. Sprache-Stimme-Gehör 16: 149–53.

Schildhammer A (1996) Einfluß eines Trainings mit Lautsprachvisualisierung auf die Sprechverständlichkeit gehörloser Kinder. Frankfurt/M: Peter Lang.

Thomas-Stonell N, McClean M, Hunt E (1991) Evaluation of the SpeechViewer computer-based speech training system with neurologically impaired individuals. J. Speech-Language Pathology and Audiology 15: 47–56.

Chapter 55
Analysis of Nasalance: NasalView (the Nasalance Acquisition System)[1]

SHAHEEN N. AWAN

Introduction

The measurement of nasalance has often been described as a useful measure in the assessment of excessive nasal resonance in speech. Nasalance has been defined as the ratio of nasal (n) to oral (o) sound pressure level, and is commonly derived via the formula $\frac{n}{n+o} \times 100$.

Studies by Dalston, Warren, and Dalston (1991), Hardin, Van Demark, Morris, and Payne (1992), and Dalston, Neiman, and Gonzalez-Landa (1993) have all indicated that measures of nasalance provide strong specificity, sensitivity, and overall efficiency when used to identify subjects with and without more than mild hypernasality in their speech. Nasalance may be considered one of our stronger objective assessment methods of the nasal speech signal since it may be derived through non-invasive and fairly simple methods. The measurement of nasalance also lends itself well to both diagnostic and therapeutic situations.

The instrumentation for the measurement of nasalance has been available since 1989 in the form of the Nasometer (Kay Elemetrics Inc., Pinehurst, NJ). The system devised by Kay is comprised of headgear (oral and nasal microphones and separation plate), hardware for the analog filtering of the acoustic signals (500 Hz centre frequency; 300 Hz bandwidth) and analog-to-digital conversion (sampling frequency = 120 Hz) and computer software for the display of nasalance (over time or as a summary statistic for a given speech sample).

Unfortunately, the use of the Nasometer presents several drawbacks to the speech clinician:

1. The use of the Nasometer has been somewhat prohibitive for most speech clinicians due to its relatively high cost. Current costs of the Nasometer and the computer required to run the system are in the

$4000 to $5000 range (costs vary depending on the computer system used). The relatively high cost of the Nasometer is, unfortunately, reflected in the statement by Hardin et al. (1992: 350) that, 'the cost-benefit ratio must be considered when adding this tool (the Nasometer) to a clinical laboratory' (pg. 350).

2. The low sampling rate and low frequency band limiting imposed by the Nasometer's design may restrict analysis of the acoustic waveforms being captured and not allow for the detailed reproduction of acoustic characteristics that may be associated with the production of hyper- or hyponasality and nasal emission.

3. The Nasometer does not allow for the storage and playback of the patient's speech productions, limiting the clinician's ability to relate perceptual judgements of the patient's speech patterns with measurements of nasality.

In an effort to address the limitations of the Nasometer, Awan (1996) has developed a computer hardware/software system called NasalView (the Nasalance Acquisition System). NasalView is a new Windows-based speech analysis system designed for the detailed analysis of resonance-based disorders. This system provides for the recording of high resolution speech signals using Windows-compatible sound cards (sampling at up to 44100 Hz at 8 or 16 bits resolution). NasalView has been designed to be a low-cost system that will aid clinicians and researchers in a variety of settings in the diagnosis and treatment of resonance disorders. Previous work by Awan (1996) has described the use of the NasalView system in the analysis of various degrees of nasal and non-nasal utterances in adults. Awan (1996) has also described the validity of the data collection procedures and computer algorithms incorporated in the NasalView system.

The purpose of this study was to use the NasalView system in the collection of nasalance data from a large group of males and females from various age groups ranging from childhood through adult age ranges. The information gathered from this study is to be used as a preliminary database to which clinicians may refer when using the NasalView system in the evaluation of patients with possible resonance disorders.

Methodology

NasalView system overview

The NasalView system was designed to run on a 486 or Pentium PC-compatible system (also requires VGA graphics capability and 4 MBytes RAM memory). The system includes the following components:

Headgear (See Figure 55.1a and b)

The key component of the headgear is a rigid plate constructed of 2 mm thick styrene, which is used to separate an oral from a nasal microphone (Model 33-1052 Realistic microphones, Tandy Corp., Fort Worth, TX). The sound separator plate is suspended from a Jackson Model 170 headgear (Jackson Products, Belmont, MI) by styrene straps. The sound separation characteristics of this plate are augmented by the addition of lightweight acoustic barrier material (Model KNM-100B Kinetics Limp Barrier Material, Kinetics Noise Control, Dublin, OH). Tests indicated that the combination of the styrene plate and the acoustic barrier material results in an effective separation of 23 dB between oral and nasal microphones.

The microphones are shielded from lateral and posterior acoustic interference by suspending them within a hard-shelled styrene plastic box, which is open at a 0 degree angle of incidence relative to the subject's mouth and nose. To further prevent the detection of vibrations traveling through the separation plate, each microphone is surrounded by a foam cushion.

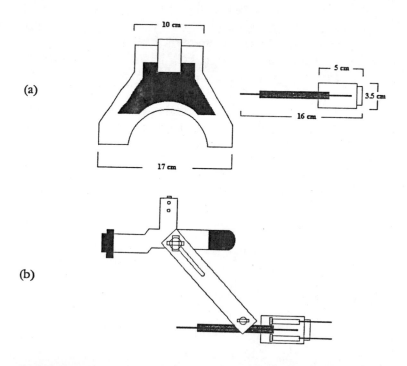

Figure 55.1 (a) Superior and lateral views of the sound separator plate used in the NasalView system; (b) The NasalView sound separator plate as attached to the Jackson headgear. Placement position of the microphones within the styrene plastic housing is also shown.

Preamplification and calibration hardware

The outputs from each microphone are preamplified using a custom-made dual-channel amplification system. The amplification unit also contains a tone-generator circuit and speaker by which calibration of the NasalView microphones may be achieved. In the calibration process, the sound separator plate is held over the speaker (approximately 7.5 cm from the speaker cone) in such a way that the microphones on either side of the separator plate are equally exposed to sound vibrations emanating from the speaker. During this process, a software routine makes any necessary adjustments to left (nasal) and right (oral) channel recording amplitudes to ensure that each channel is equally sensitive to detected sound pressure levels.

Computer hardware

The outputs from the amplification unit are then fed to the right (nasal) and left (oral) line input channels of a SoundBlaster16 or compatible A-to-D/D to A card. The SoundBlaster16 board allows for two channel recording at sampling rates up to 44 KHz; all filtering actions necessary for effective A-to-D conversion are built into the SoundBlaster16 board.

Computer software

The NasalView computer software program was written using a high-speed Windows programming language which carries out the following tasks:

1. Control the SoundBlaster16 board for both signal recording and signal playback. Each channel (nasal and oral) may be sampled at 11, 22, or 44 KHz at 8 or 16 bits of resolution. The accuracy of acoustic signal and nasalance measurement far exceeds that of the Nasometer which samples only at 120 Hz with 8 bits of resolution. The nasalance measurement used in NasalView may be referred to as a Root-Mean-Squared Nasalance (RMS Nasalance). This procedure compresses portions of the sampled data using an RMS procedure to result in RMS nasalance data that are representative of each short duration of the speech signal. Whereas an earlier version of this software applied a digital filter similar in characteristics to the analog filtering carried out by the Nasometer (Awan, 1996), the current version of the NasalView software allows the full range of frequencies reproduced by the relatively high sampling of the SoundBlaster16 board to be analysed.
2. The computer software provides a graphical output of oral and nasal acoustic signals as well as the corresponding nasalance over time

graph (see Figure 55.2). This type of graphical display is an important improvement over that provided in the Nasometer. By allowing
the clinician the ability to review acoustic speech signals and the
nasalance trace simultaneously, one can readily observe which particular speech sound or group of sounds is responsible for conspicu-
ous increases or decreases in nasalance. Whole speech segments or
individual phonemes can be played back for listener examination.
Summary statistics for the utterance under analysis are also provided (mean nasalance and standard deviation, median, maximum
and minimum nasalance, and range of nasalance). The user is also
given the capability to zoom in on particular portions of the graphical
RMS nasalance trace that may be of interest.

3. All signal files may be edited (if necessary) and stored on disk for
future analysis or pre/post-therapy comparisons.

Figure 55.2 shows an example of the results of analysis of the word
'sunshine' using the NasalView system.

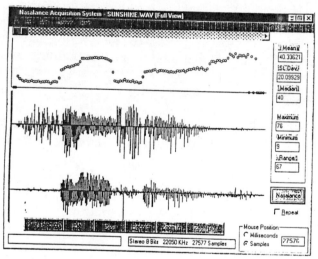

Figure 55.2. Graphical display of the RMS nasalance trace for the word 'sunshine'.
The oral and nasal acoustic signals, as well as summary statistics for the analysis are
also provided.

Subjects

The data to be discussed in this chapter will focus on speech samples
collected from groups of (a) 161 male and female children between the
ages of 5 and 14 years and (b) 20 male and female adults between the
ages of 18 and 30 years. (Total N = 181). All subjects were native
residents of the Eastern Pennsylvania region of the United States. All
subjects were assessed by a speech pathologist as having normal speech

characteristics, with no evidence of hyper- or hyponasality. Subjects who had any history of clefting or any evidence of significant nasal congestion that may have influenced their resonance characteristics were not included in this study. All subjects were also required to pass a hearing screening of 25 dB at 500, 1000, 2000, and 4000 Hz.

Speech Tasks

Subjects were asked to read the 'zoo passage' (0% nasal content – Fletcher, 1972), the 'rainbow passage' (11% nasal content – Fairbanks, 1960), and the 'nasal sentences' (35% nasal content – Fletcher, 1972) while wearing the NasalView headgear. Speech samples were recorded using a PC-compatible computer at 8-bits of resolution with a sampling rate of 22050 Hz. The resolution and sampling rate used were felt to provide adequate signal reproduction for the purposes of this study and to provide the benefit of significantly reduced datafile size.

For those young children who were unable to read the whole of a passage, recordings were made of their repetitions of the first 2 sentences of the 'zoo passage'; the second sentence of the 'rainbow passage'; and the first sentence from the 'nasal sentences'. A preliminary study computed RMS nasalance for the entire reading passages and then for the individual sentences mentioned above in a group of 60 male and female subjects between the ages of nine and ten years. Results indicated strong correlations between sentence and passage productions and small mean RMS nasalance differences:

- First nasal sentence versus nasal passage: $r = 0.92$, $p < 0.001$: mean difference = 0.63%).
- Second sentence of the 'rainbow passage' versus 'rainbow passage': $r = 0.96$, $p < 0.001$: mean difference = 0.18%).
- First and second sentences of the 'zoo passage' versus 'zoo passage': $r = 0.87$, $p < 0.001$: mean difference = 0.81%).

In addition to the speaking tasks carried out using the NasalView system, all subjects carried out similar tasks using the Nasometer (Kay Elemetrics Inc., Pinehurst, NJ).

Results

Reliability

Test-retest reliability was assessed using the 20 adult subjects speaking the complete 'zoo', 'rainbow' and 'nasal sentence' passages. Retests were taken within two days of the original test using both NasalView and the Nasometer. Results are provided in Table 55.1 and show that subjects may be expected to produce test-retest nasalance scores within 2% using the NasalView system and within 3% using the Nasometer. Slight variation in test-retest reliability occurs as a function of stimuli-type.

Table 55.1. Mean test-retest nasalance data for the NasalView and Nasometer systems on the Zoo, Rainbow, and Nasal Sentence passages. Mean differences and Pearson r correlations are also provided

Stimuli	Test	Retest	Mean Difference	r
NasalView Zoo	51.98%	50.34%	1.64%	0.82
Nasometer Zoo	61.65%	58.98%	2.67%	0.61
NasalView Rainbow	36.47%	35.57%	0.90%	0.23
Nasometer Rainbow	35.21%	33.29%	1.91%	0.64
NasalView Nasal Passages	26.48%	25.95%	0.53%	0.31
Nasometer Nasal Passages	15.29%	14.16%	1.13%	0.46

Long passages

Analysis of the reading passages was carried out with 104 subjects between the ages of seven and 14. In addition, a group of 20 adult speech samples were also included in this analysis (Total N = 124 subjects). A two-between (five levels of age; two levels of gender), one-within (three levels of passage) ANOVA revealed the following:

Within each age group analysed, males and females have similar degrees of overall RMS nasalance ($F = 0.075$; df = 1, 114; $p>0.500$). Age may influence the degree of nasalance. The seven-to-eight and nine-to-ten-year-old groups performed similarly on all three reading passages. However, significant increases in measured RMS nasalance were observed between the 11-to-12, 13-to-14, and adult groups on the 'zoo' and 'nasal sentence' passages (critical difference = 1.19%). Significant increases in measured RMS nasalance were observed between the 11-to-12 and 13-to-14-year-old groups. However, no significant difference was observed between the 13-14 year old group and the adult group ($F = 2.65$; df = 8, 228; $p< 0.01$). As expected, significant differences were observed between the three reading passages ($F = 3472.03$; df = 2, 228; $p< .001$):

- Nasal passages (Mean = 48.44%, SD = 6.00)
- Rainbow passage (Mean = 34.19%, SD = 4.69)
- Zoo passage (Mean = 24.67%, SD = 2.91)

Short passages

Analysis of the short passages produced by those children who had difficulty reading the entire passages was carried out with 57 subjects between the ages of five and seven years. A two-between (four levels of age; two levels of gender), one-within (three levels of passage) ANOVA revealed no significant effects of age or gender. As expected, significant differences were observed between the three reading passages ($F = 896.85$; df = 2, 106; $p < 0.001$):

- First nasal sentence (Mean = 42.92%, SD = 6.00)
- Second sentence of the 'rainbow' passage (Mean = 30.15%, SD = 4.69)
- First and second sentences of the 'zoo' passage (Mean = 20.65%, SD = 2.91)

Figure 55.3 shows the change in RMS nasalance across all of the age groups evaluated in this study for the 'zoo', 'rainbow', and 'nasal sentence' passages.

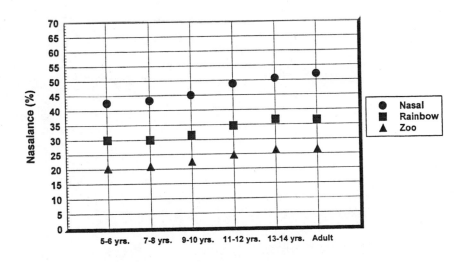

Figure 55.3. Mean RMS nasalance for the Zoo, Rainbow, and Nasal Sentence passages for various groups of child and adult subjects.

NasalView versus Nasometer

The nasalance results for all age groups were combined to produce overall mean nasalance scores for the three reading passages for both NasalView and the Nasometer. Results are provided in Figure 55.4. It is evident that the different software/hardware systems incorporated into these two systems produce substantial differences in computed nasalance. Both systems are able to differentiate between varying degrees of nasality in speech. It should be noted that the degree of deviation around the mean nasalance values is much smaller for the NasalView system than for the Nasometer. Increased homogeneity in the nasalance values of a target population should make it easier to detect true differences in nasalance that may reflect normal structural changes within the vocal tract or which may reflect mild or 'borderline' nasality problems.

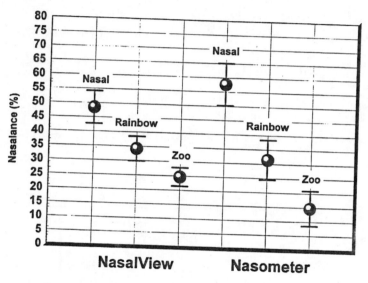

Figure 55.4. Overall mean nasalance data for the 'zoo', 'rainbow', and 'nasal sentence' passages as analysed using the NasalView versus the Nasometer systems.]

Conclusions

The results of this study lead to a number of conclusions regarding the utility of the NasalView system for the analysis of nasalance:

1. The NasalView system appears effectively to separate varying degrees of nasal speech. Although actual nasalance values differ from those of the Nasometer, these differences may be expected when one takes into account the vast hardware and software dissimilarities between the two systems.
2. NasalView provides high levels of both validity and reliability in its ability to measure RMS nasalance.
3. NasalView may have the capability to help identify age-related changes in normal nasalance that have not been previously reported or investigated.

4. The possibilities of new and important findings regarding both normal and disordered nasalance levels may be enhanced by the improved time and amplitude resolution offered by the NasalView system in comparison to the Nasometer.

The improved signal reproduction capabilities inherent in the NasalView system may be able to provide us with more detailed information on the characteristics of resonance disorders. Whereas further studies need to be conducted using the NasalView system, it appears that NasalView has the capability to be a highly effective tool for the assessment of nasalance and other characteristics of resonance-based disorders at a substantially lower cost than the Nasometer.

References

Awan SN (1996) Development of a low-cost nasalance acquisition system. In Powell, TW (Ed) Pathologies of Speech and Language: Contributions of Clinical Linguistics and Phonetics. New Orleans: International Clinical Phonetics and Linguistics Association, pp 211–17.

Dalston R, Neiman G, Gonzalez-Landa G (1993) Nasometric sensitivity and specificity: A cross-dialect and cross-culture study. Cleft Palate Journal, 30(3): 285–91.

Dalston R, Warren D, Dalston E (1991) Use of nasometry as a diagnostic tool for identifying patients with velopharyngeal impairment. Cleft Palate Journal, 28(2): 184–90.

Fairbanks G (1960) Voice and Articulation Drillbook. 2nd edn. New York: Harper & Bros.

Fletcher, S (1972) Contingencies for bioelectric modification of nasality. Journal of Speech and Hearing Disorders 37: 329–46.

Hardin M, Van Demark D, Morris H, Payne M (1992) Correspondence between nasalance scores and listener judgments of hypernasality and hyponasality. Cleft Palate Journal 29(4): 346–51.

Note

1 NasalView and NAS (Nasalance Acquisition System) Copyright 1994, 1996 S.N. Awan

Index of keywords

Abbreviations
P = entries on page given and following page
pp = entries on page given and following pages